"You'll never think about detox in the same way again after reading and experiencing *Whole Detox*. It's mind–body medicine meets nutritional detoxification through the spectrum of color. Genius, creative, and inspiring."

—Amy Myers, M.D., *New York Times* bestselling author of
The Autoimmune Solution

"*Whole Detox* offers up a comprehensive and integrative program that paves the way for reestablishing health, disease resistance, and vitality. Deanna Minich guides with knowledge, expertise, experience, and most importantly, compassion. Her dedication to the art of healing is evident in every word."

—David Perlmutter, M.D., author of the #1 *New York Times* bestsellers
Grain Brain and *Brain Maker*

WHOLE

DETOX

A 21-DAY PERSONALIZED PROGRAM TO BREAK
THROUGH BARRIERS IN EVERY AREA OF YOUR LIFE

DEANNA MINICH

HarperOne
An Imprint of HarperCollinsPublishers

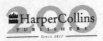

WHOLE DETOX. Copyright © 2016 by Deanna Minich. All rights reserved. Printed in the United States of America. No part of this book may be used or reproduced in any manner whatsoever without written permission except in the case of brief quotations embodied in critical articles and reviews. For information address HarperCollins Publishers, 195 Broadway, New York, NY 10007.

HarperCollins books may be purchased for educational, business, or sales promotional use. For information please e-mail the Special Markets Department at SPsales@harper collins.com.

HarperCollins website: http://www.harpercollins.com

FIRST HARPERCOLLINS PAPERBACK EDITION PUBLISHED IN 2017

Designed by Yvonne Chan

Library of Congress Cataloging-in-Publication Data is available upon request.

ISBN 9780062426802

22 23 24 25 26 LBC 8 7 6 5 4

To my father, who is healing the ancestral threads, and to my niece, Eleanor, who is creating healthy patterns for the future.

To the healing of past, present, and future generations from the effects of *all* types of toxins and with hope for a planet filled with the full spectrum of health and vitality.

You are not a drop in the ocean. You are the entire ocean in a drop.

—RUMI

CONTENTS

FOREWORD

I get the questions all the time from my patients: "Why detox?" "Isn't detoxing just a fad?" Of course, "detox" is a word that means different things to different people, which is why sometimes it can cause confusion. Most people relate detox to juicing, fasting, or eating lots of cruciferous vegetables and drinking lots of lemon water. There is definitely a food component to detox. I talk extensively about how to do a detox diet right within my book *The Blood Sugar Solution 10-Day Detox Diet*. Sure, it's taking out sugar, gluten, dairy, and caffeine. Equally important, it's about including whole, colorful foods in the diet, which are chock-full of nutrients. It's that tender balance of avoiding unhealthy foods and including nourishing foods in our everyday eating. I believe strongly in living the age-old principle of "food as medicine" and starting here first and foremost.

The other part of detox—lifestyle—gets less recognition than food, but I believe it's very important to consider. I'm a huge believer in the power of community, in sociogenomics, and in how our social networks can add or take away from our health. We need to be looking at the root of whom we are personally connected to, because as the research shows, their habits can become ours. We also need to be examining other lifestyle toxicities, like going to a toxic job every day that doesn't nourish our soul; having toxic emotions stored within, thinking recycled toxic thoughts that limit our potential; and being exposed to environmental toxins through home, school, and work.

For detox to work and take hold, it needs to address the "whole self." I've seen this time and time again in my patients. If they change their food, many times they change their lives. However, when they see detox as a temporary deprivation, only to thrust themselves back into a toxic lifestyle and do it again, then detox doesn't have the full potential it could. I am a huge advocate of lifestyle change, and I see detox as being a short-term reset button to fuel long-term changes.

I am excited to see that my colleague and friend Dr. Deanna Minich has written *Whole Detox* for this very reason. She sees detox much like I do—that it needs to focus on the whole person, incorporate whole foods, and look at the whole-systems approach we embrace within Functional Medicine. In fact, we know each other through our work with the Institute for Functional Medicine. In 2014, she collaborated with the Institute to launch and lead the seventy-thousand-person worldwide Detox Summit and then had thousands of people do the detox in the Detox Challenge. Similar to the results I find in my clinical practice, she found a 50 to 60 percent reduction in symptoms just within twenty-one days. Furthermore, she is also faculty for the Institute, teaching specifically the food and lifestyle aspects of detox.

Quite frankly, I think she is the perfect person to talk about detox in this new "whole" kind of way. Deanna is a scientist and clinician who is keen on looking at the psychology, eating, and living features of someone's life. I especially enjoy the fact that she uses so much color in her teaching and draws upon her talent as a visual artist.

It's very promising to see that we are redefining detox in the twenty-first century. The Father of Functional Medicine, Dr. Jeffrey Bland, introduced nutritional detoxification (metabolic biotransformation) in the twentieth century and brought important concepts to the foreground. Now, decades later, with the emerging areas of mind–body medicine, we've come to realize that toxins cross over between the body and the mind. Physical toxins, like heavy metals, can create psychological effects, and psychological toxins, like stress, can have physical manifestations. Truly, "detox" needs to keep up with the evolving science, and I think that's what we have *Whole Detox* here to do.

Mark Hyman, M.D.
Director of the Cleveland Clinic Center for Functional Medicine

FOREWORD

For decades, the word "detoxification" was narrowly defined to refer to pharmacogenomics, which is the manner in which specific inherited traits influence the way that drugs are metabolized and eliminated from the body.[1] In 1980, as a university professor trained in nutritional biochemistry, I started to wonder if the detoxification of drugs was influenced by the food and its associated nutrients that we ate. I had the fortune of meeting Dr. William Rea, a physician in Dallas, who had specialized in understanding the relationship between chemical sensitivity and individual differences in detoxification.[2] I began to understand that the metabolic pathways utilized in drug detoxification could be influenced by nutrients and foods.[3] For example, grapefruit juice was known to change the activity of some drugs that went through a cytochrome enzyme known as CYP3A4.[4] There were also certain herbs, like St. John's-wort, known to alter these hepatic enzymes and thus became contraindicated by pharmacists to patients if they were on specific drugs.[5]

Based on what I observed within the context of my background in nutritional biochemistry, I decided to go further down the path of exam-

1. Q. Ma and A. Y. Lu, "Pharmacogenetics, Pharmacogenomics, and Individualized Medicine," *Pharmacological Reviews* 63, no. 2 (2011): 437–59.
2. W. J. Rea et al., "Chemical Sensitivity in Physicians," *Boletín Asociación Médica de Puerto Rico* 83, no. 9 (1991): 383–88.
3. H. F. Woods, "Effects of Nutrition on Drug Metabolism and Distribution," *Comprehensive Therapy* 4, no. 10 (1978): 49–53.
4. K. Fukuda, T. Ohta, and Y. Yamazoe, "Grapefruit Component Interacting with Rat and Human CYP3A4: Possible Involvement of Non-Flavonoid Components in Drug Interaction," *Biological and Pharmaceutical Bulletin* 20, no. 5 (1997): 560–64.
5. J. W. Budzinski et al., "An In Vitro Evaluation of Human Cytochrome P450 3A4 Inhibition by Selected Herbal Extracts and Tinctures," *Phytomedicine* 7, no. 4 (2000): 273–82.

ining how nutrition, especially protein and certain plant extracts, could alter metabolism and change one's health. In 1995, I published a paper in the *Alternative Therapies in Health and Medicine* journal to detail some of our clinical research on the role of nutritional intervention in detoxification.[6] We found that patients who were chronically ill with what had been diagnosed as "chronic fatigue syndrome" and were given a medical food formulated with specific nutrients to enhance detoxification pathways in conjunction with a "clean," low-allergy, calorie-controlled diet did significantly better and had a greater reduction of health complaints (52 percent reduction) compared with those who were administered the same diet without the addition of the medical food (22 percent reduction in symptoms). We were able to show that symptom reduction was associated with the normalization of liver enzymes involved in detoxification that might have otherwise been impaired. Additionally, we were able to statistically increase reserves of sulfur and glutathione in these patients, both of which are essential compounds for biochemical pathways of detoxification. At this time, we recognized from the research of Drs. Rosemary Waring and Glyn Steventon that the onset of Parkinson's disease is often associated with insufficiencies in a patient's detoxification system, particularly in glutathione metabolism.[7]

From this beginning I came to recognize that the metabolism or detoxification of alcohol by the liver was very dependent upon nutritional status,[8] as was the metabolism of common over-the-counter drugs like acetaminophen and ibuprofen.[9]

This study sent me further in the direction of researching detoxification from biochemical and nutritional perspectives. I continued doing research into the role that various nutrients had on the metabolic detoxification processes. My colleagues and I utilized a number of specific tests to evaluate the detoxification potential of the individual, including the caffeine and

---

6. J. S. Bland et al., "A Medical Food-Supplemented Detoxification Program in the Management of Chronic Health Problems," *Alternative Therapies in Health and Medicine* 1, no. 5 (1995): 62–71.

7. Adrian Williams et al., "Xenobiotic Enzyme Profiles and Parkinson's Disease," *Neurology* 41, no. 5, suppl. 2 (1991): 29–32.

8. C. S. Lieber, "A Personal Perspective on Alcohol, Nutrition and the Liver," *American Journal of Clinical Nutrition* 58, no. 3 (1993): 430–42.

9. K. D. Rainsford and J. Bjarnason, "NSAIDs: Take with Food or After Fasting?" *Journal Pharmacy and Pharmacology* 64, no. 4 (2012): 465–69.

benzoate clearance tests.[10] In 1991 Dr. J. O. Hunter, a well-respected medical research professor at Cambridge University Hospitals, authored an article that indicated that the adverse reaction some people have to specific foods may be a result of their inability to detoxify the natural substances found in the food.[11] All of these studies proved to us that nutritional status and specific nutrient supplementation programs could have a significant influence on detoxification of both foreign chemicals and endogenous toxins produced by normal metabolism.[12]

It was at this point that I was very fortunate to have Dr. Deanna Minich join our research group at MetaProteomics in Gig Harbor, Washington. From the day she joined our research team the focus on nutrition and specific nutrients took a step forward. She was a superb researcher who helped pioneer the understanding of nutrition in supporting the detoxification processes of the body. Her work on the role of the alkaline diet in detoxification was a major advance in the development of a dietary program to support improved detoxification.[13] The recent paper on detoxification that she and her research colleague Romilly Hodges have had published is a landmark review paper that clearly defines the role of foods and food-derived components in metabolic detoxification.[14]

Over the past thirty years in the field, I have come to recognize that "detoxification" is a term that means more than nutritional detoxification. The use of the word often implies something quite different from how we had used the word within my research. The term now describes the metabolism of drugs, metabolites from gut bacteria, pollutants, metabolic byproducts, and even "toxic" experiences, relationships, and thoughts.

---

10. T. Wang et al., "Caffeine Elimination: A Test of Liver Function," *Klinische Wochenschrift* 63, no. 21 (1985): 1124–28; J. Soto, J. A. Sacristan, and M. J. Alsar, "Use of Salivary Caffeine Tests to Assess the Inducer Effect of a Drug on Hepatic Metabolism," *Annals of Pharmacotherapy* 30, nos. 7–8 (1996): 736–39; and M. Takayama and S. Yamada, "Clinical Usefulness of Benzoate Tolerance Test in Patients with Liver Cirrhosis" [in Japanese], *Rinsho Byori* 40, no. 12 (1992): 1303–6.

11. J. O. Hunter, "Food Allergy—or Enterometabolic Disorder?" *Lancet* 338, no. 8765 (1991): 495–96.

12. W. R. Bidlack, R. C. Brown, and C. Mohan, "Nutritional Parameters That Alter Hepatic Drug Metabolism, Conjugation, and Toxicity," *Federation Proceedings* 45, no. 2 (1986): 142–48.

13. D. M. Minich and J. S. Bland, "Acid–Alkaline Balance: Role in Chronic Disease and Detoxification," *Alternative Therapies in Health and Medicine* 13, no. 4 (2007): 62–65.

14. R. E. Hodges and D. M. Minich, "Modulation of Metabolic Detoxification Pathways Using Foods and Food-Derived Components: A Scientific Review with Clinical Applications," *Journal of Nutrition and Metabolism* (2015): e760689.

With this broad definition of detoxification, I come back to what we know of the relationship of diet and specific nutrients to support the specific inducible metabolic processes associated with detoxification. This concept of detoxification has become one of the seven core physiological processes within the functional medicine concept. There is now irrefutable evidence that toxic burden contributes to many chronic diseases, including type 2 diabetes,[15] cardiovascular disease,[16] arthritis,[17] and neurodegeneration.[18]

I am so impressed with how Dr. Minich has incorporated into her book *Whole Detox* the expansive, evolving science of nutritoxigenomics into a sensible program for improving the body's detoxification program that the average non-scientist can successfully apply in their own lives.

For more than ten years I have observed Dr. Minich in her role as a senior leader of our research and development team, in which she provides consultation to patients in the Functional Medicine Research Center. Deanna is not only an expert in the science of nutrition as it relates to detoxification but also a holistic systems thinker who is able to understand the broader personal and lifestyle issues related to detoxification. Her knowledge about how people develop and then respond to detoxification programs is not theoretical but rather derived from years of clinical experience with hundreds of patients. In addition to her background as a functional medicine nutritionist, she has integrated elements of personalized lifestyle medicine, determining what felt right for her patients specifically and how to tailor their detoxification to their specific needs.[19] Deanna is able to make the sometimes technical aspects of lifestyle medicine more consumer friendly through her artistic use of images and color. She teaches with metaphor and creativity, which allows for a well-rounded approach to all she does.

15. K. W. Taylor et al., "Evaluation of the Association Between Persistent Organic Pollutants (POPs) and Diabetes in Epidemiological Studies: A National Toxicity Program Workshop Review," *Environmental Health Perspectives* 121, no. 7 (2013): 774–83.

16. M. Porta, "Persistent Organic Pollutants and the Burden of Disease," *Lancet* 368 (2006): 558–59.

17. A. I. Catrina, K. D. Deane, and J. U. Scher, "Gene, Environment, Microbiome, and Mucosal Immune Tolerance in Rheumatoid Arthritis," *Rheumatology* (Oxford) 23 (2014): 469–75.

18. V. Nicolia, M. Lucarelli, and A. Fuso, "Environment, Epigenetics, and Neurodegeneration: Focus on Nutrition in Alzheimer's Disease," *Experimental Gerontology* 68 (2015): 8–12.

19. D. M. Minich and J. S. Bland, "Personalized Lifestyle Medicine: Relevance for Nutrition and Lifestyle Recommendations," *ScientificWorld Journal* (June 26, 2013): 129841.

Within this book *Whole Detox*, the reader will find the best of Dr. Minich and an opportunity to improve their health through the wisdom she provides from both her extensive research and her clinical applications. This is the book in which the approach to detoxification offers the whole picture in a program that is tried and proven to be successful.

Jeffrey Bland, Ph.D.
President of the Personalized Lifestyle Medicine Institute

INTRODUCTION: WHY WHOLE DETOX?

My patient Sandy was frustrated.

"Dr. Minich," she said, "I'm *really* hoping you can help me. I feel like I've tried every detox under the sun, and they all work, but only for a little while. I've heard that your detox does some really great things and that it will change my life, and I really hope that's true. Because, honestly, I'm starting to lose hope."

I could well understand Sandy's frustration. Like many of my patients, she was looking for a way to lose weight, feel great, and boost her energy. She was also struggling with brain fog and some mild anxiety. Some of my other patients suffer from aching joints, sleep problems, depression, list-lessness, or fatigue. For many, I'm not the first stop on the health-care trail; they've tried conventional medicine, a number of supposedly healthy diets, a wide range of fitness programs, and at least one or two cleanses. Many even improve—for a while. Then, like Sandy, they start to drift back to the same set of problems that sent them searching for help in the first place.

Does that sound like you? Are you also frustrated that those five or ten or twenty pounds keep coming back after you've worked so hard to lose them? Do you wish there was a way to regain your lost energy and sharpen up your brain? Are you struggling with sleep problems, anxiety, or depression that you'd prefer to treat naturally? Do you feel as though you keep running into the same brick wall?

If so, I hear you. I've spent enough of my life seeking answers for my own health problems to know just how frustrating and sometimes scary that can be. When I began as a functional medicine nutritionist, I was thrilled that I'd have the chance to translate my years of science and research into practical ways of giving people access to the vibrant health that is our birth-right. At that point, I had a lot of faith in good nutrition as the royal road to health—the way to living well and feeling great.

Over the years, though, I, like Sandy, became frustrated. I began to see that for many patients, the wonderful nutritional suggestions I was making simply didn't "take."

Maybe they would for a while. The patients would be incredibly excited as they finished the consultation, thrilled with their jump-start to a healthy life. They had shed pounds and lost inches. Their brain fog had cleared. Their anxiety had calmed. Their depression had lifted. Detox had given them a glimpse of just how great life could be when they felt this good, all the time.

And then a month, two months, half a year later, many of those same patients would return, discouraged, maybe even defeated. They had started to regain the weight. Their aches and pains were back. They no longer felt the energy, the hope, the vibrant health they had once enjoyed.

What had gone wrong? Why would an approach that had worked so well stop working?

I struggled with this problem for several years, and then finally I got it.

The reason most detoxes have so little staying power is that they treat only a part, but not the whole.

They deal with part of your body, not your whole body.

They tell you what to take out, but they don't focus on what to put in.

They deal only with your physical body, not with your whole self.

And as a result, they often fail.

WHY MOST DETOXES DON'T LAST

They Don't Deal with Your Whole Body

Most detoxes pick one single part of your body—your liver, perhaps, or your gut. But very few programs look comprehensively and systematically at your whole body and make sure that your entire physical self—from your feet through your belly through your heart to your brain—has every bit of support it needs to expel all your toxins.

This whole-body approach is essential, especially given that the latest developments in medicine focus on the activity and interrelationships of your body's networks: not just your gut but your digestive system; not just your digestive system but the interaction between it and every other organ and system in your body. Your liver doesn't work separately from your gut; they work together. (The scientific terms for this type of thinking are "network medicine" and "systems biology.")

They Focus on What to Take Out, Not What to Put In

Most detoxes zero in on reactive foods, industrial chemicals, and other environmental toxins. They tell you how to protect yourself from these toxins, and maybe they even offer you a few weeks' worth of meal plans. Or they focus on a few potentially toxic foods—caffeine, sugar, and gluten, perhaps, or maybe soy, peanuts, and artificial sweeteners. Some detoxes are more restrictive, with an even longer list of things to cut out. But none of these approaches gives enough attention to your whole body, comprehensively, systematically making sure that every one of your vital systems is getting the full spectrum of nutrients it needs.

They Focus on the Body, Not the Whole Self

Most detoxes tell us how to avoid reactive foods and industrial chemicals, which is great. But do they help us shed toxic thoughts, let go of limiting beliefs, or cope with the stressful situations that frequently make us ill? Not that I've seen.

Every time you encounter an upsetting relationship, a frustrating personal situation, or a depressing day at work, your body is flooded with biochemicals that have the power to sabotage your health. I'm talking about stress hormones like cortisol, which cues your body to put on the pounds, disrupt your sleep, and drive up your blood pressure, potentially sending you down the road to obesity, diabetes, autoimmune conditions, and cancer. I'm talking about the shattering experience of heartbreaking grief, which research has shown can literally disrupt the workings of your heart. I'm talking about lives that seem plagued by loneliness and boredom, which numerous studies have shown are characterized by more chronic health problems and also end sooner than lives full of passion, meaning, and community.

We now have volumes full of research showing that stress, boredom, frustration, and heartbreak aren't simply psychological states. Rather, they are *physical* conditions that profoundly affect your health: through your hormones, your blood pressure, your neurotransmitters, and, ultimately, your entire biochemistry. A happy, relaxed person is biochemically different from an angry, sad, or fearful one. Your body affects your thoughts and feelings . . . and your thoughts and feelings affect your body. This interaction is straight out of Human Biochemistry 101. It can be a significant disrupter of your health—or a profound tool for healing.

Yet most detoxes ignore this life component and stick strictly to nutritional advice. Even when they pay lip service to "stress relief" or "taking time for yourself," they fail to offer any concrete, workable program to actually get rid of your life toxins. As a result, most detoxes are sadly incomplete, because if you don't heal the whole person, you'll just see the same problems coming back again and again and again.

DETOX'S NEW FRONTIER

I didn't want my patients to keep suffering. I didn't want them to follow up the brilliant initial success of their detox with a disappointing fizzle a few weeks later. I didn't want a detox that worked only briefly, randomly, or occasionally, and I didn't want a detox that addressed the body alone.

So I began searching for a program that would allow us to remove every single toxic barrier that keeps us from total health and vital, fulfilling lives. I drew on my years doing academic and professional research into the biochemical and nutritional properties of food, and on my experience as a clinician who had worked with thousands of patients. I wanted a detox that spoke to every facet of our bodies and our lives—a clear, actionable program that even the busiest and most stressed of my patients could follow.

The culmination of this process was Whole Detox: the first comprehensive, systematic approach to breaking through *all* the toxins that hold us back. But first, I had to rethink what I meant by "toxin."

REDEFINING "TOXIN"

Okay, we all know that "detoxification" means, literally, to get rid of toxins. But what exactly are toxins? We're used to speaking of them in purely physical terms. My research and my clinical practice have taught me that they are much, much more. Toxins are better understood less as poisons than as *barriers*—obstacles to the life and health we truly want.

On a physical level, this is pretty clear. If we look at the thyroid signaling system, for example—the complex network of glands and hormones that regulate thyroid function—we see that poor thyroid function makes the whole body more vulnerable to environmental toxins, interfering with our ability to detoxify. At the same time, the increasing toxic burden disrupts the thyroid signaling system, making it more difficult for different parts of the system to communicate with one another. These toxic barriers to communication further depress thyroid function, creating a vicious cycle that can sabotage our entire quality of life. Depression, weight gain, brain fog, exhaustion, memory problems, and, potentially, heart disease are only some of the chronic conditions that can result.

Yet when you remove the toxic barriers, communication resumes. Thyroid function improves, and we suddenly have a new lease on life.

Slowly I came to see that the very same principle applies to life toxins. If mental, emotional, or spiritual challenges are standing in our way, they can block our progress—and undermine our health. I began to see that when I helped my patients release their life toxins, their health improved as well.

For example, my patient Marqueta had struggled for years with a limiting belief: she felt she couldn't be a successful, empowered woman and also retain her femininity. Marqueta's mother had grown up in a very traditional religious household, and she had tried to instill those same values in her daughter, including the notion that women were supposed to be quiet, timid, and sexually passive.

This limiting belief was keeping Marqueta from pursuing relationships with men who really interested her. Any time she found a man she liked, she worried that she was being "too sexual" and "too forward." She also worried that the man would be put off by her success as the administrator of a local hospital.

When she came to me, she was suffering from crippling menstrual cramps. She also described herself as "dried up—my brain just won't work." Once a creative, vital person, she was clearly struggling with many toxic barriers. Her physical symptoms expressed her life issues; her life issues were shaped by her physical problems.

Enter Whole Detox. I addressed Marqueta's hormonal issues in a variety of nutritional ways: healthy fats, better hydration, some herbal supplements. I also worked with her to identify the limiting belief that functioned as such a daunting obstacle. I encouraged her to foster her creativity, even in such little ways as how she dressed or how she decorated her office. I asked her to write in her journal about the women she admired and wanted to emulate, and to identify the qualities in herself that resembled those women. Through a wide variety of modalities—diet, supplements, lifestyle, self-exploration, journaling, and creative activities—I helped her get rid of the toxic barriers that were holding her back.

Once Marqueta understood how to identify and overcome all the toxins in her life—from reactive foods to limiting thoughts to frustrating relationships—she was able to reclaim her health. Because she wasn't following an abstract system but rather identifying her own personal toxins, she was empowered far beyond what partial detoxes could achieve. Thanks to the tools she had learned through Whole Detox, she would be able to target and defeat her personal toxins for the rest of her life.

Even after a few weeks, the results were astonishing. Soon after we began working together, Marqueta transformed her wardrobe from dull grays and beiges to brilliant oranges and yellows, which suited her much better. She began to feel creative and "flowing" again, no longer "dried up" and "stuck." She started a new relationship, slowly and tentatively, but with more passion and excitement than she had previously allowed herself. Her menstrual cramps disappeared. Her hormones were in balance. The culmination came at her last appointment, when she showed up with a haircut so dramatic and different from her previous style that I honestly almost didn't recognize her.

This, to me, is the essence of Whole Detox. Marqueta had broken through the toxic barriers that were limiting her life so she could finally savor the full spectrum of her whole self.

DISCOVERING WHOLE DETOX

When I developed Whole Detox, I had been working for nearly a decade as a nutritionist. I had done graduate research into the nutritional properties of the carotenoids that give foods their color, as well as into the biochemical properties of fats.

I had also explored other ancient healing arts, including Traditional Chinese Medicine (TCM), Ayurveda, and many others. A single yoga class I took more than twenty years ago first turned on the lightbulb in my head, illuminating the many healing truths available to us, even if they are often neglected by conventional practitioners.

So in my quest for detox's new frontier, I went back and searched my library for every discipline I had ever studied: nutrition, neuroscience, epigenetics, physiology, and psychology as well as yoga, Ayurveda, TCM, and traditional healing. Odd as it might sound, I also explored color and drew on my background in the visual arts. After all, color has long been associated with emotion and mood as well as with the phytonutrients that make fruits, vegetables, herbs, and other plant foods such a crucial part of our diet. Color plays a role in East Indian healing too.

Working with this rich array of influences, I came up with a new approach to detox. Its power was astounding. As I introduced this approach to my patients, I saw how deeply mind, body, and emotions all affect one another. Remove a toxic food from your diet, and you might also free yourself from depression, anxiety, or helplessness. Eliminate a toxic thought, and you might also rev up your metabolism and lose some unwanted weight. Tear down the barriers to your sense of purpose and connectedness, and you might also revitalize your immune system and restore your optimism.

The opposite was also true. Hold on to a toxic belief, and the healthiest diet in the world might not free you from troublesome symptoms. Remain mired in a stressful life, and even without caffeine, sugar, and refined flour, you might still feel wired, anxious, or depressed. A raging hunger for meaning or community might keep you dissatisfied and on edge even when your body is fully nourished.

Every one of us is a complex biochemical structure in which every factor affects every other factor in an endless synergistic loop. Sometimes this synergy works against us: Negative thoughts can impair our health; poor health can breed negative thoughts. As your health gets worse, your thoughts get bleaker; as your thoughts get bleaker, you move less, crave more sugar, and send more stress hormones coursing through your veins. You feel even sicker . . . and your thoughts spiral further down into depression. Talk about a vicious cycle!

But with Whole Detox, you can transform the downward spiral of disease into an upward spiral of vibrant health. By addressing nutrition, exercise, thought patterns, and many other factors at the same time, you can break through toxic barriers and create an energized, full-spectrum life.

WHAT WHOLE DETOX WILL DO FOR YOU

Whole Detox integrates Western science and Eastern medicine. It is a systematic way of overcoming every barrier that keeps you from health, energy, and fulfillment. So welcome to Whole Detox, because it will change your life:

- You'll begin to heal the parts of your body that are struggling under their toxic burden, including your endocrine system, digestion, heart, bones, and brain.
- You'll shed pounds, boost your energy, heal your aches and pains, and recover from debilitating symptoms, feeling calmer, more vital, and more energized than you have in years.
- You'll detoxify your relationship with your community, your family, and yourself.
- You'll detox through food and also through movement, new thought patterns, and emotional expression.
- You'll break through conflicts and creative blocks, which will free you to pursue long-deferred dreams for work, love, and personal satisfaction.
- You'll feel nourished, not deprived, because sometimes the best detox is not cutting something out but rather bringing in more of what you need!

Most important, Whole Detox is a *personalized* approach. You'll zero in on the parts of your body—and your life—that most need cleansing, healing, and revitalization. You'll also acquire the lifelong ability to target your personal barriers by using the Whole Detox Spectrum Quiz. As a result, Whole Detox is the fastest and most effective way to become your healthiest, most energized, and most fully realized self.

THE POWER OF WHOLE DETOX

To illustrate the power of Whole Detox, let me share with you the story of George, who came to me frustrated and helpless about six months after completing a detox with another practitioner. George's problem was that he couldn't sleep—an aching frustration that had been with him ever since his sophomore year in college.

Now in his midforties, he was paying a heavy price for his insomnia. He often found himself short-tempered with his children as well as his wife. Since his father had been a short-tempered, angry man, George hated the feeling that he was repeating his father's version of family life.

At work, too, George struggled to remain calm and centered. The owner of a small tech company, he frequently had to travel on business, working with clients in various parts of the country. He knew that a sleepless night before an important meeting could jeopardize a vital relationship, yet he hated to depend on sleep aids.

Sleep problems were ruining his life, he told me frankly the first time we met. His despair was all the greater because he had recently completed a detox that, for a few sweet months, had finally seemed to heal the problem. On that program, he cut out caffeine, sugar, white flour, and unhealthy fats. He drank water with lemon juice to flush the toxins out through his urine, and he took yarrow pills to support his liver's detox function. He got a water filter, an air purifier, and blackout curtains to keep "light pollution" out of his bedroom. Anything that could interfere with his sleep, he got rid of. And for a time it worked. George's sleep quality improved until finally, after less than two weeks, he was sleeping deeply throughout the night. For the next few months, he felt as though he had witnessed a miracle.

Then, slowly but surely, the old sleep problems began creeping back.

When a loud noise in a hotel corridor woke him up one night, he tossed and turned for hours. When a difficult client meeting loomed the next day, he couldn't fall asleep till nearly five A.M. When his ten-year-old daughter came down with a high fever one night, he lay rigid beside his sleeping wife, imagining all the terrible ways her illness might play out.

"What's the problem?" George asked when he eventually came to see me. "Once I started sleeping again, why couldn't I *keep* sleeping?"

"I think three things might be going on," I suggested. "First, there may be some toxins that are personal and specific to you—some reactive foods or problematic chemicals that are disrupting your body. Most detoxes are cookie-cutter—one size fits all. They can be a great first step, but they don't necessarily identify the toxins that are disrupting your system."

George nodded, beginning to look more hopeful.

"Second, although your previous detox focused on what to cut out, you didn't really find out what to put in. Healthy fats are really important for sleeping. So are complex carbohydrates. There may be some other imbalances we will discover as we work through your entire body, systems in your body that are not getting all the nourishment they need."

George nodded a second time, seeming even more hopeful.

"Finally—and maybe most important—we can't just look at your body. We have to look at your whole self."

Now George was startled. "You mean there's something wrong with me, with my personality?" he asked.

"Not at all," I said quickly. "But your body and your mind aren't really separate. They're both part of the same system. Your thoughts and feelings are biochemical events that have a profound effect on the rest of your physiology. We can work only on the body level, as your previous detox did. But this is Whole Detox, and I think it would help you to work on the life level as well."

George and I had many long talks about what might be keeping him awake. As he thought about his bad-tempered father, he recalled many late-night arguments his parents used to have. His father had worked until midnight at the restaurant he owned, and when he came home, he expected George's mother to offer a sympathetic listening ear and a plate of hot food. George's mother, for her part, was exhausted after a long day of working at an office downtown and then making dinner for her children. George's father frequently woke her up, and the two fought, waking George. The sense that night was the time to be alert, on edge, ready to protect the people he loved yet helpless to do so, had never really left George.

He had also held on to the sense that to be a truly successful business-man, like his father, he had to stay up late, worrying about his business. Without realizing it, he had adopted that same worry, as though by fall-ing into a deep sleep he was neglecting his business and letting down his clients. Of course, the exact opposite was true. His sleep problems were actually interfering with his ability to be a good family man and an effective businessman.

Certainly, he had found it helpful to cut out the foods and beverages that had disrupted his sleep, and he also benefited from adding in the supportive foods I suggested. But George was a whole person, and he needed a whole detox, one that included both health and life issues. To solve his sleep prob-lem, he had to identify all the toxic barriers that kept him up at night, not just the nutritional ones.

YOUR 21-DAY PROGRAM

The Whole Detox George embarked on with me is what you're about to begin, too.

In chapter 1, I'll give you an overview of the cornerstone of Whole Detox: the Seven Systems of Full-Spectrum Health. These are seven clusters of physical and life issues that can be supported, healed, and detoxed in similar ways.

Once you've learned about each separate system, chapter 2 will help you see how all of them work together. It's called "The Power of Synergy" because synergy—the extra benefits you get from many systems all working in harmony—is truly the force behind Whole Detox.

Then, in chapters 3 through 9, I will provide an in-depth look at every system so that by the time you begin your Whole Detox, you'll be able to see your body, your life issues, and your goals in those terms.

This approach offers you two striking advantages that make Whole Detox more effective and longer lasting than any other detox I've seen.

First, these seven systems target every aspect of your body and your life: every anatomical system and also every life issue (work, love, community, spirituality, etc.). When you target each of the seven systems, you guarantee yourself a truly whole detox, identifying every single barrier that stands between you and optimal health, between you and a wholly inspired and fulfilling life.

Second, working with the seven systems enables you to create a truly personal detox—one that zeroes in on the specific barriers that are most troublesome to you. The Whole Detox Spectrum Quiz helps you work through every one of the seven systems, identifying each specific physical, mental, or emotional issue that stands in your way. What most people discover is that one or two systems are more out of balance than the others, while one or two other systems are areas of strength and power. When you identify your strengths and weaknesses, you can find ways to immediately support the strengths and improve the weaknesses, which will improve your physical, mental, and emotional well-being.

THE SEVEN SYSTEMS OF FULL-SPECTRUM HEALTH

Here are the seven systems that encompass the health of your entire being:

The ROOT: adrenal glands, immune system, DNA, bones, skin, survival, community

The FLOW: ovaries/testes, reproduction, fertility, urinary system, colon, partnerships, creativity

The FIRE: digestive system, blood sugar, work–life balance, energy production

The LOVE: thymus, heart, blood vessels, lungs, compassion, expansiveness, service

The TRUTH: thyroid gland, throat, mouth, ears, nose, speaking, choice, authenticity

The INSIGHT: pituitary gland, brain, neurons/neurotransmitters, sleep, mood, thoughts, intuition

The SPIRIT: pineal gland, electromagnetic fields, circadian rhythms, connection, purpose, meaning

These seven systems might seem a bit counterintuitive at first—why should adrenals, the immune system, and community all be part of the first system while ovaries, creativity, and the colon fit together in the second? But I promise, by the time you've finished reading chapters 1 through 9, these seven systems are going to seem intuitive and even a little obvious. And by the time you've finished your twenty-one-day program, you won't remember thinking any other way.

As a clinician, I found that these seven systems of health were my keys to the kingdom: through them, I could see that seemingly disparate issues—usually separated into nutritional, anatomical, psychological, and spiritual—did actually benefit from being treated together.

For example, the first system of health includes, among other things, immune function, bone health, identity, rootedness, and security—all the things that ground us and define us in a physical way. I could address immune function by giving my patients an immune-healthy diet, but I could also help them to create a strong sense of personal boundaries. They could enhance their bone health through supplements but also through yoga exercises that help them feel grounded. Meanwhile, a healthy immune system and strong bones could create a feeling of rootedness, safety, and security. In other words, treating one ROOT issue opens the door to a whole new world of improvement.

During your twenty-one-day program, every three days you'll detox another system of health, starting at the ROOT and working your way up to the SPIRIT. By the end of the three weeks, you will have addressed every toxic barrier in your life.

I'll be with you every step of the way. I'll tell you exactly what to eat each day (the recipes are simple, colorful, and delicious!). And I'll guide you through each day's activities: affirmations, meditation, visualization, journaling, explorations of limiting thoughts, and recommendations for healthy movement: a whole spectrum of ways to break through your personal toxic barriers. The instructions are clear and unambiguous—all you have to do is follow directions.

I've provided every single thing you need to complete this program successfully, including mouth-watering recipes, most of which can be prepared in thirty minutes or less. I've also shared shopping lists and some suggestions for how to lay the groundwork in the week before you start.

Whole Detox may be one of the most exciting journeys you'll ever take—and it doesn't end after twenty-one days. I've also included a section on how to maintain Whole Detox for life, so you can be sure to keep removing barriers and creating fabulous results.

DETOX FOR THE TWENTY-FIRST CENTURY

I'm thrilled to share Whole Detox with you, because I think it's high time we found a new definition for "detox." We need a detox that employs the whole spectrum of ancient and modern knowledge, and one that treats the whole spectrum of who we are. As a functional medicine nutritionist, I believe that "food is medicine," but I've also come to believe that this approach is not enough. Most people cannot heal on food alone. Yes, health requires a foundation of good eating, but good eating will not necessarily solve our emotional woes or stop our limiting beliefs and toxic self-talk.

The Seven Systems of Full-Spectrum Health have been recognized by ancient healing traditions for thousands of years. They still hold true in the present day. Our physiologies are so intricate and complex, and so are the ways each of our bodies interacts with our entire being. No two of us are alike, yet each of us contains these seven systems, this spectrum of color that helps define our bodies and our lives.

Whole Detox empowers us to remove not just physical toxins but *all* the barriers that impede our growth. Whole Detox is a twenty-one-day program, yes, but it's also the beginning of a *whole* new way of life.

CHAPTER 1

WHOLE DETOX FOR YOUR WHOLE SELF

My patient Padma was confused—and skeptical.

"I came to you for nutritional advice, and to detox," she said with her faint flavor of an Indian accent. "But you are talking to me about all sorts of other issues besides food. I am a person of science—a sociologist—and I want to focus on science and the facts."

I smiled. I had heard these objections before, but seldom did my skeptical patients express their opinions so bluntly, and so soon.

By being so clear, Padma allowed me to be clear in response. "I am also a person of science," I told her. "And what I've learned in more than fifteen years of research and clinical work is that the most scientific approach to healing doesn't ever focus on just one small part of the human body, let alone ignore the role of thoughts, beliefs, and emotions in our health. You get the best results by addressing the whole person. That's what this program is all about."

Padma still looked doubtful.

"Padma," I went on, "you think that beliefs and emotions are separate from the physical body. But, in fact, every time you have a thought or feeling, it is expressed biochemically, as a cascade of neurotransmitters, hormones, or cellular responses. Therefore, your physical condition can have an enormous impact on your mood, your ability to think clearly, and your overall outlook on life—just as your mood, thoughts, and beliefs can affect your physical condition. Mind–body medicine isn't some mystical mumbo jumbo. It's Human Biochemistry 101."

Most of us are used to making distinctions between our body and our emotions. We believe that "I feel hot" or "My foot hurts" or "My doctor tells me I'm at risk for a heart attack" are fundamentally different types of statements from "I feel scared" or "My heart aches" or "If my boss keeps me late one more night this week, I'm going to go through the roof."

Of course, in some ways, those *are* different statements. While we can't measure the subjective experience of heat or pain, we can take our temperature with a thermometer, x-ray our foot for broken bones, and run a whole range of tests to assess our risk for a heart attack. Fear, grief, and anger are harder to measure. And even though we turn to physical metaphors to express our emotional states, we know we don't mean them literally. Your heart doesn't *really* ache. Your blood isn't *literally* boiling. You aren't *actually* about to explode.

Yet in a very real sense, the contrast between mind and body is what my old professors used to call "a distinction without a difference"—a distinction that, at the end of the day, isn't really very useful. Because, in fact, there isn't really any such thing as "body," "mind," "sensation," "emotion"— those are just the names we've come up with to make sense of our experience. What we *really* have, when we look at our human lives, is biochemistry: one big interactive network of hormones, neurotransmitters, synapses, and glands whose job is to respond to the challenges and opportunities of our environment. These responses all happen through electricity and chemistry, and all of them are always *both* physical *and* emotional. That is, any thought or emotion is reflected in a biochemical event, and any biochemical event has its mental and emotional dimensions.

If someone runs up to you with a knife, for example, you might experience the emotion known as fear. Or you might feel anger or determination or some other emotion. You are likely to think, *This doesn't look good* or *I wonder if I can run fast enough to get away.* Whatever thoughts and emotions you might have, you'll also experience an immediate, measurable physical response: the stress response. Your muscles will tense, your blood will begin to flow toward your muscles and away from your stomach, your heart will beat faster, your pupils will contract, your palms will sweat, and you'll start to breathe quickly. And behind both the mental and the physical responses is a flood of stress hormones—cortisol, dopamine, adrenaline, noradrenaline, and many others—triggered via a complicated chemical cascade initiated in your hypothalamus and passing on to your pituitary and your adrenals. Your mental, emotional, and physical experience—the thoughts, feelings, and sensations you experience—all show up in bio-chemical events.

And guess what? It doesn't really matter if you *actually* experience danger or if you just *think* you *might* be in danger . . . or even if you *remember* a time ten years ago when you actually were in danger. Memory, imagination, fantasy, anticipation—all of these produce the same physical response. A hypnotist can convince you that you're scared and produce in you a stress response. So can a powerful speaker alerting you to a political or social threat. So can a movie, a roller coaster, or even a really scary novel. Or a dream. You might think the attacker with a knife is real and the nightmare is unreal, and of course that *is* an important distinction, but an equally important point is the fact *your body doesn't know the difference*. The biochemical responses and electrical impulses that trigger the chemical cascade are the same whether they are generated by an actual physical event or a mere thought.

Now, what does this mean for those of us who want to lead healthy, fulfilling lives? It means we need to be aware of the complex ways in which our bodies and minds interact—in which the categories we like to call "physical," "mental," and "emotional" are often blended and blurred. If you feel depressed and I suggest you eat more fiber, and in a few weeks you've cheered up, then your body has measurably affected your mind. If you feel stressed and you then have trouble digesting your food (because, among other things, stress lowers your stomach acid), your mind has measurably affected your body.

When I realized this truth, I understood that I needed to incorporate it into my work as a functional medicine nutritionist. I couldn't just tell my patients what to eat; I had to help them detoxify from *all* the factors that might be adversely affecting their health.

This insight cut two ways. Patients with seemingly intractable psy-chological issues—anxiety, depression, stress—frequently got spectacular results from changing their diets. At the same time, patients with seemingly incurable physical issues—joint pain, cardiovascular issues, thyroid prob-lems, and ulcerative colitis, to name only a few—got their own spectacular benefits from letting go of some limiting beliefs, nourishing their creativity, and otherwise supporting their minds and emotions.

We tend to think of the boundary between mind and body as a kind of seawall—a rigid, firm barrier clearly marking out the difference between water and land, wet and dry. In reality, the boundary is more like a wide patch of damp sand over which the tide ebbs and flows: now water, now land, now a mixture of both—and constantly changing.

HORMONES: WHERE MIND AND BODY BLUR

One of the quickest ways to understand the interplay between our emotions, thoughts, and physical selves is to consider our hormones.

A hormone is a signaling molecule that helps to regulate the body's physiology and behavior. Hormones are produced by glands, which are part of our endocrine system, the system of hormones and glands that regulates immune function, stress response, fertility, digestion, circulation, metabolism, cognition, mood, the sleep–wake cycle, our circadian rhythms, and many other aspects of ourselves.

Unfortunately, hormones in popular culture have been blamed for female "craziness"—the kind of insanity that women are supposed to feel when they are PMSing, pregnant, or undergoing menopause. The fact is, we all have hormones, and every single one of us—of every age and gender—is profoundly affected by them. When our hormones are in balance, we are sexually vital, vigorous, clear-headed, calm, motivated, and energized. When our hormones are out of whack, so are we: anxious, obsessive, wired, and insomniac . . . exhausted, listless, "foggy," and depressed . . . or, for a double whammy, some of both.

Please don't misunderstand me: I am not saying that our hormones rule our lives (though it can often seem that way!). I am saying that they are the middle, overlapping ground between what we usually think of as "mind" and "body." If you are terrified by thoughts of losing your job, you'll have very high levels of stress hormones. That thought—*I'll lose my job and I won't be able to support myself or my family*—is enough to measurably alter your anatomy. (Yes, there is research in which scientists measured blood levels of hormones after asking subjects to think about upsetting situations.) If you listen to music, your stress hormones may decrease, and you may find yourself able to think more calmly and rationally about whether your job is really at risk or how you'll respond if you do lose it. (Yes, there is research about how music lowers your stress hormone levels.) If you drink caffeine, your cortisol levels will rise in response to the physical stimulus—and these rising hormonal levels might cause you to start feeling anxious about your job again. If you meditate or just breathe deeply, you might once again lower your cortisol levels and find yourself in a calmer state. Your thoughts might reflect that calm feeling, moving from *I'll never work again* to *I'll call Judy on Monday and see if she's hiring*. This positive thought might make you feel even calmer . . . and your stress hormones will fall a little bit more.

Do you see how quickly mind and body flicker back and forth? Whether the stress hormone spike is caused by something physical (caffeine) or mental (the prospect of being fired), you experience a measurable physical response (rising hormone levels). That physical response—whatever its cause—affects your mind.

Likewise, whatever caused your stress hormones to go up (caffeine or fear), you can lower those hormones through something physical (a warm bath) or mental (meditation). And when your stress hormones have fallen—for whatever reason—you will experience different thoughts and emotions.

CASE STUDY: STRESS HORMONES

What Produces Stress Hormones?

Physical: caffeine, blood sugar spikes and crashes, hunger, environments that are too hot or too cold, physical danger (facing an attacker, skydiving, bungee jumping), physical challenges (hiking rough terrain, rowing a boat, lifting weights)

Mental: a tough puzzle to solve, a difficult math problem, an unfamiliar language, note-taking as a speaker talks too fast, a phone call on a bad connection where you can't quite hear the other person

Emotional: a troubled child, a sick parent, a challenging relationship, worries about health or finances, anxiety about public speaking

As you can see, the lists under each category could go on and on. What I want you to notice is how seemingly unrelated events—bungee jumping and worrying about bills; public speaking and working out at the gym; a fight with your spouse and white-water rafting—all stimulate a release of hormones.

Now, here's where it gets even more interesting. How you think affects how you feel, and, consequently, how you feel affects your stress hormones. If you learn you are about to be fired, you might experience any of several different responses, for example:

- *I'll never get another job.*
- *There are plenty of jobs out there. Guess I'll polish up my résumé and start hunting.*

- *My family will think I'm a failure.*
- *My family will come through for me. I can't wait to see them on Sunday to tell them all about it.*

- *I really screwed up this time.*
- *Sometimes things just go wrong. This really isn't such a big deal.*

Can you guess which thoughts on this spectrum are more likely to raise your stress hormone level and which are more likely to lower it? This is why working with belief patterns and limiting thoughts is such a crucial part of Whole Detox.

The problem gets still more interesting—and more urgent—when I tell you all the ways that excessive stress hormones can adversely affect your body:

Symptoms
- Acne and skin problems
- Anxiety
- Brain fog
- Depression
- Imbalanced blood sugar
- Increased blood pressure
- Increased likelihood of PMS, menstrual problems, menopausal problems
- Indigestion
- Insomnia—can't fall asleep, can't stay asleep, or both
- Lowered sex drive and/or sexual function

Disorders
- Autoimmune conditions
- Cancer
- Cardiovascular conditions
- Diabetes
- Obesity

We've taken only a brief look and only at one group of hormones. Your body contains dozens of other hormonal groupings that profoundly affect you as well! Each time you examine one of the Seven Systems of Full-Spectrum Health, you'll learn some of the endocrine glands and hormones associated with that system. You'll be able to see in sharper detail just how your hormones mediate between your body, thoughts, and feelings. You'll realize how hormonal—and overall—health is supported by altering what you eat, yes, but also by exploring what you think, feel, and believe.

A CLOSER LOOK AT THE SEVEN SYSTEMS OF FULL-SPECTRUM HEALTH

We have just seen that our biochemistry crosses the boundaries between body, mind, and emotion. The next step is to ask how we can best treat common physical, mental, and emotional problems. That's where the Seven Systems of Full-Spectrum Health come in: seven clusters of physical, mental, and emotional issues that are best addressed together.

My notion of the seven systems is informed by science and inspired by the combined healing traditions of medicine, spirituality, and yoga. Each system is based in an endocrine gland, moving from the base of the spine up to the crown of the head, and each one represents a nexus of anatomy, physical function, and biochemistry as well as a group of emotions, thoughts, and life issues. It's a very sophisticated and elegant way of integrating body, mind, and emotions—far more nuanced and specific than any other approach I've seen.

In fact, the more success I've had with the seven systems, the more dissatisfied I've become with the notion of "body-mind-spirit." Rather than the sum of these three parts, we are a spectrum of many. Why talk about "body" in such general terms when we could make precise distinctions between the immune system and adrenals (part of the first, the ROOT, system of health), the urinary tract, kidneys, and reproductive system (part of the second, the FLOW, system), and the digestive tract plus the pancreas (part of the third, the FIRE, system)?

The Seven Systems of Full-Spectrum Health give us a way to focus our thoughts about different issues, through nutrition; lifestyle, which includes mental, emotional, and spiritual concepts; and color, which allows us to access the powerful emotional and physical effects of each color as well as the various nutritional properties embodied in the colors of food.

System	Nutrition	Lifestyle	Color
The ROOT	Red foods Protein Minerals	Identity Groundedness Family Tribe	Red
The FLOW	Orange foods Healthy fats Hydration	Creativity Fertility Letting go and being in the flow	Orange
The FIRE	Yellow foods Complex carbohydrates Healthy sweeteners	"Fire in the belly" Ambition, drive Work–life balance Self-esteem	Yellow
The LOVE	Green foods Leafy vegetables	Love Expansiveness Service Grief	Green
The TRUTH	Liquid foods (e.g., soups, stews, sauces, juices) Iodine-rich foods Moist fruits	Verbal expression Authenticity Choice	Aquamarine
The INSIGHT	Blue-purple foods Nutrients that modulate mood and cognition Foods that help with sleep	Imagination Intuition Dreams and sleep	Indigo
The SPIRIT	White, detoxifying foods Fasting Pure foods	Spirituality A sense of being part of some- thing larger than oneself Meaning and purpose	White

Using the seven systems approach gives me and my patients a powerful set of tools to identify toxic barriers and come up with solutions. If I know that you're having trouble with immune function—say, you're frequently coming down with colds and flu—that suggests you might have some toxins in your first system of health. You might need to eat more red foods or up your intake of protein and/or minerals. And/or you might need to consider your sense of personal boundaries—refusing to take on other people's problems or not allowing loved ones to blame you for their own shortcomings. And/or you might want to think about how to improve your relationship with your "tribe," the people who give you your primary sense of identity.

Likewise, if you tell me you feel "ungrounded" or you "just can't settle down to anything" or you frequently feel anxious and unsafe, I might also diagnose first system issues, which I might also address with a combination of physical, mental, and spiritual approaches. Using these seven systems allows me to get more specific than just "body," "mind," and "spirit." And when you have mastered them (and you will, I promise!), you'll be able to get equally specific and equally powerful at overcoming toxic barriers.

These seven systems may seem counterintuitive at first. You might not see why leafy green foods belong in the LOVE system along with your heart, or why blue-purple foods, like blackberries, belong in the INSIGHT system alongside the pituitary gland. But bear with me, because once you grasp the nature of each system of health, it's going to start making a whole lot of sense.

What follows is an overview so you can start to see how these seven systems account for all the physical, mental, emotional, and spiritual issues we experience. They cover the whole spectrum of human experience—another reason I call this program Whole Detox.

To ground each system for you in practical terms, I've included a few specific Whole Detox suggestions, just so you can see how these concepts might translate into real life. Don't worry about following them now or even remembering them; they're just to give you a taste of how this approach works. When you follow the actual twenty-one-day program, I will tell you exactly what to do on each day.

SYSTEM 1: THE ROOT
Adrenal Glands, Immune System, DNA, Bones, Skin, Survival, Community

The ROOT part of us represents our most basic sense of safety and survival. As psychologist Abraham Maslow taught us, if we don't meet our survival needs or feel safe, it's difficult even to think about anything else: we are constantly on edge until we feel rooted. So Whole Detox starts by addressing your ROOT, emphasizing the core elements of survival and identity, including family and community.

The ROOT also speaks to our basic identity as a physical person. If we're going to be fully present in our body, we need to feel rooted, grounded, and safe. Our adrenal glands kick into action whenever we feel threatened, releasing stress hormones at the least sign of danger. At the same time, our immune system keeps our inner boundaries secure. DNA and genetic expression—all the essential biochemistry that creates our core identity (and that is inherited from our family and community)—is also part of the ROOT. Finally, the ROOT includes the anatomical structures that define our body and keep us planted firmly on the earth: bones, feet, joints, legs, muscles, skin, and rectum.

Red is the color of the ROOT. For example, red foods, such as red bell peppers, strawberries, and tomatoes, are rich in the vitamin C our bodies need to manufacture stress hormones. Red blood cells feed on ROOT foods' iron, copper, and calcium. Proteins of all types, including animal protein like red meat and vegetable protein such as black beans, assist in stabilizing our bodies' energy by helping us to balance our blood sugar and by supplying the necessary iron for the red blood cells to carry oxygen.

When you detox your ROOT, you will focus on eliminating foods that stress your adrenal glands and immune system while eating the protein, minerals, and red foods that support all core issues of your ROOT. You will also consider your relationship to family, community, and tribe.

SYSTEM 2: THE FLOW
Ovaries/Testes, Reproduction, Fertility, Urinary System,
Colon, Partnerships, Creativity

Moving up from the ROOT, we address the second system of full-spectrum health, the FLOW. As Mihaly Csikszentmihalyi has shown in his landmark book *Flow*, being in the flow is crucial for creativity, whether we're talking about art, scientific discovery, or innovative ways to solve problems. When we enter this space, we become capable of sustaining a profound relationship with our work, colleagues, friends, and intimate partners.

Accordingly, the FLOW centers on the parts of the body that enable us to create new life—our ovaries (for women), testes (for men), and entire reproductive system—as well as our ability to produce new cells. Meanwhile, our kidneys and bladder literally govern the body's water fluxes, helping to balance our consumption of liquids and regulating our hydration. When we are in the flow, it means taking in and letting go with ease. The large intestine is also part of this system, since it allows us to pull out the water we need from the waste products we eliminate.

The FLOW also includes the still or turbulent waters to creativity, emotions, and relationships. I've had more than one patient who found herself able to become pregnant after releasing blocked emotions in a relationship or making more room for creativity in her life.

Orange is the color of the FLOW. Orange foods, like carrots and sweet potatoes, get their color from carotenoids, such as beta-carotene, which are associated with hormone levels and ovulation. Maybe that's why I've noticed that a lack of orange-colored, carotenoid-rich foods seems to be linked to infertility. Other types of orange foods, such as citrus fruits, contain bioflavonoids that keep our blood vessels open, preventing the stagnation of varicose veins and allowing our blood to flow. Finally, both carotenoids and bioflavonoids help to prevent cancer, keeping our bodies from engaging in unhealthy types of growth and reproduction.

When you detox your FLOW, you will focus on staying hydrated, removing the substances that disrupt your reproductive hormones, supporting your FLOW with healthy fats, and rekindling your creativity. You will also look at ways to keep your emotions flowing.

SYSTEM 3: THE FIRE
Digestive System, Blood Sugar, Work–Life Balance, Energy Production

Moving further up the body, we reach the glands and organs associated with the third system of health: the FIRE. Our pancreas, liver, gallbladder, small intestine, and stomach all burn the food we ingest, transmuting it into the energy we need to survive, just as a fire burns fuel to produce life-giving warmth. Accordingly, nutrient absorption, biotransformation, blood sugar balance, and digestion belong to this system of health.

The FIRE ignites our drive to work, achieve, and compete. A healthy FIRE is full of energy, power, and confidence. An overactive FIRE might lack work–life balance, losing the joy of accomplishment in the burning need to do more and more and more. An underactive FIRE might feel simply "burnt out." My research and clinical experience have shown me that this system of health tends to be out of alignment for just about everyone, with nearly 80 percent of my patients and students showing some imbalance in this system. An imbalanced FIRE is truly the bane of our busy, burnt-out modern lives!

Just as a fire must burn in balance—neither starved for fuel nor choked by too much green wood—so do our bodies need balance: the right types of food to keep our blood sugar stable; the right amounts of rest and stimulation to keep our energy stable. Likewise, we must all find the balance in our lives, between situations in which we "go with the flow" and situations in which we take charge, assert ourselves, and blaze forth with our goals, projects, and achievements.

Many of the glands and organs associated with the FIRE are located in and around the solar plexus—the area at the pit of the stomach—so I find it interesting that when we talk about someone who has a lot of energy and drive, we say that he or she has "fire in the belly." When our energy is depleted, we're "burnt out" or "fried to a crisp," possibly because we've been "burning the candle at both ends." We can also be "fired" from a job. These common expressions speak to our intuitive recognition of this third system of health, and to the way both our bodies and our life issues are components of the same system.

Yellow is the FIRE's color, and it's also the color of quick-burning refined carbohydrates. The diet that has become increasingly common in the modern world tends to include far too many of these high-energy, yellow foods, which perhaps is part of the fuel for an overactive FIRE. A more balanced FIRE is fueled by slow-burning, low-glycemic, high-fiber carbohydrates, such as those found in whole grains and legumes. The FIRE also requires a whole team of B vitamins, such as thiamin (B1), riboflavin (B2), niacin (B3), pyridoxine (B6), folate (B9), and cobalamin (B12), all of which are crucial for generating a healthy metabolism and extracting energy from our foods.

Detoxing your FIRE has you loading up on high-fiber carbohydrates and fiery yellow foods, such as ginger and turmeric. You'll also look at how to create your own personal version of work–life balance and harness the "fire in your belly"—your ambition, energy, and drive.

SYSTEM 4: THE LOVE

Thymus, Heart, Blood Vessels, Lungs, Compassion, Expansiveness, Service

Moving up from the belly and into the chest, we arrive at the LOVE, the fourth system of health, which resides in the kingdom of the heart and lungs. Here we open up to compassion and service as well as expansion, in the way that love in all its forms makes us feel larger, more generous, a "bigger person," someone whose warmth and good feeling radiate outward into the world. The LOVE can also expand through an embrace, an apology, a feeling of gratitude, or the simple, comforting touch of a loved one's hand. Central to this fourth system is the thymus, the organ that governs our adaptive immune system. Also central is the magnificent heart, which is far more than just a pump. Science suggests that it is also a neuroendocrine gland, affecting hormone balance as well as blood flow.

Just as love and compassion enable us to respond to a wide variety of threats, so do the thymus and heart help the body distinguish between various challenges. Meanwhile, the blood vessels, lungs, and lymphatic system serve us by spreading nourishment and oxygen throughout the body, while the lymph carries toxins away. You might see the LOVE organs as providing compassion and self-care to our entire being while helping us overcome the obstacles to growth and healing.

One of the challenges of the LOVE is to make sure that we are giving it to ourselves. Many of my patients find that their LOVE has become imbalanced, always expanding out to children, parents, friends, spouses, and perhaps even clients or colleagues, but rarely directed inward toward themselves. Forgiveness—of both ourselves and others—is an example of a way to balance the LOVE. The Western tradition associates love with the heart, while TCM views the lungs as the seat of grief. Indeed, when the LOVE is out of balance, it often manifests as overwhelming grief—"heartbreak" that refuses to heal. Too much pain can also cause us to shut down our hearts, closing off our urge toward compassion, service, and love.

Green is the color of the LOVE. The color green represents healing and nourishment, so it's no wonder that green foods are "heart-healthy." All green foods contain chlorophyll, which acts as an antioxidant and blood purifier, promoting robust circulation. Green detox foods include spirulina, chlorella, leafy greens, and cruciferous vegetables like broccoli, Brussels sprouts, and kale.

Detoxing your LOVE focuses on green leafy vegetables and expansive aerobic movement, which allows your cardiopulmonary system to function at its best. You will also consider how to expand your sense of compassion, gratitude, generosity, and self-love.

SYSTEM 5: THE TRUTH
Thyroid Gland, Throat, Mouth, Ears, Nose, Speaking, Choice, Authenticity

From the heart, we go up to the throat area, where both the voice box (larynx) and the thyroid gland are located. Now we are in the fifth system of health, which I call the TRUTH.

The TRUTH includes an array of sensory organs that provide us with inputs to integrate: ears, nose, throat, and mouth. We need to take in information and choose what to do with it—decide what's true and what isn't, make authentic decisions, and truthfully express our responses. Listening and speaking are therefore part of the TRUTH.

Smelling and chewing are also integral to this system, along with the thyroid gland, which helps us metabolize the food we take in, finding the body's authentic rhythms and, ideally, its healthiest weight.

The TRUTH also guides the image you present to the world—your sense of who you are. Words like "authenticity," "choice," and "voice" are all part of the TRUTH—"voice" in both the physical sense of speaking and the metaphoric sense of your unique self-expression. If you can tell the world your truest thoughts—if you can share your most genuine and authentic self—you have taken a powerful step to support your TRUTH.

Many of my patients struggle to face their personal truths and express them to the world. People who feel their metabolism "won't let them" lose weight are often afraid to speak their truth. Maybe they've been told all their lives to shut up, to be polite, or to lower their voice, literally or metaphorically. Maybe they don't believe they have anything important to say. But I'm struck how finding the voice to speak your own truth can be a powerful, liberating force for thyroid function and the creation of a healthy metabolism, especially when you are also supporting your thyroid gland with the right foods and supplements.

Aquamarine is the color of TRUTH. When you detox your TRUTH, you'll consume delicious sea vegetables and lubricate your throat with fruits, soups, sauces, and juices. You'll bring more awareness to your daily habits so you can begin to make the choices that serve you best.

SYSTEM 6: THE INSIGHT
Pituitary Gland, Brain, Neurons/Neurotransmitters, Sleep, Mood, Thoughts, Intuition

The sixth system of health—the INSIGHT—includes your pituitary gland, which some consider the "master gland." The pituitary is like a busy train station, constantly receiving and transmitting signals throughout the entire brain and body. This central hub of your physiology and psychology is well recognized in ancient traditions of healing as a pivot point for meditation.

The pituitary is also sometimes called the inner eye, as it maintains surveillance over a wide range of activity throughout your entire biochemistry. Your physical eyes belong to this system too. In other words, both outer and inner sight are part of the INSIGHT. Similarly, the INSIGHT includes all your neurons, neurotransmitters, and brain cells, which process and interpret what you see, perceiving metaphorical and abstract truths as well as literal, physical ones.

Mood, thoughts, and sleep are all part of this system of health, as are visualization, imagination, reflection, and intuition. If you've ever felt that a bad night's sleep, a foggy brain, or a depressed mood was keeping you from seeing things clearly, you've experienced how crucial this system can be.

And if you've ever felt that your vision cleared after a good night's sleep, a nourishing meal, or a comforting talk with a friend, you know the potential of detoxing the INSIGHT and seeing truly once more.

When I treat patients whose INSIGHT needs Whole Detox, I marvel at the deep, intimate relationship between body, thought, and emotion. You simply can't think clearly when you're getting the wrong foods, and you're all too likely to be depressed, anxious, or overly emotional as well. Likewise, when you see the world clearly, you have the passion and energy to commit to your health, because you understand better what your body needs.

Indigo is the color of the INSIGHT, so we support this system of health with blue and purple foods: blueberries, blackberries, purple kale, purple asparagus, purple cauliflower, purple grapes. Berries and grapes in particular are good sources of resveratrol, the powerhouse antioxidant that helps protect your brain and nerves. Blue and purple foods also promote neuronal plasticity, which is the scientific way of saying that they improve your brain's ability to create new pathways, improving your cognition, learning, and memory.

Detoxing your INSIGHT involves loading up on blue and purple foods, keeping a dream journal, and learning to listen carefully to that "still small voice" within. You will support both your brain matter and the workings of your mind.

SYSTEM 7: THE SPIRIT
Pineal Gland, Electromagnetic Fields, Circadian Rhythms, Connection, Purpose, Meaning

Finally, we come to the seventh system of health, the SPIRIT, which includes some of the biggest issues we ever wrestle with: connection, purpose, and—for want of a better term—what we might call soul. This system enables us to experience that we are both microcosm and macrocosm, both individual beings and indistinguishable from the whole, both individual drops of water and participants in one big ocean. The SPIRIT is where you connect to meaning in your life, to your life's calling, to the values, beliefs, and activities that most profoundly embody what you consider important.

Grounding the SPIRIT in the body is the pineal gland—a receiver within our brain that distinguishes between light and dark, day and night, sunlight and moonlight. If your circadian rhythms are off—if you can't get into a regular sleep pattern, if you can't make an easy transition between seasons, if you can't function optimally while doing shift work, or if you feel lost and disconnected—your seventh system needs Whole Detox.

This is the system in the body that regulates your vitality and your ability to age gracefully. When you feel you are declining in health faster than most or you are aging too fast, it's often your seventh system—governing your "life force"—that could use some support. You might need more time in the sunlight, some nutrients to help your cells remain vital, or perhaps a different room in which to sleep. You might even be feeling drained because you don't know your life's purpose—you don't have a reason to get up in the morning. A sure sign of a "toxic" seventh system is feeling out of touch with the significance of events and commitments that get you through the day.

White foods help cleanse and clarify the seventh system. When you think of the color white, you might think of purity or clarity. This system holds within it the high path of enlightened, good clean living. Sometimes it's not as much about what we eat as the manner in which we eat, at what time we eat, and whether we eat too much. That's why one element of the SPIRIT is abstinence of food through a variety of fasting approaches.

Now, let's be clear: "White foods" doesn't mean processed foods full of white flour or white sugar. When it comes to the SPIRIT, it refers to foods that embody the ultimate healing properties for multiple organs: ripe pears (especially good for moistening the lungs), cauliflower (cleansing for the liver), coconut products (an accessible energy source for the intestines), onions and garlic (cleansing for the blood and liver), cabbage (cleansing for the liver and, when fermented, excellent for the gut), and white beans (high in fiber).

The SPIRIT detox focuses on naturally white foods, healing light, and journaling about your life's purpose. You will also have the opportunity to reflect on the "miracles" in your life—the tiny bits of awe that keep you feeling the juice of what it means to be alive.

WHOLE DETOX IN PRACTICE

When you go through your twenty-one-day program, you'll look at each system of health separately, so you can make sure to fully address each one. But as you carry Whole Detox into your life, you'll work with the whole spectrum, just as I do with my patients. To give you an idea of how Whole Detox and the full-spectrum approach works in real life, let's go back to my patient Padma.

Padma taught urban sociology at a university, a job she generally enjoyed but also found rather stressful. During her first year of college, she suffered from crippling panic attacks as well as stress-related headaches. An M.D. prescribed some antianxiety medication, which Padma used very judiciously, fearing she would become addicted. As she saw that she was capable of getting good grades and pleasing her professors, she became less anxious and was able to stop taking the meds.

Now, however, her panic had returned, set off by rumors of funding cuts at her university. Although she was one of the senior members of her department, she was beset by fears that her research funding would cease. Although she wasn't having panic attacks, she did feel far more anxious than she would like, and her headaches frequently caused her to miss classes and appointments.

As with all my patients, I looked at the full spectrum of Padma's physical, mental, and emotional life. When she told me that she drank several cups of coffee throughout the day, I knew that was at least partly responsible for both her anxiety and her headaches.

But Whole Detox delves into more layers. I wanted Padma to identify her own personal toxins, whether in the form of food, relationships, thought patterns, or other issues, so she could either remove them or develop the strength to live with them more gracefully. I knew that, either way, Whole Detox could allow her to find the vitality and resilience she needed to overcome any barrier that held her back.

I began by giving Padma the Spectrum Quiz I give to all my patients. (You'll get to take this quiz too.) As we analyzed her results, we discovered that she had weaknesses in three systems of health: the ROOT, the FLOW, and the TRUTH.

As a child of immigrants, Padma had always felt a kind of disconnect between her Indian identity and her American one. Although she admired innovative thinkers, she always felt too fearful to let her own creative impulses flow or to "think outside the box." She felt nervous, too, about expressing her true opinions, for fear of alienating others who already saw her as foreign and perhaps a little strange.

At the same time, she tended to eat irregularly, and not in a particularly healthy way. A vegetarian, she wasn't making sure to get the full spectrum of vitamins and minerals her body needed. Instead, she lived largely on lentils and rice, with few fresh, moist fruits or vegetables. She rarely drank water or even tea, which meant she was fairly dehydrated. She was beginning to develop a thyroid condition, which was at least partly responsible for her anxiety and her headaches, and was at least partly caused by an iodine deficiency.

Here are some of the ways Padma's problems manifested across the spectrum:

	Physical symptoms	Nutrition	Lifestyle
The ROOT	Headaches	Too much caffeine Not enough protein Not enough minerals Not enough red foods: beets, cherries, water- melon	Struggles with ethnic identity while living in a foreign country A feeling of unground- edness Uncertainty of her tribe
The FLOW	Anxiety	Not enough fluids Not enough orange foods: carrots, sweet potatoes, oranges/citrus	Not allowing herself to be creative A feeling of being "out- side the flow of life"
The TRUTH	Thyroid dysfunction	Not enough iodine Not enough ocean foods: sea vegetables Irregular eating	Fear of "speaking up" Not wanting to appear different Reluctance to present new ideas

Diagnosing Padma's concerns was not a simple matter of cause and effect. Anxiety, poor thyroid function, low iodine levels, and a reluctance to speak her truth—Padma struggled with all these issues, and who is to say which had come first or which were most important? The bad news was that they were all making each other issue worse. The good news was that any steps Padma took—even small changes—could create a healing momentum that might operate on many levels at once.

Accordingly, I encouraged Padma to undertake a spectrum of physical, emotional, mental, and social activities:

- cut back on caffeine;
- hydrate regularly throughout the day;
- eat more sea vegetables in soups and broths, more protein, more fresh fruits and vegetables;
- do some grounding yoga poses; and
- spend some time journaling about what "speaking her truth" meant to her.

This last point was not completely clear to Padma, so I asked her to think of some people in history or in her life who spoke their truth—who made it clear through words and deeds exactly what they believed in and what they stood for. Padma identified Gandhi, the writer Toni Morrison, and Marisa, a friend from childhood with whom she was still close. "You always know where they stand," she told me. When I asked her whether that was true for her as well, Padma slowly shook her head. "I am more secretive," she told me. "I don't want people to know so much about what I believe." I asked her to think about whether that was something she might want to change, and, if so, to imagine how she might make this shift in her life. I also suggested that Padma explore ways to identify her tribe—whether culturally, by being part of an Indian community, or professionally, by finding social scientists she respected and with whom she felt safe expressing her ideas. As you can see, the full-spectrum approach allows for a wide variety of responses to a problem while helping each response enhance the others.

Sometimes we need to detox by letting go of foods, habits, or relationships. Sometimes we need to get more of something. Padma, for example, had to let go of excessive caffeine while also getting more iodine, protein, and fresh produce. She had to let go of her fears of what others might think while also enriching her life with more community, rootedness, and connection.

Within a few weeks, she began feeling the benefits of Whole Detox's full-spectrum approach. She looked better, felt better, thought better, worked better. She enjoyed the glow of health. She celebrated the richness of her complex identity. She slept better. She spoke out more at faculty meetings. She had more energy. She began to write an article that she felt was much closer to her "true voice" than any of her previous publications. "I can feel the barriers melting away," she told me on our last visit. It's a thrilling feeling—and one that I want for you too!

Let's get started. The next seven chapters will take you, one by one, through the Seven Systems of Full-Spectrum Health. The more you get acquainted with each one of them, the more clearly you'll be able to see how these systems operate in your life and how to make Whole Detox work for you. As soon as you begin your twenty-one-day program, you'll realize how quickly Whole Detox pays off. The great thing is, it just keeps getting better and better.

THE WHOLE DETOX SPECTRUM QUIZ

Welcome to your Whole Detox Spectrum Quiz! You will have the opportunity to focus on each system of health, targeting the physical, mental, and emotional barriers that are holding you back from optimal health and a wholly fulfilling life. In each system, you will identify the issues in five areas: two relate to food and your bodily symptoms, and the other three concern life issues.

These questions and categories may seem powerful and exciting, or they may not seem to make much sense. You may find it inspiring to answer these questions, or perhaps you'll find yourself feeling anxious, sad, or even a little angry. Many of my patients feel some or all of these things as they move through each question.

Whatever your responses, I promise that you will learn a lot, and you will set yourself up for a powerful detox journey. Go ahead and fill out the quiz. Allow yourself at most about ten to fifteen minutes to complete it, so that you don't belabor any one question but rather go with your first impulse. When you've finished, I'll tell you how to make use of the results.

I recommend doing the Whole Detox Spectrum Quiz three times within three days under different circumstances. For example, on Sunday, when you might be relaxed and not working, then again on Monday, perhaps during the day or during a break you have at work, and then finally on Tuesday evening, when you come home from work. Having three points of reference will help you see what is consistently imbalanced rather than a simple situational response.

For each statement, answer either *yes* or *no*. When you are done, tally the number of *no* responses for each system. Write down the number in the box provided at the end of the quiz.

THE WHOLE DETOX SPECTRUM QUIZ

THE ROOT

Do you feel "comfortable in your own skin"?	Y N
Do you feel it's acceptable to say no to others?	Y N
Do you feel safe in your body?	Y N
Do you feel safe in your home?	Y N
Are you free from pending danger or harm?	Y N
Do you find it easy to deal with daily stressors?	Y N
Are you capable of working well under pressure?	Y N
Is surviving in your everyday world easy?	Y N
Do you go with your instincts?	Y N
Do you trust others?	Y N
Do you spend quality time in supportive communities?	Y N
Could you go to your community for help when you need it?	Y N
Are your social networks positive and uplifting?	Y N
Are your family and/or close friends supportive?	Y N
Are you in harmony with your family of origin and/or upbringing?	Y N
Do you remember to eat when stressed?	Y N
Do you eat protein with most meals?	Y N
Do you avoid foods that disagree with you?	Y N
Do you eat natural, whole foods that are red in color (e.g., apples, cherries)?	Y N
Do you feel grounded after eating?	Y N
Do you have a strong constitution?	Y N
Are you usually "the last one to get sick"?	Y N
Are you at a healthy body weight?	Y N
Is your skin clear?	Y N
Are you free of joint pain and inflammation?	Y N

THE FLOW

Do you express your emotions to others with ease? Y N
Do you readily go with the flow? Y N
Do you express yourself when you feel something is "off"? Y N
Do you refrain from eating emotionally? Y N
Are you generally in touch with your feelings? Y N
Do you take a creative approach to life? Y N
Do you generally put your ideas into action? Y N
Do you have unique perspectives on situations? Y N
Do you have a healthy "creative side"? Y N
Do you enjoy being your creative self? Y N
Do you make time for play? Y N
Do you consider yourself playful? Y N
Do you aim to have fun in all you do? Y N
Are you comfortable with your sexuality? Y N
Are you able to create a healthy, fulfilling partnership with another person? Y N
Do you eat some healthy fats and oils every day? Y N
Are you eating natural, whole foods that are orange in color (e.g., carrots, pumpkin, oranges)? Y N
Do you regularly eat tropical fruits (e.g., mango, papaya, coconut)? Y N
Do you drink purified water? Y N
Do you drink fluids throughout the day? Y N
Is your sex drive good? Y N
Are your bowel movements of a normal consistency (no diarrhea or constipation)? Y N
Do you feel adequately hydrated? Y N
Do you engage in activities that make you sweat? Y N
Are your hormones balanced, to the best of your knowledge? Y N

THE FIRE

Do you think you have a good energy level? Y N
Does your daily life energize you in a healthy, stimulating way? Y N
Does being around people give you energy? Y N
Do you feel energized after eating, as though you are full of energy to be active and to move? Y N
Do you take on a reasonable number of goals without overreaching? Y N

Are you confident yet not egotistical?   Y N

Are you ambitious in achieving your goals yet never lose sight of priorities in your
personal life?   Y N

Are you focused on your goals but also flexible in your process to achieve them?   Y N

Do you feel satisfied with your performance on projects or tasks?   Y N

Do you keep your ambitious goals in check with enjoying life?   Y N

Do you maintain work–life balance?   Y N

Do you make time to have fun away from work?   Y N

Are you realistic about taking on work that you can reasonably do?   Y N

Do you handle a busy schedule without fretting?   Y N

Do you only say yes to things you can comfortably do?   Y N

Do you avoid consistently eating sweets or desserts?   Y N

Do you avoid consistently eating meals high in processed starchy foods
(e.g., breads, pastas, pretzels)?   Y N

Do you avoid quick-energy, caffeinated drinks?   Y N

Do you avoid overeating when you are stressed?   Y N

Are you more likely to take time to prepare meals than eat out?   Y N

Do you digest your food well?   Y N

Do you have healthy blood sugar levels?   Y N

Are you free of digestive complaints or conditions?   Y N

Does your stomach feel comfortable after eating?   Y N

Are you trim in your belly area?   Y N

THE LOVE

Have you been able to release past events that hurt you?   Y N

Are you able to easily let go of grief?   Y N

Are you quick to forgive?   Y N

Are you able to give to and receive from others equally?   Y N

Is your heart open but with select boundaries that are healthy?   Y N

Are you physically active?   Y N

Are you physically fit?   Y N

Do you make time to be in nature?   Y N

Do you breathe deeply?   Y N

Do you do some aerobic activity on a regular basis, such as walking, biking,
or running?   Y N

Do you make time for *you*?   Y N
Do you let others help you if you are in need?   Y N
Do you take care of yourself to the same extent you are able to take care of others? Y N
Are you living out your heartfelt passions?   Y N
Are you routinely setting aside time in your schedule to do what you *feel* like doing
    rather than do what you feel obligated to do?   Y N
Do you eat plant-based foods every day?   Y N
Do you eat cruciferous vegetables (e.g., broccoli, kale, Brussels sprouts, cabbage)
    at least three times per week?   Y N
Do you eat leafy green salads at least every other day?   Y N
Do you feel grateful for your daily meals?   Y N
Do you love eating vegetables of all types?   Y N
Are your hands and feet comfortably warm?   Y N
Can you breathe without difficulty?   Y N
Is it easy to breathe while you exercise?   Y N
Is your blood pressure normal?   Y N
Is your heart rate normal?   Y N

THE TRUTH

Are you true to yourself no matter what?   Y N
Do you enjoy your uniqueness?   Y N
Do you feel free to be you?   Y N
Are you consistent in living according to your values?   Y N
Do you feel open in giving your opinion when asked?   Y N
Do you speak your truth in a clear and conscientious way?   Y N
Are you comfortable expressing yourself verbally?   Y N
Do you find it enjoyable to converse with others?   Y N
Do you enjoy talking things out as a way of processing an event or issue?   Y N
Do you speak up if there are issues you feel strongly about?   Y N
Are you confident in your decision-making ability?   Y N
Can you easily make a decision even when there are many choices?   Y N
Are you able to choose what is important to you?   Y N
Do you usually walk away knowing you made the best choice you could?   Y N
Are you comfortable making decisions?   Y N
Do you chew your food well?   Y N

Do you eat an adequate amount of food (not too little, not too much)?   Y N
Do you have a normal, healthy appetite?   Y N
When you eat, do you only eat and not multitask?   Y N
Do you choose foods you know are healthy for you?   Y N
Does it seem that you have a normal metabolism?   Y N
Is your thyroid healthy, to the best of your knowledge?   Y N
Does your throat stay moist and free from soreness?   Y N
Do you have healthy teeth?   Y N
Is your jaw loose and relaxed?   Y N

THE INSIGHT

Do you consider yourself to be smart or able to easily understand concepts?   Y N
Are you good at solving problems based on what you know?   Y N
Compared to most people, do you consider yourself a "thinker"?   Y N
Do you like learning new things?   Y N
Are you a quick learner?   Y N
Do you consider yourself intuitive?   Y N
Do you get impressions about things yet to happen?   Y N
Do you have a good sense of discernment?   Y N
Do you listen to your inner knowing?   Y N
Do you allow your intuition to help guide you through life?   Y N
Do you sleep all through the night?   Y N
Do you regularly sleep seven to eight hours per night?   Y N
Do you have a consistent, healthy sleep pattern?   Y N
Do you fall asleep easily without the use of sleep aids?   Y N
Do you wake in the morning feeling refreshed?   Y N
Do you avoid drinking too many caffeinated drinks?   Y N
Do you avoid eating too much chocolate?   Y N
Are you free from food addictions?   Y N
Do you abstain from drinking excessive amounts of alcoholic drinks?   Y N
Are you able to focus your attention without relying on external substances
   (e.g., caffeine, alcohol)?   Y N
Are you able to clear your mind before bedtime?   Y N
Are you attentive to tasks on hand and mindful of your actions?   Y N
Is your memory good?   Y N

Are your moods stable? Y N
Do you meditate or engage in a mindful practice of some sort? Y N

THE SPIRIT

Is your life full of meaning? Y N
Do you feel connected to life in ways that invigorate your spirit? Y N
Are you concerned with greater planetary causes (e.g., ending hunger, world peace)? Y N
Do you feel you have a special mission or a calling by which you live? Y N
Do you find yourself inspired to commit to changing the world? Y N
Do you live a spiritual life? Y N
Do you have faith that everything works out as it needs to? Y N
Do your spiritual views direct your life decisions at a high level? Y N
Do you feel strengthened through your spirituality? Y N
Do you believe in something greater than yourself? Y N
Do you have regular exposure to sunlight? Y N
Do you feel that you radiate an inner glow? Y N
Do you sleep during the nighttime hours and stay awake during the daylight hours? Y N
Do you have access to bright white lights in your living space? Y N
Does life feel "light and wonderful" rather than "heavy and dark"? Y N
Do you regularly detox your body? Y N
Do you regularly eat certain foods that are known to be good for detoxification? Y N
Do you eat fresh organic food over fried food? Y N
Do you avoid plastic containers (e.g., for food, water)? Y N
Do you avoid using toxic personal care products (e.g., chemical-laden lotions, hair-care products, makeup, deodorant)? Y N
Do you take precautions in minimizing your exposure to excessive electromagnetic fields (EMFs)? Y N
Is your nervous system healthy (e.g., no pain, numbness)? Y N
Are you resilient and recover quickly from any illness? Y N
Do people say that you look younger than your age? Y N
Do you think that your life force, or constitution, is stronger than most others? Y N

SCORING YOUR QUIZ

Note the number of *no* responses within each system:	
The ROOT	
The FLOW	
The FIRE	
The LOVE	
The TRUTH	
The INSIGHT	
The SPIRIT	

INTERPRETING YOUR SYSTEM SCORES

- If you answered *no* to fewer than ten questions within any system, this system is likely to be balanced.
- If you answered *no* to between eleven and fifteen questions within any system, you have a *moderate* imbalance of that system.
- If you answered *no* to more than fifteen questions within any system, you have a *severe* imbalance of that system.

Your scores help you identify systems that include your core strengths as well as systems that are out of balance. You'll learn more about each system in the next several chapters, and in your twenty-one-day program, I'll work with you in detail to heal each one.

You might be tempted to skip right to a particular system, but I urge you to read through every chapter. Every system works with every other system—that is the power of synergy—and to heal one, it helps to understand them all.

For any system where you have a strong imbalance, take a look at the questions to which you answered *no* and see whether you can detect a pattern or similarity. For example, if your *nos* in the ROOT all relate to food, you should pay particular attention to proteins, minerals, and red foods. Or if all your *nos* in the TRUTH concern your voice and self-expression, you'll know to pay special attention to those issues and how you can speak your truth more fully and easily. One of the wonderful things about Whole Detox is the way it allows you to target personal concerns and fine-tune your responses. Remember that no matter which system you focus on, you are focusing on the whole of who you are. Everything is interconnected, as I explained earlier.

What if your scores indicate that *all* your systems are balanced? Well, that may happen, similar to when you get your blood work done and find that your number fit within the range of what is considered healthy. For example, your thyroid hormones may check out normal, but you still have issues of thyroid imbalance. I would encourage you to look at the scores in a more personalized way: you might be at the top or bottom of that range. If all your scores come in as balanced, you have two ways to target your personal barriers and take advantage of opportunities for growth. You can do either or both:

- Pick the system with the most *nos* and focus some extra attention there. For example, maybe your FLOW is balanced with fewer than ten *nos*, but out of all your systems, it's the one that has the most number of *no* responses. That would indicate you need to put your energy here. Even if you are generally balanced in that system, a single *no* indicates a potential barrier that might be keeping you from enjoying your fullest spectrum of health, wellness, and fulfillment.
- Scan the questions and note the *nos* to which you have the most intense, anxious, or sad response:
  - *Oh, I could never do that!*
  - *I wish I could do that, but it's not gonna happen.*
  - *Other people can do that, but not me.*
  - *I don't even want to do that—why are you asking me about it???*

If you had a strong reaction to a particular question, that might indicate a barrier that is holding you back. As you move through your twenty-one-day program, be open to the possibility of removing or overcoming that barrier.

Whatever your score, it is essential to think about how each system operates in your life. Continue to ask yourself how you can make the most of your current strengths. What can you do to remove your current barriers? And, most important, what can you do to make sure each system helps you achieve your overall purpose, bringing you to a richer and more inspired life?

CHAPTER 2

THE POWER OF SYNERGY

Before you look at each of the seven systems separately, I want to introduce you to the synergy that animates each system and binds all seven systems together. This is your chance to think further about how Whole Detox affects your body and your health. What does a healthy balance look like for you?

Because each of us is a unique individual, your healthy balance will look different from mine. Because you are on a lifelong journey, each system will likely take on different meanings at different times in your life. And because life resists simple solutions, your greatest strength may resemble your greatest weakness.

The one constant in this process is *synergy*: different elements working together to create a whole that is greater than the sum of its parts. Synergy can work negatively, as when excess weight, a struggle with anxiety, a stressful job, a neglected love life, and an overwhelming sense of perfectionism all make each other worse. (Can you see that these elements are all part of an imbalanced third system—an excess of the FIRE that has quickly led to burnout?) Synergy can also work positively, as when high-fiber carbohydrates, a joy in work, some refreshing meditation, and a self-loving attitude create a steady supply of fuel to support your health and well-being.

In fact, the greatest strength of Whole Detox is the way it reverses negative synergy and replaces it with positive synergy. This is why my patients enjoy such swift and powerful results. Each element of Whole Detox—food choices, exercise, affirmations, journaling, and other activities—works in concert with the others to create an ever-widening upward spiral: a veritable healing cyclone!

So in this chapter you're going to take a closer look at synergy: within each system, between all seven systems, and throughout the course of your life. This perspective should enable you to further personalize your approach to Whole Detox as you identify and overcome the barriers in your life.

WHEN YOUR STRENGTH LOOKS LIKE YOUR WEAKNESS

Roberto is the kind of solid, reliable guy everybody can depend on. He married his college sweetheart, went into the family business, and is raising two children, who are doing well in school. He lives just a few miles from his parents, and most Sundays he and his family join his relatives for a big, raucous dinner with everybody's favorite foods and long games of touch football, soccer, or cards.

Roberto is proud of his work and family. Sometimes, though, he wonders whether his life lacks adventure. And while he knows his marriage is stable, he has the feeling that his wife would like a little adventure too.

———

Zenia has had, by all accounts, an extraordinary life. A talented photographer, she has spent most of her life traveling from one assignment to another: a battle in rural Afghanistan, a presidential inauguration in Buenos Aires, an art opening in Stockholm, a fashion show in Milan. She has always had an unusual ability to adapt to whatever circumstances in which she found herself, and now, in her sixties, she can look back upon an impressive body of work, several satisfying romances, and a network of friends and colleagues around the globe.

In this latest phase of her life, however, Zenia is beginning to crave a little stability. She wonders whether her scanty savings will be enough for her old age. Does she need a new retirement plan? She wonders, too, whether it's time to pick a home and put down roots, maybe even look for someone steady in her life.

———

Jared has a forceful, fiery energy that has taken him to the top of his marketing company in a remarkably short time. He works long, hard hours and is amazingly productive. He loves his work, is proud of his accomplishments, and, in his midthirties, looks forward to more.

But Jared frequently feels stressed and burnt out. His long-suffering girlfriend has just given him an ultimatum. And he wonders where he could make room in this demanding life for the children he has always wanted.

———

Leah has the gift of empathy. Close friends, new acquaintances, and even total strangers seek her advice, her listening ear, her open, loving response. She always seems to know what another person might think or feel, and she has a seemingly boundless ability to step up with comfort or help.

But Leah finds it so easy to see another person's point of view that she often loses sight of her own. And she is so willing to give to others that she finds it challenging to nurture herself.

———

Brandon is a truth teller. A natural leader, he has the ability to take charge of a situation, speak honestly about what the problems are, and offer workable solutions. His colleagues, employer, friends, and family all depend on him to cut through the "noise" with clear, useful answers.

Sometimes, though, Brandon is so preoccupied with his own vision of the truth that he forgets to listen to others. Or maybe he doesn't *forget*; he might simply not see the need. As a result, he occasionally makes mistakes that might have been avoided—and he sometimes alienates those who feel ignored.

———

Solange is one of the most intuitive, insightful people her friends have ever met. If you have a problem that makes no sense to you, Solange is the one to speak with. She has the uncanny gift of seeing through the surface and penetrating right to the heart of a matter.

Sometimes, though, Solange feels overwhelmed by her own mind, buried under all the thoughts and insights that seem to keep coming and coming and coming. Although she usually enjoys her insightful vision, she does sometimes wish she could just empty her head and give her mind a rest.

———

A calm and generous professor of religious studies, Matthew is considered by his community to be very spiritual. He always seems to be operating in another dimension, inspired to a higher purpose and connected deeply to his students, his research, and his ascetic lifestyle.

One winter, however, Matthew picks up the flu and he just can't seem to shake it. When he comes to me, I realize that Matthew is severely malnourished and underweight. Although he has been feeding his soul, he has neglected his body, with potentially dangerous consequences for the future.

These seven portraits all illustrate the challenges of creating a positive synergy and a balanced, healthy life. In every case, the person's greatest strength is also their "fatal" weakness; their heroic achievement is also their tragic flaw.

I share these stories not to criticize these seven people, all of whom I appreciate and admire. Rather, I want us all to see how hard it can be to make the most of our gifts, each of which has both a bright and a dark side. As you take your own journey through the seven systems, I hope you will treat yourself with patience and compassion, recognizing that there are no easy answers and no one right way of navigating these dilemmas. Instead of pursuing one final resolution, I invite you to view these contradictions as opportunities for growth.

System	Positive attributes	Negative attributes
The ROOT	Steady, solid	Stuck, stagnant
The FLOW	Creative, expressive	Dramatic, chaotic
The FIRE	Ambitious, achieving	Workaholic, perfectionistic
The LOVE	Caring, compassionate	Self-sacrificing, people pleasing
The TRUTH	Authentic, free	Resistant to authority, paralyzed by choices
The INSIGHT	Intuitive, intellectual	Moody, thought-obsessed
The SPIRIT	Purposeful, seeing the big picture	Fragmented, languishing in the physical world

A LIFELONG JOURNEY

One powerful way to view the seven systems is as a lifelong progress, with each system characterized by the issues of a different phase in life:

1. The ROOT: As infants and children, we seek stability and rootedness in our family, our community, and our tribe. We are primarily preoccupied with issues of safety and identity, wanting to know at the most basic level who we are and how we can protect ourselves (or who will protect us). A solid ROOT enables children to explore and grow, venturing beyond the security of the family circle and out into the wider world. An unstable ROOT can create a lifelong quest for identity, safety, and/or a primary family.

2. The FLOW: As teenagers, we enter into the turbulent FLOW of hormonal life, feeling creative, sexy, generative, and ready to go where life takes us. Our identities are fluid as we explore the possibilities that have newly opened up, and we meld into the networks formed with friends and peer groups. Although many adolescents yearn for solidity and certainty, the teenage years are almost inevitably a time when everything is uncertain, open, and flowing, and the best we can do is accept the instability, embrace the excitement, and enter into the waves of emotions.

3. The FIRE: In our early twenties, we burn with drive and ambition, on fire with the desire to make our mark on the world. Youth is as restless as a runaway fire, reaching as high as a leaping flame. For those young people who have chosen a life's work or profession, youth can be a time of burning joy as well, in which every new achievement explodes like a burst of fireworks, lighting up the night and illuminating the way ahead.

4. The LOVE: Our late twenties and thirties are often a time for focusing on the heart, as relationships turn into marriages and twosomes turn into families. This is a time to nurture our partners and our children, expanding into a love and service that go deeper than any we have yet known.

5. The TRUTH: In our forties, we have begun to understand our own truth and to find our own voice. At the halfway mark in our lives,

we have reached the time for big decisions and clear choices. Do we continue on our present course or switch to a new way of life? Either decision is momentous and requires a clarity about our inner truth and our path.

6. The INSIGHT: Turning fifty brings a new depth of wisdom and understanding, the chance to see the world in our own way and to make sense of all we have learned. "Insight" is the watchword for this half-century mark, as we finally learn to trust our intuition and inner knowing.

7. The SPIRIT: In our sixties and beyond, we begin to think more of the spirit than of the body; we become preoccupied with meaning, connection, and our place in the larger scheme of things. As we grow older, we prepare to leave behind our bodies and the physical world, embracing the spirit as the next phase of our existence.

In this view of the seven systems, the synergy emerges over time. Each system modifies and deepens the ones that came before it as wisdom deepens and perspective grows. From this viewpoint, a lifetime is not enough to make use of all the seven systems have to offer. But at each stage of life, we can appreciate where we are now, what has come before, and the new stage that is still to come.

BALANCE ACROSS THE SEVEN SYSTEMS

One of the challenges of Whole Detox is for each of us to customize our own approach, pursuing our unique goals in our own special way. The point is not for all of us to end up with identical versions of health and wellness but rather for every one of us to craft a unique path.

Here are three examples of patients who created lives that worked for them, each with a different balance among the seven systems:

- Leila is an ambitious professor of literature who works slowly but steadily toward her goals. In her midforties, she has published two books—about average for her field.

  Leila wonders if she might accomplish more if she put more

time and energy into her work. But she is unwilling to focus on work at the expense of the other things she enjoys: attending yoga classes, cooking healthy meals, and sharing a warm, close relationship with her husband.

———

Danny married his high school sweetheart as soon as they both finished college, and he never looked back. Together they have four children, and while life is hectic sometimes, they both really enjoy their family life.

Danny works as a CPA in a local accounting company, a job he doesn't love but doesn't mind. His favorite thing about it is that he's able to finish at five P.M. each day, so he can head home to spend time with his family.

Recently, he has started volunteering at a local homeless shelter. He gets a lot of satisfaction from helping people who really need it, and sometimes he convinces one of his kids to come with him and give a few hours as well. Danny sees his highest purpose on earth as taking care of others—whether his clients at work, his family at home, or the folks at the shelter. Sometimes he's bored, and sometimes he's frustrated, but mainly he's satisfied.

———

Kira has been a dedicated tennis player since she was a little girl. Every spare minute goes into improving her game, and her professional results bear witness to her impressive efforts. Now she is approaching the age when she'll have to step back from the highest levels of the game, and she's trying to decide what she'll do next. Coach? Start a sports-related business? Take some time off and travel the world? Kira has been focused on tennis for so long that she has no idea what her next move should be.

Leila, Danny, and Kira are each trying to craft a life that fits them—a life that balances all the different things they want. If we look at each life in terms of the Seven Systems of Full-Spectrum Health, we might come up with something like this:

	Leila	Danny	Kira
The ROOT	Strongest	Very strong	Weak
The FLOW	Moderate	Weak	Weak
The FIRE	Moderate	Weak	Strongest
The LOVE	Very strong	Strongest	Weak
The TRUTH	Moderate	Weak	Weak
The INSIGHT	Moderate	Weak	Weak
The SPIRIT	Moderate	Moderate	Weak

What conclusions can we draw from these three very different people?

First, it's nearly impossible to end up with strength in all seven systems. We just don't have the time and energy. You can have moderate strength in many systems or outstanding strength in a few systems or another balance of weakness and strength, but there simply isn't room in a single human life to have strength in all seven systems at the same time.

Second, each of us has different needs and capacities, and our systems reflect that. To Leila, living a balanced life is very important, so perhaps it is not coincidental that all of her systems translate into being rather equal. Even though she doesn't achieve exact strength in all seven systems, she comes close. Kira, by contrast, is happiest focusing all her attention on the FIRE. If her single-minded focus on tennis ends, she'll have the chance to decide whether she'll direct her FIRE toward another goal, go with the FLOW for a while, commit to the LOVE or the SPIRIT, or make a completely different type of choice. These choices would leave Leila and Danny feeling adrift and dissatisfied, but they work for Kira.

Finally, as we have already seen, things change over a lifetime. Having established a strong family life and a well-balanced LOVE system, Danny has the room to strengthen his SPIRIT system. Having spent many years focused on the FIRE, Kira might be ready to experiment with a different type of life. Leila might at some point decide to put more energy into her work or to open up her life still further and find new ways to go with the FLOW. Different choices are right for different times.

AWARENESS IS YOUR FIRST STEP

My goal in teaching you about Whole Detox and the Seven Systems of Full-Spectrum Health is not to prescribe a certain type of life for you or even a certain route to health. Rather, it's to give you the tools so you can make the choices that are best for your life and your health. If something isn't working—if you're struggling with toxic barriers that are creating symptoms, frustration, or pain—it's often helpful to look at which system or systems are out of balance or perhaps need more attention. But if your life is fulfilling and your health is optimal, that's an excellent sign that you're following the path that's right for you.

My guidance to you is to be aware of all the possibilities and to not sell yourself short. Far too many people live lives of quiet desperation, resigned to borderline health, frustrating jobs, and unsatisfying relationships. If something in your life isn't bringing you joy, you can use Whole Detox and the seven systems to diagnose where the problem is and come up with a solution. If something that worked for years has now stopped working, you can use the principles of Whole Detox to figure out where to go next. And if you know something is wrong but you can't quite put your finger on what, Whole Detox is there to help you find awareness.

That's why I'm excited to introduce you to the Seven Systems of Full-Spectrum Health. When you've understood each one, you'll have a very real and concrete sense of the possibilities in life—how good you can feel, how fulfilled you might be. In that sense, Whole Detox is a great adventure, inviting you to celebrate the full spectrum of life. So turn the page and let's get started! A rainbow of opportunity awaits.

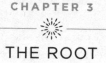

CHAPTER 3

THE ROOT

Consider a tree for a moment. As beautiful as trees are to look at, we don't see what goes on underground—as they grow roots. Trees must develop deep roots in order to grow strong and produce their beauty. But we don't see the roots. We just see and enjoy the beauty. In much the same way, what goes on inside of us is like the roots of a tree.

—JOYCE MEYER

UNDERSTANDING THE ROOT	
Anatomy	Adrenal glands, immune system, DNA, skin, bones
Functions	Identity, defense, fight-or-flight response
Living	Safety, survival, community, tribe
Eating	Protein, minerals, red foods

THE SCIENCE OF THE ROOT

The ROOT includes a number of seemingly disparate concepts: immune system, adrenal glands, protein, community, and tribe. Intriguingly, a growing body of scientific research associates these issues as well. As you will see, the elements of the ROOT concern our core identity plus our sense of safety, self-defense, boundaries, and belonging.

- Our *immune system* protects us from foreign invaders, such as bacteria and viruses, and helps us restore body integrity after an injury or a wound. It distinguishes between self and non-self at the most basic level.
- Our *adrenal glands* protect our survival by triggering the fight-or-flight response—our body's primary reaction to any type of challenge, including illness, stress, and danger.
- *Protein* is a building block of our whole structure, from our DNA and enzymes to our bones and muscles to our skin, hair, and nails. Protein is fundamental to our physical self. It also provides our adrenal glands with balanced fuel during a stressful event and can assist us in feeling stabilized.
- *Community* and *tribe* help create our understanding of who we are and whom we "belong to" ("an American," "a Southerner," "a New Yorker," "a Catholic," "half Portuguese, half Italian," "a member of the Rodriguez family," "a Green Bay Packers fan").

Many of us are used to thinking of these elements separately. But each affects the others, in both negative and positive ways. Excess stress on the adrenals can weaken the immune system. Loneliness and isolation lead to stress. Having a strong tribe can make us more able to resist both stress and illness. All of these ROOT issues affect our sense of identity and well-being, and when we deal with them together, we can unleash a powerful synergy.

Let's take a closer look.

IMMUNITY AND STRESS

Many of us think of immunity and stress as separate issues, but in fact, they are closely intertwined. When you experience stress—whether physical (a wound, an illness) or emotional (a deadline, an argument), your immune system frequently takes a hit. When you experience constant stress—again, either emotional or physical—your immune system is significantly challenged. Understanding the biology of how stress and immunity affect each other will help you better care for your ROOT.

Let's begin by looking at the stress response, which is generated by your adrenal glands. In fact, stress is one of the biggest toxins we confront on a daily basis. When you face a challenge of any type—physical, mental, or emotional—your body triggers a cascade of energizing chemicals that fire you up, make you more alert, and help you mobilize your resources for the task at hand. One of these stress chemicals is cortisol, which is great at the right levels but becomes a huge health hazard when your levels are chronically elevated.

Healthy cortisol levels leave you feeling energized and focused. When levels are too high, too low, or fluctuate in unhealthy ways, you might feel wired, anxious, sleepless, and jumpy; drained, exhausted, foggy, and unfocused; or a confusing mixture of both. This is known as adrenal dysfunction, though some of us just call it exhaustion!

If you have one single challenge to face in a day, you can often rise to the occasion, mobilize your resources, respond appropriately, and then relax. One stress at a time, followed by a period of relaxation, allows your adrenals to remain healthy and strong because you haven't overloaded them and you've given them time to recover.

However, in our modern world, many of us live with continuous stress. Some of us face major challenges that never seem to go away: a sick parent, a troubled kid, a debilitating relationship, a frustrating job. Others face a set of smaller challenges that also never seem to subside: constant errands, never-ending housework, driving the kids from lesson to lesson, a job that never seems to leave you time for lunch or even a coffee break.

Continuous stress is where the problem begins, because that type of stress creates chronically high levels of cortisol and adrenaline. These high levels of stress hormones affect you in all sorts of ways—often unhealthy—including an overactive immune response. After all, stressors mean challenges, and challenges often mean danger. So when your cortisol levels are chronically high, your immune system responds with alarm, resulting in inflammation.

Unfortunately, the same problem can result when your cortisol levels are chronically low. At this point your immune system sees that you don't have enough cortisol to respond to a challenge—those times when you feel foggy, exhausted, and seriously in need of a break—and once again, it mobilizes a protective response, i.e., inflammation.

When your chronically unbalanced cortisol gives rise to chronic inflammation, and this chronic inflammation in turn alarms your adrenals, it triggers yet another flood of cortisol. Thus a vicious circle is born, as these two integral aspects of the ROOT work to undermine your health:

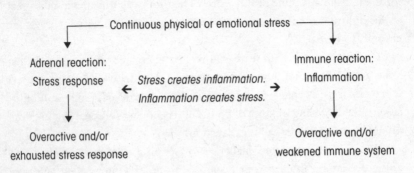

Continuous physical or emotional stress

Adrenal reaction:
Stress response

Stress creates inflammation.
Inflammation creates stress.

Immune reaction:
Inflammation

Overactive and/or
exhausted stress response

Overactive and/or
weakened immune system

Stress weakens the immune system in a number of ways. When pregnant mothers are stressed, for example, the immune systems of their offspring suffer, making them more susceptible to infection. Children from families in which there is a lot of psychological stress show low immune activity, and they tend to overreact to the toxins in some vaccines compared with those who are not stressed. A person who faced traumatic stress in childhood is more likely to be hospitalized with an autoimmune disease later in life.

If you have an autoimmune condition, you may already have discovered that daily stressors can play a role in setting off your symptoms. That's because of the way cortisol and inflammatory chemicals interact: excess cortisol triggers an inflammatory response, which in turn produces symptoms. Even if you don't have an autoimmune disorder, excess cortisol can trigger a whole host of symptoms, from acne to achy joints to PMS / hot flashes to sexual dysfunction to frequent colds and flu, as well as more serious disorders and risk factors (see page 60).

Fortunately, healing your ROOT with Whole Detox can help you reverse this process, creating a healthy synergy between your stress response and your immune function and supporting your optimal survival in the physical world.

IMMUNITY AND COMMUNITY

Stress isn't the only factor that affects your immune response. So does your community and your tribes. In fact, several studies have shown that people with strong social networks tend to be hardier and more robust. Most clinicians will tell you that people who feel supported by their social networks experience a greater sense of safety and enjoy generally lower stress levels. As a result, their immune systems are far less challenged by continual bursts of cortisol.

By the same token, people who have weaker social networks tend to be more stressed—and less healthy. Research done with university students found that those who reported themselves as lonely and those with smaller social networks tended to have lower immune function as measured in their response to a vaccine. Loneliness was also associated with a number of other symptoms, such as less quality sleep—and higher circulating levels of cortisol. As we just saw, constantly high blood levels of cortisol are very bad for your health, disrupting a number of other organs and putting you at risk for a wide variety of disorders.

One of my favorite studies was conducted in 2003 and published in a journal called *Psychological Science*. A group of 334 healthy men and women were exposed to the virus for the common cold and then monitored for symptoms. The volunteers who described themselves as "most sociable"—who spent the most time with people and seemed to have the closest social relationships— were far less likely to come down with the cold. To me, this study makes a lot of sense when you know that community and immune function are both part of the ROOT, both part of what keeps us feeling safe and secure.

THE POWER OF RED

Research associates the color red with some attributes related to the ROOT:

- Alertness
- Anger and aggression related to survival and danger
- Avoidance of a threat
- Self-control, ego
- Vigor

For example, a 2014 article published in the conference proceedings of the Engineering in Medicine and Biology Society found that when participants were put in a room with red light, they had a higher level of brain activity associated with "alertness, agitation, mental activity, and general activation of mind and body functions." They also were more likely to feel anger and "vigor."

A 2015 study reported in the *Personal and Social Psychology Bulletin* associated red with anxiety, to such an extent that reading words in red type—or even the word "red" printed in black type—could "impair cognitive performances." In other words, red stressed people so much that they had trouble focusing on their reading.

An article in a 2014 edition of *PLoS ONE*, the journal of the Public Library of Science, intriguingly titled "Red—Take a Closer Look," suggested that the color red made people more attentive to both happy and angry facial expressions; that is, red made people more alert to the possibility of either reward (a happy expression) or threat (an angry expression). A 2013 study in *Emotion* came to a similar conclusion: in the words of the article's title, "Red Enhances the Processing of Facial Expressions of Anger." In the study, when subjects viewed faces on a red background, they were more easily able to identify angry facial expressions. Once again, it seems that the color red has a subtle but striking effect upon our adrenal system, which alerts us to potential threats and danger.

A 2012 study discovered that red plates and cups actually caused people to eat and drink less than when the plates and cups were blue or white; the authors suggested that the color red acted as a subtle stop signal. Or perhaps, on a subconscious level, the color made the subjects more alert and aware of what they were eating. When we don't notice our food, it's much easier to overeat. Red can wake us up to attend to our surroundings and ourselves.

Now that you're aware of the power of red, how can you take advantage of it? I'll tell you what I tell all my patients and students: Start tuning in to the effects of the color red (and all other colors) upon *you*. Notice what you choose to wear and ask yourself if you've chosen those colors for a particular reason. Become sensitive to the ways the colors in a room affect you: the colors of the walls, the curtains, the tablecloth, the plates. Does red rev you up to feel alert and focused? Does it provoke your anxiety or perhaps your sense of excitement? Does it help you to feel grounded, rooted, more down to earth?

One of my patients told me that when she's feeling "up in the air," she wears a red T-shirt to bed, "so I can get grounded while I sleep." Another patient who had systemic inflammation didn't realize that she was wearing the color red all the time—as far down as her underwear and as far up as her lipstick. When I asked her if her clothing was reflecting what was happening on the inside of her body, she had an aha moment. She began wearing light blues and greens to create a different experience in her everyday life, one that was more calm and relaxed.

Her experience was supported by the comment of a dermatologist who knew nothing about my Whole Detox approach. He once said to me, "Why is it that women that come to me for inflammatory skin conditions like acne and rosacea seem to also be wearing red much of the time?" I don't know whether the color expresses the problem, causes it, or both, but I do know that color can have a powerful healing effect. Becoming aware of how color affects *you* is an eye-opener within Whole Detox, as you learn to invite all the colors of the spectrum into your life.

GET TO KNOW YOUR ROOT

Identity and the Immune System

As we just saw, the ROOT represents our relationship to the physical world: how we distinguish self from non-self and how we respond to threats to our physical survival—safety, home, food, and money. Because our immune system defines our boundaries—what we let in, what we reject—you might say that it represents our identity: who we are within a complex environment. If we don't have a basic sense of self—what's good for us, what's bad for us, what supports our body, and what threatens it—it's very difficult to feel safe.

The immune system defines us and protects us by identifying threats and developing responses. Of course, your immune system is constantly encountering entities it doesn't recognize, most of which are harmless. So your adaptive immune system learns to identify the threats and then develops antibodies—biochemicals that signal your immune system to go on alert when a previously identified danger enters your body.

Some of these dangers are toxic bacteria. That's why, after you've been exposed to a bacterium—either through actually getting sick or via a vaccine—you have antibodies that alert your adaptive immune system to keep that bacterium from attacking you again.

But sometimes your immune system overreaches, tagging common foods like milk, cheese, eggs, bread, pasta, and soy as dangers. This reaction can occur because of a common disorder known as leaky gut, when the lining of your intestinal wall becomes permeable, depriving your immune system of a safe boundary. Instead of tightly holding in all the food you're trying to digest, that permeable lining allows some partially digested food to leak through. Your immune system fails to recognize this undigested food and may come to consider it a toxic invader, tagging it with antibodies. Then the next time you eat that type of food, your immune system produces its standard defense: inflammation.

As we saw earlier, inflammation is intended to be a healing response, but it does have side effects. And when inflammation is chronic—when your immune system is continually responding to invader foods—you get symptoms:

- Anxiety
- Brain fog, trouble focusing
- Depression
- Digestive issues: reflux, nausea, feeling too full, indigestion/ heartburn, constipation, diarrhea
- Frequent colds, flu, sore throat
- Headaches
- Listlessness
- Muscle and/or joint pain
- Restlessness
- Skin problems: acne, rosacea, eczema
- Sleep problems

This is why Whole Detox begins at the ROOT, pulling out all the foods that might be causing this type of immune system response:

- Alcohol
- Caffeine (chocolate, coffee, soft drinks, tea)
- Dairy products (cheese, milk, yogurt)
- Eggs

- Gluten (barley, spelt, wheat, and, in some cases, oats)
- Peanuts
- Processed carbohydrates
- Processed meats
- Shellfish
- Soy
- Sugar and sweeteners (includes artificial ones)

After a twenty-one-day Whole Detox, your immune system calms down, many antibodies disappear, and you can reintroduce foods back into your diet. Some people never really lose the antibodies and will have to keep some foods out permanently. Other people can eventually reintroduce foods after several months. When you have finished your twenty-one-day program, you'll learn how to figure out which foods you can reintroduce (see chapter 12).

Self-Defense and the Adrenal Glands

If the immune system takes care of your *internal* response to danger, the adrenal system manages your *external* response. Your adrenal glands are designed to put you on high alert whenever your body perceives a potential threat. If your immune system interprets partially digested food as a threat, your adrenals will be on high alert far too much of the time.

As we have seen, your adrenal glands generate your body's response to stress—anything that challenges you to greater exertion. Stress can be physical (hiking, working out at the gym, lifting your groceries up onto the counter) or it can be emotional (a sick child, a difficult boss, a troublesome relationship). Stress can also take the form of minor but significant demands on your body—the kinds of little things we tend not to notice but that nonetheless take their toll:

- Exposure to toxins—the kinds normally found in our external environment: air, food, water, and items found in our homes, including many types of furniture, carpet, cleaning products, and personal-care products
- Inflammatory foods—the ones that challenge our immune system
- Lack of sleep

All of these forms of stress trigger an adrenal response: the body mobilizing itself to respond to danger.

Ideally, your stress response is followed by a "relaxation response," allowing your mental and physical resources to restore and replenish before the next big challenge. But when the stress never really stops, you never get enough of a relaxation response. Instead, you get more or less constant stress—and your adrenal glands start to feel the strain.

Constant stress can come from a state of mind: you're always worried about work, family, relationships, or life in general. It can also come from physical stressors: you never quite get enough sleep, you're eating too many foods that stress your body. For many people it's both. This unremitting stress creates a constant drip, drip, drip of stress hormones into your system. As a result, you often feel edgy, anxious, wired. You might have trouble sleeping. You might also have the opposite reaction: feeling draggy, listless, unfocused. Some people have both reactions: sometimes feeling wired, other times feeling exhausted. Often, sleep cycles get messed up, so that you're wide awake late at night but can't keep your eyes open in the afternoon.

Some version of this adrenal distress happens to many of us, as we skimp on sleep, stress over grades or job performance, or worry about career and security. These are all ROOT issues: adult identity, financial safety, ability to survive independently, and ability to take care of our loved ones.

Although we may not be in any actual physical danger, our adrenal glands know only one response to stress: the fight-or-flight mode, during which a cascade of stress hormones gears the whole body up for danger. And because we aren't countering that stress response with a relaxation response, our adrenals start working overtime.

Luckily, with Whole Detox, we have a number of ways to support our adrenals:

- Addressing issues of identity, family, and survival
- Finding ways to relax
- Getting enough sleep
- Supporting adrenals with clean proteins and red foods
- Removing problem foods

BALANCE YOUR ROOT

Our goal with Whole Detox is to achieve a kind of balance—not necessarily "more" of the ROOT but rather "the right amount" of the ROOT.

Of course, "imbalance" can mean either too much or too little. A person with an underactive ROOT might be anxious, spacey, or ungrounded. A person with an overactive ROOT might be stubborn, a creature of habit, or stuck in a rut.

The right amount of ROOT will look different for each of us. For one person, it might mean going to work in the same place at the same time, day after day. Another person might flourish in a community of friends who are available by phone, e-mail, or Skype. For yet another person, it's about staying close to their biological family in the town where they grew up. The right amount of ROOT might also look different at different points in our lives, as our need and capacity for different types of stability evolves.

We are also complex creatures who often possess many contradictory traits. As you look at the following lists, you may find indications that your ROOT—or that of someone you know—is sometimes balanced, sometimes overactive, and sometimes underactive.

So, bearing in mind that these indications are provisional—meant to point you toward your own definitions rather than simply adopting mine—here are some portraits of ROOT balance and imbalance.

A person with a healthy ROOT
- has a well-functioning immune system, with no autoimmune issues and rarely, if ever, gets colds or flu;
- has a strong social network of friends and/or family members;
- is free of adrenal issues, feeling neither tired nor wired, with a deep reserve of energy to respond to the stresses and challenges of their life;
- feels "at home" in their body, rarely, if ever, feeling physically unsafe or threatened;
- eats moderate amounts of protein throughout the day to stabilize their blood sugar, support their body, and fuel their energy;
- feels comfortable and settled yet also flexible and able to move out of habitual ruts if needed; and
- eats a variety of red foods to support immune and adrenal health.

A person with an underactive ROOT

- frequently gets colds and flu, and might suffer from an autoimmune condition;
- struggles with adrenal issues, frequently feeling tired, wired, or both;
- eats little protein but a lot of carbohydrates, especially refined carbohydrates, perhaps to compensate for the low energy that results from exhausted adrenal glands;
- feels easily thrown or bowled over by the stresses of daily life;
- feels a deep sense of insecurity about their physical safety;
- has the uneasy sense that they don't have a right to exist like everyone else, that their very survival is a burden or at risk;
- has trouble "settling down," whether in a home, a relationship, a career, or simply to focus on completing a task;
- feels "lost" without a tribe or community to support their identity;
- feels isolated, exiled, outcast, or emotionally homeless;
- might have given up on their physical survival, might neglect themselves physically;
- might be struggling with challenges to their survival, such as homelessness or unemployment;
- might be or have been anorexic; or
- might be fragile, thin, and jumpy, feeling that life is always "coming at me" in insurmountable ways.

A person with an overactive ROOT

- has difficulty adapting to change of any kind;
- seems stuck in a rut or set in their ways;
- takes everything literally;
- feels heavy and stuck in their life;
- stubbornly resists changing a custom or long-standing way of doing things;
- rarely changes their opinion;
- can't imagine making a decision or even having an opinion that might upset their family or go against their community;
- can't imagine an identity separate from their family or community;
- might eat too much red meat;

- might be overweight and/or thick in their lower body;
- might have varicose veins or hemorrhoids;
- might have gout, arthritis, or joint inflammation;
- might say yes to every potential moneymaking endeavor because they never feel they have enough money to survive;
- is on constant alert, possibly paranoid about issues of privacy or being controlled; or
- might stock their kitchen pantry full of food because "you never know when disaster might strike."

RE-GROUND YOURSELF:
HOW THE ROOT DETOX WORKED FOR ROB

My patient Rob was struggling. A law student in his midtwenties, he had always been ambitious and hardworking. He'd gotten top grades at a top college, won admission into a prestigious law school, and become an editor of his law review. Thanks to his commitment and dedication, his future seemed assured.

Then, suddenly, Rob was plagued with a set of mysterious symptoms. He was drained of energy, listless, and unmotivated. He either felt so exhausted that he had to take an afternoon nap or so wired that he couldn't fall asleep till the sun came up. Previously able to depend on his laser-sharp mind, he suddenly found himself unfocused and foggy.

He also had the feeling that, as he put it, he just "couldn't settle down to anything." When he tried to read, he couldn't finish an assignment. When he began to write, he had trouble completing a thought. When he started work on one class, he found himself switching to the assignment for another. "Whatever I'm doing, it seems like I should be doing something else," he explained. Underlying this restlessness, he noticed a kind of creeping dread, as though something was really wrong that he just couldn't put his finger on.

He was at his wit's end, so he began to look for help. His first stop was to see a doctor, who suggested a combination antidepressant/antianxiety medication. But Rob was fairly certain he wasn't depressed, just tired and foggy. And while he often felt anxious, he hated the idea of taking a medication to, as he put it, "erase my feelings."

Then his mother, whom he described as "sort of a health nut," suggested that he eat more fresh vegetables. Rob tried to remember to grab some lettuce from the salad bar and to snack on carrots and celery while he studied, but he didn't really notice much difference.

His girlfriend thought maybe he needed to see a therapist to work on whatever psychological issues were dragging him down. But somehow, that idea just didn't click with Rob, who couldn't really believe that the problem was "all in my head."

When Rob came to me, one of my first thoughts was how piecemeal and partial the other responses had been. Conventional medicine, nutrition, and psychology can all be extremely helpful, but none of these disciplines typically treats the whole person. We need a comprehensive, systematic approach. In most cases, you can't just add a few things into your diet and hope that fixes the problem. And while therapy can open up important areas for exploration, it might miss some nutritional issues that are helping to create the problem. By contrast, Whole Detox addresses the whole person.

Rob's inability to settle down and focus, as well as his lack of motivation, led me to believe that he might be wrestling with his ROOT system. I wondered if he was questioning his identity in some way. Maybe some of his lack of focus and motivation had to do with a feeling of being ungrounded—being literally unable to "settle down."

It turned out that Rob's parents had recently retired, selling the house he'd grown up in and moving into a nearby retirement community. Somehow, the loss of those childhood roots threw Rob into a state of confusion. When his family home was intact, he had felt grounded and settled. Having a firm foundation had freed him to pursue his goals. But with the loss of that grounding, his whole identity seemed "up in the air." He began questioning what he was doing in law school, whether he had chosen the right path for himself or whether he had forged forward on this path because of ingrained, early-imprinted family stresses around being successful and having enough money. He worried about paying back his huge loans after he graduated and whether he could create for himself the life he wanted. With his parents moving on to a different stage of their lives, he realized that he, too, had arrived at a new stage, and he felt overwhelmed by his new adult responsibilities.

At the same time, he wasn't getting the nutrients he needed to support him in this struggle: the grounding, energizing support of healthy proteins and red foods. The immune system and the adrenals are the foundation for the ROOT, and I knew that Rob's brain fog, anxiety, listlessness, fatigue, and sleep problems were common symptoms of immune/adrenal issues.

Using a Whole Detox approach, he could address the full spectrum of his ROOT: the diet, lifestyle, and psychological exploration he needed to feel grounded and well defined once more. Let's take a closer look at the ROOT and see how I helped Rob through the first system of health.

PROTEIN TO SUPPORT YOUR ROOT

When I think about identity and defense, I immediately think of protein. We are literally made of protein. Our bodies, after all, are made of a protein-based structure, and our systems run on the proteins known as enzymes. And our DNA, the core genetic material that makes up our identity, is composed primarily of protein. When our DNA is activated by an outside signal—such as food, sunlight, toxins, or stress—it starts to churn out proteins that act as messengers in our body.

The protein matrix of the bones is packed with sturdy minerals to give us our defining structure and the bulk of our being. Our muscles hug our bones tightly, enabling us to move and function. On a finer level, our skin, which gives us physical boundaries, is made of proteins like collagen.

Even deeper within the body lie the building blocks of protein, the amino acids, which we need to fortify our immune responses. Protein is also crucial for the effective function of our adrenal glands and its production of hormones.

As you can see, protein literally constitutes our identity. Protein is who we are at the most fundamental level of our existence.

Protein also is crucial to our liver, which needs a constant supply of quality proteins in order to rid our body of toxins. Without protein, we simply can't get the poisons out of our body.

Not surprisingly, then, protein is our primal defense—our ancestors' go-to food to defend against starvation and loss of body fat. Early humans might often have been desperate for a bit of meat or fish to build up their body fat against the long, cold winters or to sustain them in treks across the desert. Even now, when we don't feel safe, most of us turn to protein, the food that originally made us feel grounded and secure.

While I don't want to encourage you to overconsume protein, as so many of us do, I do want you to remember this simple equation: protein equals survival. If you ever find yourself craving an extra-big helping of meatballs, a thick, juicy hamburger, or a succulent steak, you might well ask yourself, "Am I feeling threatened?" or "Do I feel the need to be more 'rooted' in this moment?" Certainly if you want to feel grounded, go for a high-protein food rather than one high in carbohydrates or sugars. Protein will stabilize your blood sugar and give you the sensation of satiety deep within.

In recent years, between the Paleo movement and committed vegans, it has become rather difficult to talk about protein. Some people maintain that animal proteins are best suited to the human physiology; others insist that animal proteins are unhealthy and perhaps even immoral. Since you know I'm an advocate of personalized medicine, it probably won't surprise you to learn that I won't choose sides! Some people do better with animal protein; others do better with a vegetarian or vegan diet. Be open to choosing whatever you need at any particular moment rather than following a generic diet. Your body will change over your lifetime, so what works at one time might change at another. Only you know what works best for you—and the more grounded in your ROOT you are, the better you will know. Some people do well with lots of animal protein, some with moderate amounts, some with none. While legumes are healthy choices for many, some people simply do not do well on them, even if they soak and treat them overnight, perhaps because of various phytochemicals, such as lectins, or maybe because their digestive system is not working optimally.

However, if you do eat meat, don't overdo it: no more than once a day for animal proteins and no more than once or maybe twice a week for red meat, unless you are able to find high-quality, grass-fed sources. Overeating poor-quality meat can create inflammation, which once again stresses your immune system and overworks your adrenal glands. Do your very best to eat clean meats, from animals that have been fed organically grown food and been pasture raised. Factory farms are full of industrial chemicals and antibiotics, and inhumanely raised meat is loaded with toxic stress hormones.

One potential health concern with meat is the way heterocyclic amines—a type of carcinogen—form during the cooking process. You can offset that danger by including green leafy vegetables rich in chlorophyll with your meal. In other words, make sure you prepare a hearty spinach salad (with an avocado for some extra healthy fat!) to accompany your grilled grass-fed buffalo burger.

On the other hand, if you're a vegetarian or vegan, make sure you're not skimping on the vegetable protein and you're supplementing properly with B12 if your levels are low.

Whether you prefer animal or vegetable protein, you do need protein, no ifs, ands, or buts! Besides acting as one of your body's building blocks, protein also helps to stabilize your blood sugar. Think of how quick-burning refined carbohydrates throw you onto a blood-sugar roller coaster. When you're constantly careening from sugar high to sugar crash, you feel flighty, dreamy, out of your body. Solid, healthy proteins—lentils; beans; wild-caught fish; organic, grass-fed, pasture-raised meats—keep you anchored in your physical body in a healthy, grounded way.

HEALTHY PLANT-BASED PROTEINS FOR YOUR ROOT

Different types of proteins contain different amino acids, and your body needs all of them. That's why I highly recommend that you frequently change up your protein sources, especially if you're a vegetarian or vegan. Here are some plants that are rich sources of protein:

Food	Serving size	Protein (grams)
Lentils	1 cup, cooked	18
Black beans	1 cup, cooked	15
Chickpeas	1 cup, cooked	15
Kidney beans	1 cup, cooked	15
Hemp seeds, shelled, whole	¼ cup	10
Quinoa	1 cup, cooked	8
Almonds	1 ounce	6
Brown rice, long grain	1 cup, cooked	5
Spinach	1 cup, cooked	5
Chia seeds	1 tablespoon	3

METALS VS. MINERALS

Heavy metals are a huge source of toxic trouble, whereas minerals are vital to our detox—and to our overall health. I've found that many people become confused about the difference, so let me set the record straight.

"Heavy metals" generally refers to those metals that result in health problems for humans, chiefly aluminum, arsenic, cadmium, lead, and mercury. While we want minerals to ground us and support our ROOT, heavy metals ground us too much, creating a host of problems that undermine our health and well-being.

WHERE DO HEAVY METALS LURK?

- Dental amalgams, which contain mercury
- Drinking water, which is often contaminated with a variety of metals
- Certain types of fish, which contain mercury
- Impure fish oils, which contain mercury
- Food that has been contaminated with pesticides and/or grown in contaminated soil
- Hijiki, a type of seaweed, which may contain arsenic
- Certain types of rice, particularly brown rice and rice grown in Arkansas, Louisiana, or Texas, which are high in arsenic; brown or white basmati rice grown in California, India, or Pakistan and white sushi rice contain far lower levels of arsenic
- House dust, which has a wide variety of contaminants
- Some red lipsticks as some of them are known to contain lead
- Some deodorants that contain aluminum

Heavy metals are established carcinogens that bind to different proteins in our body, preventing them from proper function. They tend to accumulate in the kidney, liver, bone, and brain, where they can produce neurological problems: tremors, trouble focusing, and other nervous system disorders. They can also disrupt gastrointestinal and cardiovascular function. Even small increments of lead in the bloodstream can raise your blood pressure, while heavy meal toxicity can also alter your white and red blood cell counts. Finally, heavy metals can create skin lesions or hyperpigmentation—a bluish or darker skin tone.

How should you protect yourself? Here are a few suggestions:

- Have any mercury-laden dental amalgams replaced by a dentist who understands the correct, nontoxic procedure for removal.
- Test your drinking water or check with your local area's water department to see if test results are available, and then, if necessary, install a water filter (see Resources).
- Keep your house as free as possible of dust.
- Choose lower-mercury forms of fish and only pure fish oils.
- Choose organically grown foods.
- Choose a natural, aluminum-free deodorant and organic cosmetics.
- If you think you are suffering from heavy metal poisoning, get a blood test and, if necessary, work with a functional medicine practitioner to detoxify your system (see Resources).

Minerals, by contrast, are crucial detox elements that help ground, strengthen, and protect us:

- Zinc is a constituent of a protein known as metallothionein that helps to upregulate this protein, which in turn binds heavy metals and helps facilitate their removal from the body.
- Selenium is required for the efficient function of glutathione, a major antioxidant and detox compound.

You can take supplements of these two minerals, or for your selenium, you can eat Brazil nuts (best source!), seeds, fish, grass-fed meats, and eggs, and get your zinc from some of the same sources: nuts, seeds, seafood, and grass-fed meats. You'll note that all of these sources will also provide you with another ROOT essential: protein.

RED FOODS AND YOUR ROOT

The ROOT represents the red segment of the spectrum. While I didn't make that association myself—I got it from East Indian medicine—I was fascinated to discover the wealth of science anchoring the color red to the ROOT.

As we saw in the beginning of this chapter, the color red provokes urgency in our survival, revving up the stress response and gearing us to fight or flee. Besides the four studies I quoted, other researchers have found that the color red triggers our stress response in various other ways. Because red captures our attention, setting off the heightened alertness that is part of the stress response, it's a useful color for stop signs, danger warnings, and other situations in which we need to focus quickly.

The scientists who made this association might have been interested to learn that certain red foods are full of vitamin C, which properly balances the production of the stress hormone, cortisol. In other words, without vitamin C, we can't mobilize a proper stress response. We also need this important vitamin for proper immune function—to defend against colds, flu, and more serious ailments. These vitamin C–rich foods include red bell peppers, chili peppers, strawberries, tomatoes, cranberries, watermelon, goji berries, raspberries, and cherries.

Red apples provide vitamin C too, along with other nutrients. They also contain the phytonutrient quercetin, which bolsters immune function and reduces inflammation. Just remember that apples are one of the most pesticide-laden fruits, so buy the organically grown variety!

Red teas are another great way to detox your ROOT. Herbal teas are one of my favorite beverages for a detox, with a lot of pivotal research suggesting that teas support our detoxification pathways. My red-colored favorites are rose hip, hibiscus, and rooibos teas, all of which have minerals, flavonoids, and other phytonutrients to help reduce inflammation and improve immune function.

Iron is essential for the ROOT since it is one of the central components of red blood cells, which carry oxygen and give us the energy to exist. Of course, the most abundant source of iron is red meat. Iron can be both good and bad for us. In the right quantities, iron stabilizes our red blood cells for better oxygenation, helping us to feel invigorated and alive. However, too much iron can be toxic and cause a form of rancidity or rusting to occur in the body, known as oxidative stress. To keep your iron levels optimal, you'll want to balance plant and animal sources of red foods, both during and after your detox. You'll get a feel for how to do this in the first three days of your Whole Detox, which should help you balance your red foods afterward.

Another type of red food nutrient is lycopene, a red carotenoid found in tomatoes, pink grapefruit, and watermelon. Recent research shows that lycopene is a strong supporter of your ROOT, helping to build strong bones, with possible protective benefits against cancer, heart disease, and other age-related disorders.

MAKE THE MOST OF YOUR TOMATOES

Cooking your tomatoes is a nutritious choice, because you make the lycopene more "bioavailable"—that is, more available to your biochemistry. In other words, when you eat raw tomatoes, your body absorbs less lycopene than when you eat them cooked or processed. And if you cook them with olive oil, you get even greater benefit. Cooked tomatoes are likewise superior to raw because the heat makes it easier for you to absorb phytonutrients like naringenin (a potent antioxidant, especially for liver health) and chlorogenic acid (which positively impacts sugar and fat metabolism).

So besides adding protein to your diet, add some red foods of all types: a healthy ROOT likes variety! Choose beets, cherries, red apples, pomegranates, strawberries, raspberries, goji berries, watermelon, and some red herbal teas, and watch your immune system and adrenal glands flourish.

SUPPORT YOUR ROOT WHILE YOU EAT

We will fully address ROOT issues during the first three days of the twenty-one-day program. But if you're feeling in the need for some immediate support for your ROOT, here are a few quick tips on how to cultivate rootedness while you eat:
- Eat on the floor rather than in a chair.
- Eat with your hands or use wooden or ceramic utensils rather than silverware.

- Eat in nature, outside on a sunny day.
- Eat barefoot, with your legs uncrossed.
- Follow your instincts on food choices.
- If you are having trouble making healthy choices, ask your body what it needs in that moment.
- Do a simple guided imagery to get rooted in your body before preparing or eating food.

GET GROUNDED—LITERALLY

A number of studies have discovered several benefits In making direct contact with the earth, by walking barefoot outside or, if that's not possible for you, being mechanically wired to a device that transfers the earth's electrons into the body. This practice, known as earthing or grounding, seems to decrease pain and inflammation, improve sleep and mood, and reduce blood viscosity and clumping. As Dr. Gaétan Chevalier and his research team have said, "The research done to date supports the concept that grounding or earthing the human body may be an essential element in the health equation along with sunshine, clean air and water, nutritious food, and physical activity."

Since grounding is so beneficial, why not find as many ways as possible to maximize the connections between your body and the earth? As I mentioned above, you might want to try eating barefoot, close to the ground, using your hands rather than silverware. When the weather is nice, maybe take your meal outside and enjoy it under a tree.

LIFE ISSUES: IDENTITY, SAFETY, SURVIVAL, COMMUNITY

Let's return to my patient Rob and what he needed to do to strengthen his ROOT. On a physical level, his body perceived that his safety and survival were at risk; hence, the overreaction of his immune system (to defend him from "dangerous" foods) and his adrenal glands (which kept putting him in fight-or-flight mode in response to the "danger"). This affected his psychology as well. You can't have your body in a fight-or-flight state and not feel anxious, revved up, on edge; that's what that state is for. So if you frequently find yourself feeling anxious and on the brink of feeling like you are falling apart, you might consider whether there are physical or nutritional reasons for your stress as well as psychological ones.

Of course, Rob was also facing a number of stressful issues. His parents had sold his childhood home. He was in a challenging program, about to face a highly competitive career. For the first time in his life, he would be responsible for his own finances, and he was taking on that responsibility while saddled with an enormous amount of debt. There were very good reasons for him to feel at risk.

On the other hand, the stress response—preparing for a fight-or-flight situation—isn't always upsetting. Sometimes it's exciting, thrilling, or full of pleasurable anticipation. A team getting ready to play a big game, a musician about to perform a major concert, a person about to go on a romantic date—all of these people are stressed in a physical sense, but they experience those stress hormones as positive, even enjoyable. So one of the ways I worked with Rob was to see if he could reinterpret his feelings of dread and unsettledness as excitement and anticipation. Yes, his identity was changing rapidly. Now, instead of being a child who lived with his parents, he was an adult preparing for an adult career. That certainly might seem scary, but wasn't it also an adventure? After all, he had chosen this career, he'd done very well at school, and he'd been quite excited about becoming a lawyer. We worked in various ways on his choice to perceive "unsettled" and "uncertain" as potentially exciting states as well as frightening ones.

Besides the challenges in his work life, Rob faced challenges to his core sense of self. When his parents sold his childhood home, his very identity seemed to be in question—his primary relationship to his community. Instead of being a son, a child, someone to be cared for, he was about to become an adult, a man, an independent person. Instead of his primary tribe being other young people his age—the friends he hung out with, the girlfriend he dated—he was about to join a new tribe: lawyers. So we worked on helping him to further define his tribe and his new identity, as a lawyer, as an adult, as a man in a serious relationship with a woman, as the adult child of aging parents. Yes, he was losing one identity, but he was also forging another. Focusing on his new identity helped him feel less "unrooted" about losing his old one.

At the end of an extensive ROOT detox, Rob felt focused, clear, and determined. While he couldn't eliminate the uncertainty in his life, he could shift his relationship to it, celebrating what he was going *toward* even while, perhaps, mourning the stage of life that he was leaving. He could support himself with the kinds of foods that kept him grounded, alert, and best able to handle stress. He could avoid the foods that made his life challenges more difficult, and he could make sure to get the sleep and relaxation he needed.

Rob also liked knowing that he had learned so much about himself and his ROOT. He knew that if he ever again felt unsettled and ungrounded, he had the tools to identify what was going on and to remove any barriers in his way.

DETOXING YOUR ROOT: WHAT TO CHOOSE
- Clean, lean proteins to support your adrenal glands and immune system
- Organically grown red fruits and vegetables, such as beets, cherries, apples, pomegranates
- Body awareness to balance your stress response and keep yourself in the moment
- Community—contact with people who reinforce the identity you have chosen

DETOXING YOUR ROOT: WHAT TO AVOID
- Toxins that stress your immune system, such as heavy metals, genetically modified organisms (GMOs), artificial dyes, foods with additives or preservatives
- Foods that cause your immune system to be reactive—maybe take a temporary break from dairy, gluten, eggs, and soy
- Situations in which you often feel you have to defend yourself
- Situations that stress your adrenals, such as when you do too much, say yes when you'd rather say no, or lose your sense of healthy boundaries
- Negative attitudes and limited beliefs about safety, survival, and money, for example,
    - *If I don't have a lot of money, I'll never get anywhere.*
    - *It's a man's world—a woman might as well give up before she starts.*
    - *There's no room in this world for someone like me.*
    - *I can never survive without my family's support.*

STRENGTHEN YOUR ROOT

I'm excited for you to go through the twenty-one-day program of Whole Detox—the same program I've shared with thousands of students and the same approach I use with my patients.

But to me, Whole Detox is just the first step. The real benefit is how the program helps you become aware of the role each system of health plays in your life and the ways in which each color affects you. The more you learn about Whole Detox, the more options you will create to support your health—and your life.

We could easily spend an entire book just on the ROOT, but I want you to get to know the other six systems of health as well! So let's move on to the second system of health: the FLOW.

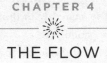

CHAPTER 4

THE FLOW

Life is a series of natural and spontaneous changes. Don't resist them—that only creates sorrow. Let reality be reality. Let things flow naturally forward in whatever way they like.

—LAO TZU

UNDERSTANDING THE FLOW	
Anatomy	Ovaries/testes, large intestine (colon), urinary system
Functions	Fluid balance, reproduction
Living	Emotions, creativity, partnerships, sexuality
Eating	Healthy fats and oils, water, orange-colored foods

THE SCIENCE OF THE FLOW

The ROOT is all about grounding to the earth and anchoring ourselves in the physical world. The FLOW, by contrast, represents our fluid, flowing, dynamic emotions. The FLOW calls upon us to let "e-motions" (energy in motion) move freely through our bodies so they don't stagnate and end up diseased.

If you feel "stuck," "dried up," or "blocked," chances are that something has disrupted your FLOW. Likewise, if you feel "swept up" in your feelings, "flooded" with emotion, "dissolving" in grief, or emotionally out of control, you might be struggling with an overflow of the FLOW. Whenever you feel moody, overly emotional, numb, infertile, or uncreative—and especially if you are having problems with sex or reproduction—you would do well to take a Whole Detox approach and consider your FLOW.

On a physical level, the FLOW refers to the parts within the body that help water ebb and flow: our cellular fluid, urinary system, and large intestine, which controls the uptake of water from the undigested matter running through us.

The urinary system is what enables us to balance the fluid in the body. It's a complex array of organs, including the bladder, which holds the urine; the ureters/urethra, which channel urine out from the body so it can be excreted; and the kidneys, which govern the whole process.

Most of us don't think twice about urination unless something goes wrong, but in fact, it's a hugely important bodily function. Throughout the day, we accumulate physical toxins—from food, air, water, home items (furniture, carpet, mattresses), cleaning products, and personal-care products (shampoo, moisturizer, cosmetics). Getting rid of those toxins on a daily basis is a crucial factor in our health.

The body has natural ways of getting physical toxins out: through urine, bowel movements, tears, and sweat ("pee, poop, cry, and sweat," as I usually say to my patients). If we can't properly excrete toxins through our urine, they build up inside us with problematic consequences, including weight gain, fatigue, and other symptoms: headaches, skin problems, digestive issues, and frequent colds, flu, and infections. In some cases, the toxic buildup causes even more serious problems, making us vulnerable to autoimmune conditions and cancer. Keeping our FLOW in good shape is one way to stay healthy and strong.

What's the best way to support your urinary system? I can tell you in three words: hydrate, hydrate, hydrate. Take half your body weight, convert it to ounces, and drink that much purified water every day throughout the day. If you drink coffee, tea, or any other caffeinated beverages, add some more water to cover the diuretic (water-releasing) effects of caffeine. If you're physically active or live in a hot climate, add several more ounces to cover that too.

Most of my patients are dehydrated when we start working together,

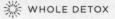

usually without even realizing it. Our thirst monitors—evolved during a prehistoric era when we couldn't be certain of getting clean water on demand—tend not to kick in until we're already well past the point of dehydration. In other words, by the time you feel thirsty, you've already stressed your body—and your urinary system. Remember in chapter 3 when I told you that chronic stress can result from not sleeping enough or eating too many inflammatory foods, and that this stress can have terrible consequences for your adrenals and immune system? Well, dehydration is another type of chronic stress that can burden your body, so you may be surprised to discover what a calming, healing effect proper hydration can have. Your goal is to drink enough water to prevent yourself from ever getting thirsty.

If you're not used to drinking lots of water, you might have a little trouble at first getting yourself to drink enough. Within two or three days, though, you'll find yourself naturally craving the water your body needs. You'll know that you're drinking enough water when your urine always comes out light yellow or almost clear, even first thing in the morning (unless, of course, you are taking certain vitamins, which can turn your urine yellow).

The Creative FLOW

We've looked at the physical FLOW, but there are other considerations as well. One is creativity, evoking our playfulness, openness, pleasure, and sensuality. Our reproductive organs—ovaries and testes—help us create life, making them part of this second system of health. The FLOW is also associated with each cell's ability to replicate and grow.

Our physical creativity depends upon our ovaries (if we're female) or testes (if we're male). Whole Detox is crucial to support these glands, which are under an increasing amount of pressure from the environment, thanks to the ever-growing number of toxins to which we are exposed. I'm saddened but not surprised to see that we have a growing infertility epidemic among both men and women. After all, plastics contain toxins that are endocrine disrupters; that is, chemicals that disrupt our endocrine system, or our hormones. (These toxins are often referred to as "xenoestrogens," from the prefix xeno, meaning "foreign.") Endocrine disrupters can block or alter pathways in the body that are regulated by estrogen, creating hormonal imbalances in both sexes. It can also cue both men and women to manufacture too much estrogen, leading to a condition known as estrogen dominance: basically, when you've got too much estrogen relative to your other reproductive hormones.

Estrogen dominance can have disastrous results for both men and women. Females with too much estrogen suffer from menstrual and menopausal issues as well as weight gain, mood swings, and other symptoms. Men don't have the menstrual problems, but they do face all the others. And both sexes struggle with sex drive and fertility.

Infertility can also result from stressful emotions, and infertility can lead to emotional distress. As we discussed previously, stress—especially extreme stress and most especially continuous stress—produces an excess of stress hormones, particularly cortisol. Cortisol, in turn, disrupts male and female hormones, which, when you think about it from a biological perspective, makes sense. For our ancestors, stress meant either starvation or life-threatening exertion—treks across the tundra, enduring the arctic cold or the desert heat. Those were hardly the times when the community would be served by the birth of new members. The resources of the body were thus directed not toward conception, pregnancy, and breast-feeding but toward basic survival and caring for the children they already had. In our own time, we see this phenomenon when young female athletes lose their periods or never get them in the first place—another example of the body's primal effort to hoard its resources for survival in the face of "life-threatening" exertion.

Now you can see why Whole Detox begins at the ROOT. Before we can meet any of our other needs, we need to know that basic survival has been assured and the needs of the community have been met. Frequently, when someone comes to me with a fertility or hormonal issue, I'll make sure we address the ROOT as well as the FLOW, so the two systems of health are not working at cross purposes.

Another factor in sexuality and reproduction is a person's own attitudes about being a man or woman. We live in a society with very firm and even rigid ideas about what male and female is. Many of us don't fit the ideal we've been given, and as a result, we might run into physical problems as well as psychological ones.

While I don't have scientific research to support this, I do have my own clinical observation and that of my fellow practitioners. We often see situations in which someone comes for treatment about a sexual or reproductive issue and is helped by diving into their own sense of being masculine or feminine.

For example, I've observed many women who feel they have no time to be feminine or they don't even know what it means to be a woman other than being stressed and juggling multiple roles. I've actually struggled with these notions myself, and I know that in both myself and my patients, female struggles can manifest in "female problems," including difficult menstrual cycles, challenging entry into perimenopause or menopause, infertility, and endometriosis.

Another common result of female stress is polycystic ovarian syndrome (PCOS), a syndrome in which women who are highly driven in a stressful environment develop high cortisol and high testosterone. This hormonal imbalance produces a number of symptoms, including irritability, hirsutism (the growth of hair), and an ovary that isn't quite fertile.

Men also wrestle with gender identity. Our culture equates manhood with violence, overwork, and competitive sports. Men pursuing an alternate version of masculinity—supportive, nonviolent, collaborative, with the goal of becoming a leader who inspires and empowers—might encounter ridicule, harassment, or even physical aggression.

Whole Detox, with its full-spectrum approach to the second system of health, can help to resolve these issues in both physical and emotional ways. When our creative FLOW is released, we can enjoy a rich fertility, as when a river overflows its banks to nourish the surrounding soil.

Another dimension of creativity, of course, is nonbiological: the creation of art, stories, new ideas, interesting ways of preparing a meal or arranging a room. Looking at the FLOW in all its dimensions, we can see that being creative is a healing force, helping us to resolve biological issues as well as emotional ones. As you'll learn later in this chapter, many of my patients have renewed their FLOW—biologically and emotionally—by giving themselves permission to be creative. And many who had felt their creativity was blocked have recovered their inspiration and creative vision by addressing the physical nature of the FLOW.

In all of these voyages toward healing, color is extremely important. The color orange has a remarkable ability to unlock biological fertility as well as intellectual and emotional creativity.

THE POWER OF ORANGE

The science on the color orange is fun and fascinating. A wide variety of research has linked orange to the FLOW via its relationship to fertility and hydration.

First, it seems that orange is a mating color, one that alerts members of the animal kingdom to go with the flow of their reproductive urges. Researchers in the Department of Marine Ecology at the University of Gothenburg, Sweden, found that when some fish engage in courtship—including when females are competing for the attention of males—"a rapid increase in orange coloration . . . gives the belly an intense 'glowing' appearance" that attracts potential mates. A study from the Department of Ecology and Evolutionary Biology at the University of Toronto found that certain guppies are so attracted to the color orange that prawns have developed orange spots on their pincers to entrap the sexually excited fish with a "sensory lure." Moreover, as scientists from the University of Padua have discovered, orange correlates to guppies' fertility, specifically "with faster and more viable sperm . . . suggesting a possible link between dietary carotenoid intake and sperm quality." Thinking about the FLOW, I like to remember that what we're talking about here is the ability of sperm to swim, to negotiate the reproductive fluids that enable the creation of new life.

The color orange is linked to reproductive health in birds as well. According to a group of Swiss researchers at the University of Bern, male birds with brighter plumage have sperm that is better protected against oxidative stress. Researchers wondered whether beta-carotene—the compound that turns foods orange—offers that protection. Their hypothesis was confirmed when they gave less colorful males carotenoid supplements and improved their sperm quality. Of course, you don't have to take carotenoid supplements; you can just eat more orange foods!

Another fascinating area of animal research indicates that beta-carotene concentrates in the corpus luteum (a developing egg in the ovary), where it may play a role in ovulation by assisting with the production of progesterone. Animal studies likewise suggest that beta-carotene supplementation supports ovarian activity and progesterone synthesis in goats. As I've said, I've noticed a similar effect in my human patients, who sometimes seem to have hormonal shifts when consistently increasing their intake of beta-carotene-rich, orange-colored foods. Indeed, Polish scientists have discovered that uterine tissues contain beta-carotene, while a 2014 study published in the journal *Fertility and Sterility* suggests that when women boost their beta-carotene intake, their chances of becoming pregnant seem to improve.

Finally, a study in the *Journal of Urology* found that men who drank orange juice enjoyed a reduced risk of kidney stones, linking orange both to kidneys and to the image of fluids freely flowing through the urinary system. After all, aren't kidney stones a particularly painful form of stagnation that impedes urinary flow?

To bring of the creative flow of orange into *your* life, try drinking your water in an orange-colored glass. Place an orange-colored object in any space where you'd like to ramp up your creativity: your workspace, your home office, perhaps even your kitchen. And on days when you'd like to generate more inner flow—emotional, creative, or relational—slip into an orange sweater or put on a pair of orange socks or earrings. Your FLOW will love you for it.

GET TO KNOW YOUR FLOW

The FLOW of Relationship

The FLOW represents the relationship between opposites—the movement that flows back and forth between male and female, mind and body, yin and yang. Just as the ROOT brings out the need for community, the FLOW allows us to appreciate the need for another person. Thus we can see the power of the FLOW in our partnerships or the relationship between two people. In any important relationship—work and friendship as well as romantic—we are always growing and creating through the dynamic dance with others. Sometimes we have blocks to commitment and we flow from one relationship to another, never quite arriving at what we need. Other times we begin to stagnate within the framework of a comfortable relationship that might not suit who we are, yet we don't feel like we have an escape available.

The FLOW teaches us both the beauty and the bane of interdependence. In a healthy relationship, the FLOW creates enhanced personal growth for each individual. In an unhealthy relationship, we encounter the shadow of codependence as each partner leads the other into a downward spiral of fear, anger, and pain, bringing out the worst in each other and moving each other in a negative direction.

The FLOW reminds you to ask how your relationships and choices are creating who you are in every moment, for better or for worse. When my patients reach this phase of Whole Detox, I see them questioning their toxic relationships, marriages, and business partnerships. They begin to see that the FLOW offers them possibilities and potential. The FLOW is a constant reminder to avoid the stagnant water of unhealthy partnerships and move into those that bring us into the rushing current of life, where creativity is always possible.

FLOWING WITH SMALL MOVEMENTS

A Native American teacher once told me that when we stop dancing and telling stories, we stop living—that is, we cease feeling full of life. Life is movement, and when we are not tapping into our gift to move, we stagnate. Our chi, prana, or life force starts to create stagnant pools in various parts of our bodies—often in our joints or muscles, which ache from the toxic accumulation. This type of stagnation can cause pain and lack of function in organs as well.

Luckily, we can start our bodies flowing again by embracing movement, even seemingly small and insignificant movement. Walk a few steps farther in the parking lot instead of parking close to the entrance of a building. Take the stairs instead of the elevator. Every hour or two, walk briskly to another floor in your office building or grab a ten-minute walk on your lunch break.

You can also embrace therapeutic movement. If you choose a type of movement that you feel passionate about, you will most likely stay in the flow, so experiment a bit and find something you really enjoy. Here are some moving ideas to start you flowing:

- An afternoon walk in the park
- Gardening
- Yoga of all types: hatha, kundalini, Bikram, ashtanga, etc.
- Tai chi
- Qigong

- Aikido and other martial arts
- Kayaking and water sports—especially great for flow because of the water element!
- Dance classes: Zumba, ballet, free form, Nia, etc.

The Emotional FLOW

The physical FLOW, the creative FLOW, and the relating FLOW regulate our urination, reproduction, and relationships. For the FLOW to operate freely, however, we need to consider one final dimension: the emotional.

Water has long been a symbol of emotions in many mythologies and many types of traditional medicine. And no wonder. When we are flooded with grief, water comes out of our bodies in the form of tears. When we are awash with fear, water comes out of us as urine and watery diarrhea. The moon—which both science and mythology link to emotions, mood swings, and periods of "lunacy"—has the magnificent ability to shift large bodies of water on our planet. Emotions bring together the symbols of water, urination, fertility, and creativity. And, indeed, when our emotions are unexpressed, fertility and creativity are frequently blocked as well. Biologically, we can imagine that stuck emotions are stressful—either caused by or causing stress, or both—and that the excess stress leads to too much cortisol, which disrupts mood, cognitive function, and, as we've just seen, our ability to feel sexual and to reproduce.

Problems can result from unfelt emotions and thwarted creativity, including unwanted creative proliferation within our bodies. Perhaps unhealthy bacteria or yeast will multiply in the gut, creating digestive problems. Maybe emotional distress will lodge in the gut, creating diarrhea, irritable bowel syndrome, Crohn's disease, and related disorders. We might even view cancer as the overproliferation of cells in response to a physical or emotional obstacle that the body could not overcome or release.

Whenever I think of the emotions, I also think about food, which is one of the most emotional issues I know. If one of my patients feels their eating is out of control, the FLOW is where I always start. Indeed, experts estimate that as much as 75 percent of overeating can be attributed to emotions, since when we feel unable to process our emotions, many of us are tempted to stuff them down with food.

What's exciting about these findings is the multiple solutions they allow us to consider: hydration, nutrition, emotion, creativity, or some combination of these. Addressing each of the issues supports the others, toward an end result of greater health, freer emotions, unblocked creativity, and greater sexual and reproductive function. Whole Detox draws much of its power from the power of synergy: the way each feature of a system of health supports and heals every other one.

Support Your Flow by Crying and Sweating

As we release water through our eyes or our pores, we often release emotion as well: sorrow or joy with our tears, anxiety or excitement with our sweat. Both the physical and the emotional release can have highly beneficial effects.

Crying is a form of detox in which we let go of our stored emotions and inner pain. It also literally eliminates inflammatory compounds: cytokines and chemokines. People who cry easily in response to emotion might even have fewer symptoms and better health than those who restrain their tears. Interestingly, healthy fats that embody a fluid, flowing structure—the omega-3s—can help heal dry eye, suggesting an additional close partnership between the characteristics of this second system.

Sweating is another primary way to release toxins, including PCBs, phthalates, bisphenols, and other compounds. In some cases, sweating is an even more efficient form of elimination than release via blood or urine. That's why I want you sweating through physical activities or in a sauna during your Whole Detox. Keep those toxins flowing out so you can allow more of the healthy creative FLOW in.

BALANCE YOUR FLOW

Balancing each system of health can be tricky; sometimes you may have "not enough" and sometimes you may have "too much." Everyone has their own personal definitions for "not enough," "too much," and "just right," and these definitions will likely change over the course of a lifetime. But again, bearing in mind that these are just provisional images, let's consider what balancing the FLOW might look like.

A person with a healthy FLOW

- has a healthy reproductive system, with the ability to be fertile at the appropriate age;
- has a healthy urinary system and the ability to resist urinary tract infections and other urinary problems, such as stones and inflammation;
- is able to excrete fluids effectively by sweating, urinating, and crying;
- has healthy levels of gender- and age-appropriate hormones, such as progesterone for women and testosterone for men;
- feels open to "going with the flow," remaining unconstricted when things don't go their way;
- has a creative approach to living, responding to challenges with some innovative solutions;
- has the capacity to be playful and open;
- can accept the ups and downs—the "flow"—of life;
- accepts his or her sexual orientation and gender identity, whatever they define it to be;
- is open to partnerships and relationships of all types—sexual, creative, emotional—and
- is comfortable eating healthy fats, chooses a healthy variety of fats, and avoids unhealthy or excessive fats.

A person with an underactive FLOW

- has edema or swelling somewhere in their body;
- might be going through premature menopause;
- might be prematurely infertile due to low levels of hormones;
- might have reproductive issues that involve stagnation or blocks, such as a blocked fallopian tube (hydrosalpinx), vaginal dryness, or impotence;
- might be losing their vitality at an early age, such as declining testosterone in men or declining progesterone in women;
- might avoid consuming dietary fat because they think they will get fat;
- might believe they are fat when they are not;

- might have issues with codependence;
- might have difficulty expressing or even realizing their emotions;
- might have difficulty "going with the flow" and/or might appear overly serious; or
- might be constipated or have infrequent or hard bowel movements.

A person with an overactive FLOW

- might be overly dramatic and emotional;
- always comes up with new ideas, but rarely puts them into motion;
- is prone to emotional eating;
- has many fleeting relationships with partners but is unable to sustain them;
- has high body fat relative to muscle mass for their age and gender;
- has reproductive issues that involve overactivity or inflammation, such as heavy cramping or bleeding with periods, prostatitis, cysts, or fibroids;
- has high levels of estrogen;
- has high exposure to xenoestrogens / endocrine disruptors;
- excessively urinates or feels the urge to urinate;
- has frequent bouts of diarrhea;
- is constantly thirsty;
- eats salty foods;
- eats high-fat foods; or
- indulges excessively in life's pleasures.

FIND YOUR FLOW:
HOW THE FLOW DETOX WORKED FOR MY PATIENTS

Because the FLOW manifests in so many different ways, I'd like to share with you five seemingly diverse patient stories. Each of them, however, has one thing in common: they all relate to an imbalance of the FLOW.

Merissa felt out of sorts and, as she approached her midforties, she began gaining weight. Her hormone levels were starting to decline, and she suffered from vaginal dryness, painful periods, and almost a complete loss of interest in sex. She was also frustrated by mood swings, which seemed to come at her "out of the blue," and depressed by the thought that her sexy, sensual self had, as she put it, "sort of evaporated." "I feel like I've just dried up and I have nothing to offer anymore," she told me.

She clearly needed some support for her hormonal imbalance—more healthy fats and orange foods; fewer unhealthy fats; a cleaner diet, generally; and some FLOW-inducing exercises of the type you'll be doing in days four through six of your twenty-one-day program. But Merissa also needed support for her sexuality and creativity.

We started gradually, with a class in water aerobics and one in Zumba to get her flowing in the water and in her body. But I also suggested that she try dressing differently. Every time I saw her, she was in the same old sweats and T-shirt with a messy ponytail on the top of her head. Her outward appearance reflected her inner doldrums.

When it's difficult to change the inside, what I like to do is change the outside. So I asked her to treat herself to a little shopping spree, even at a secondhand store. Her eyes somewhat lit up at the idea, and when I saw her next, she wore gold bracelets, her hair was flowing over her shoulders, and she was all decked out in a flowery dress! She was smiling and loving her new look, clearly radiating her beautiful feminine energy. Whole Detox had affected both her inner and outer being—through nutrition, yes, but also through helping Merissa renew her relationship with her feminine self.

———

Although Jorge was a successful accountant, he harbored a deep frustration: he had always wanted to be an artist. In college, he had studied graphic design and dreamed of working in that field full-time, but his father, a struggling small businessman, had urged Jorge to choose a more secure life, "where you work for someone else and always have bread on the table." Jorge had come to me because his wife was concerned that, as he told me, "I just sort of shut down. I feel numb all the time, like I just can't feel *anything* anymore. I'm doing fine at work, the bills are getting paid, nothing is really *wrong*, exactly. But I'm just going through the motions."

Like Merissa, Jorge benefited from eating orange foods and healthy fats. But he also needed to come to terms with his personal creative flow, which he had more or less dammed up after graduating college in order to placate his father. As Jorge came to realize how deeply he longed for a more creative and authentic life, he found the courage to leave his profession and commit to his once-abandoned life as an artist. Taking a huge leap of faith, he started a graphic design business, which to his great delight became a successful enterprise. He was thrilled to discover that his emotional life opened up at the same time, allowing for better communication— and better sex!—with his wife.

————

Ariana is one of those people who seem to live at the center of a perpetual drama. A highly emotional person, she feels everything deeply. She explained to me that she struggled with irritable bowel syndrome (IBS), which she had noticed was likely to flare up at her most intensely emotional times, hitting her with severe bouts of watery diarrhea.

"I feel like my emotions just wash through me and sweep me away," she told me, dabbing at her eyes. "I don't want to be one of those people who keeps it all inside, like my husband. What is life if you can't feel anything? But I don't want to keep getting sick either."

What Ariana really needed was to work not just on her overactive FLOW but also on her underactive ROOT and lack of boundaries. I could clearly see that she needed some quality protein to feel more stabilized and she needed to take out the sugar that was contributing to her ups and downs. I also encouraged her to map out her emotions each day, using my simple Whole Detox Emotion Log (see pages 381–83).

Through her work with the Whole Detox Emotion Log, Ariana discovered that she was not just overly emotional; she was very, very sad. Her sorrow stemmed from her pain over her mother's death, made even more painful by Ariana's unwillingness to deal with the full spectrum of her emotions about her mother. Since these emotions had not been resolved before her mother had died, Ariana was left with a potent cocktail of rage, guilt, and grief, and so her sorrow continued to bubble up again and again, a wellspring that refused to be suppressed.

When we realized this, I asked her to create a grief timeline that might help us identify her unresolved sorrow. We also looked at how she had subtly but continually changed her eating habits and lifestyle after each grief event.

Whole Detox helped Ariana begin a long process of recovery, which included additional counseling as well as nutritional support. Now, years later, she is still a deeply emotional being, but she has much better boundaries and far more effective coping mechanisms to still the turbulent tides within her.

———

At age forty-two, Chuck had what he considered a deeply shameful secret: he suffered from erectile dysfunction and, as he told me, "couldn't perform as a man." This was a relatively recent problem; throughout his twenties, he had had an active sex life, which he told me was satisfying sexually although, he later revealed, not so satisfying emotionally. Two of his girlfriends had cheated on him, and one had been so withholding that "I felt like I could never do anything right." He owned a small marketing company, and he was concerned about his work life also. "I feel like I've just run out of ideas," he told me. "Like the well has just run dry."

Like many of my other patients, Chuck's issues were both nutritional and something more. His diet was certainly lacking in good-quality fats and oils. He tended to eat carelessly and even to skip meals if no food was easily available. Although he had been an avid runner and weight lifter in his twenties, he had long since stopped exercise of all types.

His FLOW was gone because he was not flowing: no food or poor food, and little exercise. He needed some basics, so I got him going with regular vegetable and fruit smoothies every day, with plenty of orange fruits and vegetables along with healthy fats. He wasn't so thrilled with this new concoction at first, but then he started to get into the groove of his morning smoothie. The energy they gave him inspired him to start running again, until gradually, he was running several miles and feeling fit.

Fitness and energy helped make Chuck more confident, and so he began flowing at work too. He landed some new projects he was really excited about, and he felt encouraged by his success.

Months later, he met Lorraine, a wonderful woman who valued and supported him in every way. With Lorraine, he was able to heal the sense of his doing nothing right that his previous girlfriends had reinforced, and also to develop a satisfying sexual life. Together, they have taken up a daily running practice, keeping each other motivated and on track.

———

Elaine was a financial analyst in her midthirties who showed up at our first meeting in a sober gray suit and white blouse. "It's my work uniform," she told me, making a face. "If I didn't dress like this, they wouldn't take me seriously, but I do get tired of it sometimes."

During this first visit, Elaine told me that she was frustrated, almost desperate: after two years of trying with her husband, she still hadn't gotten pregnant. The tests on both of them hadn't turned up any problems, but for some reason it just wasn't happening. Neither one was open to the idea of IVF or other fertility techniques, but they did want to conceive their own child. "Is there anything I can do to get things moving?" Elaine asked me.

Elaine was one of those perfectionists who always did everything "right." She had already been to all the well-known functional medicine practitioners, followed all the diets, and taken all the supplements. She was whip smart and determined to do whatever she needed to, but for the first time, her determination just wasn't paying off.

I saw at once that she was a high achiever, used to achieving her goals through sheer determination and will. Her testosterone was up, from working in a corporate environment full of competitive men. She was trying to blend in, but she was missing something. She had lost her sense of being feminine. She never indulged in anything fun. And the last thing on her mind was being creative, which she considered "a waste of time."

As with Merissa, I knew we had to take it one step at a time. First, I suggested that she take a leisurely Hawaiian vacation with her husband. Reluctantly, she agreed, but she returned from her trip more open and relaxed.

Then I asked her to sign up for a creative journaling class. "I don't have the time," she snapped.

"Okay," I answered. "Then let's dial it down. Do something creative just five minutes a day. After all, it's for your health. And it's just five minutes."

She let out a sigh of irritation but agreed to try.

A few weeks later, Elaine showed me a collage of images that represented her goals. I was excited to see that the collage was filled with color, flowers, and positive words. This small movement in the direction of her creativity opened her up to other endeavors, and eventually, she began writing poetry.

She had made peace with the idea of not having biological children, so she and her husband eventually adopted Khloe. Six months later, Elaine was ecstatic to find out that she had gotten pregnant! Getting back into the FLOW had brought her a sense of fun, creativity, and joy.

HEALTHY OILS AND FATS TO SUPPORT YOUR FLOW

You stabilized the ROOT with protein and red foods. You will nourish the FLOW with the right balance of quality oils and fats as well as orange foods.

I love encouraging my patients and students to reintroduce healthy fats into their diet, not least because I spent four years studying essential fatty acids as a doctoral student, and I'm always amazed at what an enormous boost the right types of fats can provide. Essential fatty acids come by their name honestly: they are literally essential to every cell in our bodies. Our cell walls are made of fat, meaning that we need fat to enable nutrients to flow in while toxins and waste products flow out. Moreover, our brains are mainly composed of fat, so we desperately need healthy fats to think clearly and balance our emotions.

I've noticed over the years that many of my patients become emotional about eating fats. They believe that fats are not good for them and that eating fats will make them fat. This thinking has been fostered both by conventional medicine and by poorly informed journalists, but it is a toxic notion that creates more problems than it solves. What we're after is *balance*: not no fat or too much fat, but the right proportions of the right types of fats. Your goal is to load up on the healthy fats while letting go, as much as possible, of the unhealthy ones. You also need to balance your intake of different types of healthy fats.

Reproductive health also depends on healthy fats. Animal studies have shown that unsaturated fats in the right proportion are associated with fertility. In humans, omega-3 fatty acids are important nutrients in the growth, development, and health of the fetus and newborn infant. Including high-quality sources of omega-3s in the diet, such as wild-caught salmon, and perhaps also taking purified omega-3 fish oil supplements might be helpful for increasing healthy fats in the newborn, leading to reduced inflammation and allergies.

SYMPTOMS FROM NOT CONSUMING ENOUGH HEALTHY ESSENTIAL FATS

- Cognitive and mood imbalances
- Dry skin—lack of hydration and flow
- Hair loss
- Infertility
- Inflammation—too much heat without the cooling watery flow

Two types of healthy fats are known as omega-3 and omega-6. Omega-3s are typically found in plants, nuts, seeds, and fish, while omega-6s are found in meats as well as in some types of plants, such as avocado. Grass-fed meats, dairy products, and eggs also contain some omega-3 fats.

The typical modern diet—heavy on the corn-fed meats and animal fats; light on the fish, nuts, and seeds—contains far too many poor-quality omega-6s. Compounding the problem is the way that body fat—whether animal or human—becomes a toxic sinkhole for all those fat-loving industrial chemicals like PCBs, which dissolve in fat and are stored there. So when we consume too much animal fat—especially from factory-farmed animals—we end up with an overdose of toxins.

There's another type of fat problem that applies to both animal and vegetable fats: metabolic endotoxemia. Basically, whenever we eat a high-fat meal, we get a loosening of the tight junctions that hold together the cells of our intestinal wall. The result is the leaky gut we talked about in chapter 3—a version of too much FLOW as partially digested food passes through our gut walls.

To make matters worse, excess fat stimulates our gut bacteria to produce toxic substances that can then leak into the blood ("toxemia" literally means "toxic blood"). If you feel nauseous, gassy, or bloated after a high-fat meal, it's at least partly due to the unhealthy bacteria dumping their toxic products into your blood via your leaky gut. Yuck.

If you get your fat from olive oil, fish, and avocados, you're far less likely to encounter this ugly effect than if you consume the unhealthy trans fats and industrial oils that are part of so many packaged, processed, and fast foods. It's a lot easier to overdose on the unhealthy fats too, since they saturate the chips, French fries, and pizza that so many people snack on, as well as lurk in many other store-bought and restaurant foods spreading in popularity around the globe. No wonder we are looking at a worldwide fat and oil problem!

The solution? Here are a few suggestions:

- Avoid processed, packaged, and fast foods unless you know they contain only healthy fats.
- If you eat fish, choose wild-caught.
- If you eat animal meats or animal products, choose organic, humanely raised, and free-range or pasture-raised.

- If you eat dairy products, choose organic and those free of hormones and antibiotics.
- Moderate your consumption of animal and dairy products, and make sure to balance them with omega-3s, from fish, flaxseed meal, green leafy vegetables, nuts, and seeds.
- Consider supplementing with omega-3 fats, such as two fats that are found in fish: eicosapentaenoic acid (EPA) and docosahexaenoic acid (DHA). Make sure, however, that you buy only the cleanest fish oils, or you'll just end up with concentrated mercury.

Two other categories of fat are saturated (usually solid) and unsaturated (usually liquid). Every cell in your body contains a fat layer around its perimeter. As you might imagine, the composition of this fat layer determines how the cell functions: the nutrients and other substances it takes in and toxins and waste it lets out. Adding these precious unsaturated, flowing fats to our diet can lead to significant changes in the fluidity of our cells and their ability to receive and transport more efficiently when it comes to detox.

FISH AND WATER

If you're looking for the perfect FLOW food, you couldn't do better than the slippery, silver salmon: it lives in water, has a brilliant orange color on the inside, and is rich in omega-3 healthy fats. Also, salmon is relatively low in mercury compared with other fish choices, which, as we saw in chapter 3, is a major health hazard.

Regrettably, methylmercury is frighteningly common in seafood. If you want to learn more about the healthier choices at the fish market, check the Resources section for websites that can keep you current.

The Environmental Working Group can also help you find a filter for your water source so you can hydrate in peace of mind (see Resources). Meanwhile, avoid plastic containers for water as much as possible, since the plastic likely contains substances that disrupt your creative reproductive hormones. Stick with glass and stainless steel.

WHICH FISH HAVE THE HIGHEST LEVELS OF THE FLUID OMEGA-3 FATS?

Food	Serving size	EPA (grams)	DHA (grams)
Crab, Dungeness, raw	3 ounces	0.24	0.10
Herring, Pacific, raw	3 ounces	1.06	0.70
Salmon, Chinook, raw	3 ounces	0.86	0.62
Salmon, sockeye, raw	3 ounces	0.45	0.60
Sardines, Pacific, raw	3 ounces	0.45	0.74

BE FLUID IN YOUR FAT CHOICES

Have you ever noticed how people start to think that if a food is good for you, then you need to have more of it? For some time everyone seemed to focus on extra-virgin olive oil. Now coconut oil is all the rage. Coconut this, coconut that. After being told for years that coconut oil was bad for us, we now understand that it is quite healthy—but we need to consider the overall quantity. I am sure the tide will shift again at some point. Changing up your oils is your best alternative, and you will see several different types of oils in my Whole Detox recipes.

Meanwhile, check out some of my favorite fats for you to focus on:

Essential Fatty Acids

- *Sesame* oil is naturally rich in sesamin, a plant compound that improves your liver's fat-burning efficiency.
- *Hempseed* oil contains a mixture of both omega-3 and omega-6 fats. It is also rich in an anti-inflammatory fat called gamma-linolenic acid (GLA).
- *Flaxseed* oil is an abundant source of one of my favorite omega-3 fats, alpha-linolenic acid (ALA).
- Fish oil is another great source of omega-3s and essential fatty acids, especially when you take it in concentrated form as a supplement.

Helpful Fats

- Coconut oil isn't an essential fat, but it provides an abundant source of short- and medium-chain saturated fatty acids, which your liver and gut can quickly burn for energy. I've incorporated coconut oil into your Whole Detox to give your liver, gut, and brain the energy boost they need. Some newer research on coconut suggests it is also beneficial for giving the brain fuel, in addition to being antifungal, antiviral, antiparasitic, antimicrobial, and protective for the liver.

- Extra-virgin olive oil is known to contain some potent phytochemicals that act as antioxidants and anti-inflammatories. Plus, it's delicious! When you purchase olive oil from the store, look for not just "cold-pressed" or "extra-virgin" on the label but also "unfiltered" so you are getting the dense, cloudy oil full of those medicinal agents.

- Avocado oil is a relatively new oil that is good for cooking at higher heat. It has some health benefits, such as improving the function of mitochondria, the energy-producing organelles in the cell.

Packaging Matters

When thinking about fats and oils, don't forget how they are stored! Go for glass or stainless steel containers, and avoid plastic if you don't want endocrine-disruptive plastic molecules to migrate into your food. Fats and oils go rancid in heat, light, and oxygen, so make sure the container lids screw on tight and that you're keeping everything far away from the heat of the stove as well as from direct sunlight. Consider storing oils that you don't use very often in the refrigerator to extend their freshness. And of course, make sure to cook each fat at its correct temperature, or you will have toxic fats in your meal.

GO NUTS!

A super way to support Whole Detox is to eat nature's own combination of protein and healthy fats: nuts and seeds. Not only do you get lots of healthy omega-3s but you also combine the grounding of the ROOT protein with the FLOW of healthy fats. Your liver needs protein to properly rid your body of physical toxins, while your cells need healthy fats to defend against toxins and to excrete any waste and toxins that make their way into the cells.

Nuts and seeds give you a two-for-one that is especially important for vegetarians, who need to work a bit harder than carnivores to make sure they consume enough balanced protein and fat. Nut butters are an excellent way to add some protein and healthy fat to your smoothies as well.

Of course, many people can't digest nuts and seeds, responding with allergies or food sensitivities. If that's you, try rotating them every three or four days, which might enable you to tolerate them better. In fact, this type of rotation is a healthy choice even if you're not intolerant.

If you have difficulty digesting nuts, you may want to try sprouting them or soaking them in purified water for four to six hours before eating. Allowing their structure to soften means they can flow more efficiently because your digestive tract breaks them down more easily.

Several of the recipes on your twenty-one-day program call for nuts, especially on the vegetarian track. Please avoid them if you have an allergy or sensitivity.

ORANGE FOODS AND YOUR FLOW

Ah, the wonders of orange foods, from the deep sunset-colored blood orange to the pale, creamy orange of a slice of cantaloupe. Some orange foods are sweet, some tart, and some savory, but they have one important thing in common: the carotenoids that give them their color. I spent years studying this class of plant-based compounds during my graduate research at the university, which has given me an abiding appreciation for their contributions to our health and the FLOW, with particular admiration for their role in ovulation and hormone levels.

Just as fats can go rancid on your kitchen shelf or on the stovetop, so can they go rancid within our bodies, but this process is impeded by the carotenoids, which make their way into our cells. Some animal research suggests that beta-carotene—which converts to retinol, or vitamin A—also concentrates in the corpus luteum, the developing egg in the ovary. There it may play a role in ovulation by assisting with the production of progesterone, a hormone that is vital to fertility, a smoother menstrual cycle, and overall hormonal balance.

Insufficient progesterone results in estrogen dominance as well as a number of other mood and cognition problems: brain fog, mood swings, anxiety, depression, and sleep problems. Eating orange foods and healthy fats makes you feel better in so many ways!

ORANGE FOODS THAT NOURISH YOUR FLOW

- Apricot
- Bell pepper
- Cantaloupe
- Carrot
- Curry powder
- Kumquat
- Mango
- Nectarine
- Orange
- Papaya
- Peach
- Persimmon
- Pumpkin
- Squash (acorn, buttercup, butternut, kabocha)
- Sweet potato
- Tangerine
- Turmeric powder, turmeric root
- Yam

Beta-carotene dissolves in fat, so if your body is going to absorb it properly, you need to consume a little fat with your orange foods. Some research also suggests that heat might be essential to ensure that the fibrous structure of a plant breaks down enough to let the beta-carotene flow and become available for absorption.

What's your takeaway? Add some fat to your orange fruits and vegetables—just a bit—and, if possible, cook them lightly.

COMBINING ORANGE FOODS AND FATS: A FEW SUGGESTIONS

- Sauté your orange bell peppers in sesame oil at a very low heat until they are just slightly softened.
- Add a light coating of extra-virgin olive oil to some steamed squash, maybe with a touch of lemon or vinegar.
- Cut your carrots into matchsticks and steam them lightly in some coconut milk or clarified butter, until just slightly soft.
- Dress your baked or steamed sweet potatoes with a bit of coconut milk and a dash of ground nutmeg.

I've noticed that many infertile women don't seem to be getting their daily dose of orange foods, which means they're probably not getting enough beta-carotene. Could this be why they have trouble with ovulation and conception?

Other orange foods contain different types of phytonutrients, such as the bioflavonoids we find in oranges and tangerines. Getting a wide variety of bioflavonoids is helpful for keeping our blood vessels wide open, so they easily accommodate blood flow, keeping blood from stagnating into varicose veins and similar conditions. Finally, carotenoids and bioflavonoids have been shown to help prevent cancer—imbalanced FLOW triggering the body's excessive creativity, perhaps?

TROPICAL FOODS TO SUPPORT YOUR FLOW

Have you ever lived in the tropics or been there on vacation? Why are these glorious destinations where people often choose to relax? The sunshine, warmth, and foods embody the elements of relaxation, delight, joy, pleasure, and freedom. Bringing more of these foods into our lives, especially when they are in season, can enhance our playful inner child, who wants to have fun with food, as well as our adult self, who wants to tap into sensuality. Banana, coconut, fig, kiwi, mango, orange, papaya, and pineapple are all luscious options.

SUPPORT YOUR FLOW WHILE YOU EAT

You'll learn all about how to get yourself flowing in days four through six of your twenty-one-day program. But here are a few quick tips to get you started. Use any that appeal to you and keep the rest in reserve for a day when you'd like to get things moving:

- Drink enough water so your hunger and thirst signals are not mixed. Sip fluids throughout the day.
- Drink some warm water seasoned with cooling herbs like fennel and mint.
- Pay attention to how you feel when you eat. If you're blocking your feelings, ignoring your food, or eating while stressed, you'll lose the flow of hunger and fullness, making you vulnerable to emotional eating.
- Give your inner child time to create a meal, playing with the experience, making full use of colors and textures, and experiencing your emotions about cooking and sharing food.
- Sip some coconut water, eat some young coconut meat, or take a spoonful of coconut butter to satisfy hunger urges.
- Create some playful, colorful water by adding slices of lemon, lime, strawberry, fresh mint leaves, or cucumber, or drink some orange-infused water.
- Eat high-water orange fruits, like melon, papaya, and mango.
- Make a meal of an "avocado taco": cut the avocado into two halves, pry out the pit, and with each half, squish the meat up from the skin. Mmmm, healthy, filling fats and a delicious taste besides!
- Drink smoothies containing carrot, mango, tangerine, and/or orange juice instead of soft drinks.
- Choose an orange-yellow yam over a white baked potato.
- Add turmeric powder into smoothies, into a vegetable stir-fry, and into hamburger meat patties.
- Enjoy an apricot, cantaloupe slice, clementine, kumquat, orange, tangerine, nectarine, or peach as a snack.
- Prepare puréed carrots, butternut squash, and/or pumpkin.
- Make a tropical fruit smoothie containing frozen, cubed mango, papaya, and orange in a base of coconut milk and topped with ground cardamom and cinnamon.

- Put together a trail mix by blending different nuts (cashews, almonds, walnuts) with dried orange-colored, non-sulfated fruits (apricots, mango, papaya).

DETOXING YOUR FLOW: WHAT TO CHOOSE
- Healthy fats and oils, such as extra-virgin olive oil, sesame oil, flaxseed oil, hempseed oil, coconut oil, avocado oil, fish oil, wild-caught fish
- Nuts and seeds as a source of protein, rotated frequently to avoid triggering intolerance and sensitivity
- Orange foods, such as carrots, mangoes, melons, orange bell peppers, oranges, tangerines, sweet potatoes, yams
- Tropical fruits, such as banana, coconut, fig, kiwi, mango, orange, papaya, pineapple
- Purified water
- Emotional "flow," nurturing your full emotional range without feeling emotionally out of control
- Creativity, expressing yourself in your own way
- Sensuality and sexuality, allowing your sexual, sensual side to emerge and "flow" freely

DETOXING YOUR FLOW: WHAT TO AVOID
- Impure water
- Water and foods in plastic containers
- Excessive amounts of animal fats, such as fatty meats, butter, and cheese
- Unhealthy fats, such as trans fats
- Storing emotions within rather than expressing them creatively and freely
- Repressing or denying creative expression

DIVE INTO YOUR FLOW

My patients tend to make two unhelpful assumptions when it comes to the FLOW.

One is that emotional expression and FLOW involves always expressing every single emotion or telling every person close to you exactly what you are feeling at all times. This is not at all what I mean by letting your emotions flow! Often—perhaps even most of the time—sharing our feelings instantly and unedited is not the best idea. In some relationships, tact, silence, and detachment might be much better choices than free expression. In just about every relationship, it's usually better to express your emotions when you have some mastery of them, especially if you're angry, anxious, or feeling needy. Giving yourself some time to think about your feelings and make rational decisions about how to share them is frequently the best plan.

Regardless of how you choose to express your emotions to others, however, you can always choose to let them flow freely within yourself. Knowing what you feel and allowing your feelings to bubble up without censorship or control is often a good first step. If you're in a situation in which you need to be more guarded, make sure you give yourself some space later on or at the end of the day to cry, laugh, shout, write out your feelings, or otherwise feel what you feel. And of course, in many intimate relationships, it is important to express anger, fear, and grief as well as to let other emotions flow freely "in real time" rather than controlling their expression. You've got a lot of choices about how to behave with others; just always make sure to let your emotions flow for yourself.

Second, with regard to creativity, I've noticed that many patients and students hear that word as meaning "being an artist." On the contrary, you can be creative about how to be creative! Sure, creativity can express itself through writing, music, painting, sculpture, or dance. But it can also come out through creative problem solving, a new way to arrange your furniture, or an impulsive day of unexpected adventure. Any time you come up with something new, you've tapped into your creative side—and you have found your FLOW.

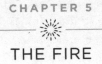

CHAPTER 5

THE FIRE

The most powerful weapon on earth is the human soul on fire.

—FERDINAND FOCH

Success isn't a result of spontaneous combustion. You must set yourself on fire.

—ARNOLD H. GLASOW

UNDERSTANDING THE FIRE	
Anatomy	Digestive system: pancreas, stomach, liver, gallbladder, small intestine
Functions	Digestion, assimilation, transformation
Living	Energy, empowerment, achievement, ambition, work–life balance
Eating	Carbohydrates (simple sugars and complex grains), fiber, yellow-colored foods

THE SCIENCE OF THE FIRE

The FIRE is one of the most challenging systems of health for just about everybody I work with. At least 80 percent of my patients and students struggle with an imbalanced FIRE, most commonly feeling burnt out with too much stress.

Another huge FIRE issue is unhealthy foods—the fast-burning refined carbohydrates and sugary sweets that set us up for a huge flare-up of energy followed by a swift, exhausting burnout. Think about the way a carefully tended fire blazes sky-high when you throw paper or dried leaves on it—and how that quick-burning fuel seems to be gone in an instant, leaving your flames starved and exhausted. That's exactly what happens when you eat refined carbohydrates and sweets: a rush of quick-burning energy followed by an exhausted crash and the desperate need for another quick burst of fuel.

Whether the problem is too much work or too many carbohydrates, imbalanced FIRE energy creates blocks and imbalances, resulting in belly fat, obesity, and type 2 diabetes—health challenges that are nearly as common among my patients as stress and burnout.

The FIRE and Your Digestion

The stress that comes from overwork creates a "fire in the belly" that ravages our delicate internal ecosystem. Increased stress depletes the digestive enzymes we need to absorb nutrients from food. With poor digestion, we can become malnourished even as we continually overeat, consuming nourishment we cannot receive.

Stressful jobs and imbalanced lives also disrupt our microbiome, the community of microscopic creatures living in our intestines and throughout our body. The microbiome is a crucial factor in our health, playing an important role in mood, mental focus, and energy levels as well as in digestion, heart function, and many other systems. Just twenty-four hours of stress can alter the composition of this bacterial community, transforming it from a friendly, positive presence into a source of toxins and inflammation.

What happens when too much work and too little play disrupt our enzymes, our microbiome, and our gut? We lose our fire, burn out, and flame out, feeling uninspired, unmotivated, and exhausted. We also set ourselves up for a host of disorders, including obesity, high blood pressure, diabetes, and metabolic syndrome.

The link between belly fat and a stressful job has been dramatically demonstrated in a number of large-scale population studies conducted in England and Japan as well as many smaller-scale studies around the globe. Time and time again, researchers came to the same conclusion: working at a high-stress job was a significant risk factor for obesity—specifically, larger waists and belly fat ("abdominal adiposity"). The association between an imbalanced work life and the belly—the center of the third system of health—couldn't be clearer. And when you throw in "fiery" yellow foods— processed carbohydrates, sugar, and fried foods—the triangle is complete.

The FIRE and Diabetes

Another intriguing body of research suggests that pressures at work are linked to diabetes in both men and women. A 2014 study published in *Diabetes Care* found that "job strain is a risk factor for type 2 diabetes in men and women *independent of lifestyle factors* [emphasis added]." In other words, even when you're not eating high-carbohydrate and high-sugar foods, a difficult work life creates blood sugar issues and an imbalanced FIRE.

A similar study in *Psychosomatic Medicine*, covering more than 5,300 workers aged twenty-nine to sixty-six in Augsburg, Germany, found that "men and women who experience high job strain are at higher risk for developing [type 2 diabetes mellitus] *independently of traditional risk factors* [emphasis added]." Once again, a problematic work life seems to create the conditions for diabetes even apart from poor diet. Several other studies come to similar conclusions.

Tending Your FIRE

By contrast, work–life balance can keep your FIRE burning with a steady, warming glow—and certainly, the right foods can help. When you bring food into your stomach, it's like making an offering to your internal altar. The flames of digestion gradually transform the food into the energy you need while your mitochondria—the powerhouses located in each cell— create cellular energy. This slow, healthy burning creates good digestion and a healthy weight.

Every one of us has a FIRE within. Sometimes it burns brightly enough to shed light on our goals, lighting up the areas where we need to put our energy. Other times, we overextend ourselves and burn out. Or perhaps our FIRE rages out of control with too much to process: information overload, racing thoughts, overthinking, a tendency to overpromise and underdeliver. The result is often chaos.

Yet it is possible to keep our FIRE burning at an even flame. Once we cherish that spark of willpower that originates in our solar plexus—the original "fire in the belly"—it can keep us moving joyously forward toward our goals, on a journey where both process and destination are bright with meaning.

THE POWER OF YELLOW

Strikingly, a number of studies bear witness to the power of yellow generating energy. A study conducted in Oxford, England, found that yellow mustard bran helped a group of young, active men have a better post-meal response to glucose after eating potato and leek soup compared to eating the soup by itself. Likewise, a Canadian study found that whole yellow pea flour—a complex carbohydrate—helped overweight people improve their use of insulin.

You can find lots of ways to brighten up your life with yellow. If you work in an office with fluorescent lights, see if you can bring in your own lamp with a soft yellow bulb, so you can enjoy the cheery and balancing effects of yellow. When you need a break or a moment to balance work and life, try lighting a candle—perhaps even a yellow candle—so you can focus on the slow, steady yellow flame and enjoy the healing, energizing properties of fire. You can also decorate your workspace with yellow, uplifting images, like a yellow smiley face, to remind you of work–life balance and to steer you away from burnout. Open yourself to the joys of yellow as you seek to balance your own personal FIRE.

GET TO KNOW YOUR FIRE

Burning Ambition

We live in a power-hungry, stress-filled society that is always expecting us to give more and more. Our ability to maintain balance in the midst of chaos becomes increasingly difficult when demands and responsibilities begin to pile high. We try to accommodate and stay in control by saying yes when we really mean no, and after a short while, we feel burdened with life, while everyday events become drudgery. Finally, we collapse in utter exhaustion, unable to integrate all that fiery energy into our core self.

Yet when we can harness the power of burning ambition, we can achieve great feats! The FIRE energy helps us reach our goals, fueling our drive and commitment. Besides food, many things can fuel the FIRE energy: conversations, inspirational movies and TV shows, dreams of achievement, visions of greatness.

The third system of health is also associated with the ego—our sense of self. An unhealthy or imbalanced ego is either overconfident or under-confident, sometimes both. A healthy ego, by contrast, is fueled by confidence and empowerment. Think of the powerful, almost glowing presence of those charismatic leaders who exude certainty and inspire an eager, productive response. Their radiant energy is lit by an inner FIRE—and it often ignites the FIRE of others.

IMPROVE YOUR DIGESTION

If you're having trouble with indigestion or struggling with blood sugar spikes and crashes, try eating smaller meals and snacks. Think of a fire that has become overloaded with fuel: it can't burn properly if it's smothered in green wood. Eat less, or if you want to keep eating large portions, eat slowly, so your stomach has time to empty itself.

I also suggest making your meals less complicated, containing perhaps just one or two foods. And please make sure you're not stress eating. The more relaxed you are when you eat, the better your ability to digest carbohydrates. Besides, people who are more anxious tend to reach for food in times of stress, and stressful eating can result in craving more sugar.

Burning Out

When we pursue our goal with energy and excitement, we make good use of "fire in the belly." But when we "burn the candle at both ends," we run the risk of burnout: feeling uninspired, overwhelmed, or "blah."

Many of us labor under the idea that we can keep putting out more and more energy, that it's just a matter of willpower and our limits are self-imposed. But our bodies, minds, and emotions do have natural limits, and if we don't respect them, our FIRE runs out of fuel. I was fascinated to read a series of psychological studies that measured the effects of stress. The studies showed that psychological energy—the energy we use for self-control, for example—is a limited commodity, in much the same way that physical energy is. Just as you can't lift an infinite amount of weight or lift weights for an infinite amount of time, you can't exert an infinite amount of psychological or mental energy.

For example, if you have to cope with a rude clerk in a coffee bar, you might normally be able to brush off the annoying treatment and respond politely. But if you've been stressed by a major deadline, an uncooperative coworker, or a sarcastic boss, your resources for coping with the clerk might be depleted. The more demands you have on your energy, focus, and self-control, the fewer resources remain. People who are trying to raise families while working at demanding jobs know from experience that there is only so much energy to go around. If work is taking too much of it, the rest of your life is bound to suffer.

Of course, to some extent, challenges provide a kind of self-sustaining fuel: the more challenges you face, the greater your energy becomes to deal with them. That happens in physical situations too: the harder you exercise, the more strength and energy you develop. However, in both cases there comes a point of overload, where too much exercise exhausts you and too many mental or emotional demands deplete you. Many of my patients have reached the point where their work and life are seriously out of balance, where the demands of their jobs begin to undermine their ability to savor the joys of life.

Over the years, I've seen the issues of overload and burnout grow almost exponentially. To some extent, the problem is economic: the work week is getting longer, vacation time is getting shorter, and many people feel so anxious about being replaced that they don't even take the vacation they do have. To some extent, the problem is electronic: e-mail, social media, and the omnipresent cell phone mean that we're on demand 24/7, overloaded with work obligations, messaging friends, keeping up with a constant stream of information. At what point are you off duty? When do you turn inward instead of outward? A fire that never stops burning is in genuine danger of running out of fuel.

Often I see a close tie between burnout and unhealthy eating habits. When too much work seems to have drained life of all its sweetness, you might want to reward yourself with a sugary treat. But when sugar becomes a compulsion and perhaps even an addiction, you can lose the joy in sweetness too.

Whenever I see someone with a roll of fat around the middle, I know they've got a FIRE imbalance that is disrupting their metabolism, along with elevated blood sugar levels and unhealthy body fat. I can almost see the stagnant energy and congested fire that come from not fully digesting food, metabolizing glucose, and transforming dietary nutrients into energy. The saddest thing is when people are overweight yet their bodies believe they are starving—because they are not able to get fuel into their cells for energy, a condition known as being overfed and undernourished. Hunger for what we really need keeps us eating, even as our weight creeps up to an unhealthy level and our blood sugar rises into the danger zone.

One of my patients, Mollie, exemplified this problem. Feeling that her life had been drained of sweetness, she turned to sugary treats and eventually developed type 2 diabetes. Working two jobs and raising five kids, she felt fried by the effort of juggling all her competing obligations. "I need something sweet to keep me going, to give me energy—just a taste of something good," she told me. I wanted to help her find more sustainable fuel—and more sustainable sweetness as well. Later in the chapter, I'll tell you more about how I was able to help her find her own personal "sweet spot."

A Burning Joy

I've been speaking of work, drive, and ambition as sources of depletion, but I want to acknowledge that they are also sources of joy. When you love your work so much that you can't wait to get back to it, that's a brightly burning fire that warms you, energizes you, and lights your way forward. When a job is exhausting but also inspiring and fulfilling, you can discover new reserves of energy, like a phoenix rising from the ashes. When you love the journey as much as the destination, even a grueling work session can be illuminated by joy.

Of course, the most joyous work requires some kind of balance. You need downtime, sleep, relaxed meals, time for your body, mind, and emotions to recover from the fiery exertions that consume you.

But if you can find the sweetness in your work and your obligations, if you can feel the spark of inspiration or the flames of desire as you go about your daily routine, then you have found a remarkable resource indeed. When you are able to maintain a healthy balance of energy taken in and energy expended, you generate the radiance of "presence." When you are the master of your own energy, you can enjoy confidence, endurance, empowerment, and achievement in their highest forms.

BALANCE YOUR FIRE

Healthy FIRE energy will look different for every one of us, and it will probably look different to you at different times of your life. Still, we can set out some general guidelines that are clues to "too much," "too little," and "the right amount" of the FIRE.

A person with a healthy FIRE
- has a robust digestion so they can eat almost anything and feel energized afterward;
- has a healthy functioning pancreas that is able to produce adequate levels of enzymes to properly break down foods and enough insulin to take care of all the sugars they eat;
- has a normal blood sugar level;
- uses carbohydrates to sustain themselves rather than as a quick fix;
- feels inspired by goal setting and the prospect of achieving their goals; and
- strives to be their best without giving up if they can't "do it all."

A person with an underactive FIRE
- prefers spicy foods;
- selects warm or hot foods over cold foods;
- avoids cold drinks;
- often lacks an appetite;
- might end up snacking through the day since larger meals tend to deplete their energy;
- often gets tired after eating;
- has blood sugar that runs low;

- has a slightly inverted belly due to a concave, hunched posture;
- often has a sluggish liver and problems with detoxification;
- frequently has undigested food in a stool;
- may struggle with poor self-esteem;
- often shows a lack of initiative and might be perceived as unmotivated or even lazy;
- is less interested in work than in personal time;
- might feel that they can't keep up with competitive, ambitious people, so they just give up;
- might settle for being average;
- might be resentful of those who are successful and see them as "selling out";
- might have a victim mentality, feeling that someone else is responsible for their situation in life; or
- might feel that life is unfair and therefore gives up easily.

A person with an overactive FIRE
- binges on sweets or has a sweet tooth;
- needs to be in charge or in control almost all the time;
- tends to be excessively busy;
- may be overly confident of their abilities, perhaps arrogant or egotistical;
- is often fiercely competitive;
- might be a perfectionist;
- fixates on his or her goals to the exclusion of almost everything else;
- must be a high achiever in almost anything they undertake;
- refuses to accept failure even when energies would be better served elsewhere;
- has difficulty balancing work and life, is a classic workaholic;
- says yes to everything because they believe they can "do it all";
- is tightly wound with high expectations of themselves and others;
- is overly concerned with work and social status;
- is bombarded with too much information;
- overthinks and ruminates over everything;

- might have excess weight in the upper belly area or a distended, protruding abdomen;
- might have metabolic syndrome or type 2 diabetes, or be taking medication to lower their blood sugar;
- might have overactive liver dysfunctions or be on medications for liver-related issues, such as high liver enzymes, hepatitis, fatty liver, high triglycerides;
- is plagued by fiery digestive complaints after a meal or emotional events, such as ulcers, an acidic stomach, an upset stomach, esophageal reflux, GERD, or burping;
- feels hot or flushed after eating;
- forgets to eat due to being busy;
- eats sweet foods as a reward for working hard;
- eats on the run whatever is convenient and accessible;
- eats based on their work schedule, often rushing or working through meals;
- might be a stress eater;
- often multitasks while eating;
- eats when triggered by energy crashes;
- eats foods high in sugar and simple carbohydrates;
- might not eat enough fiber;
- often adds sugar or artificial sweeteners to foods;
- eats highly processed, convenient foods and/or fast foods;
- is sensitive to spicy foods;
- might consume energy drinks or caffeinated beverages;
- tends to prefer cold drinks and foods; or
- is drawn to sweet and refined yellow foods, such as bananas, corn, corn chips, or popcorn.

BURN BRIGHTLY: HOW MY PATIENTS HAVE USED THE FIRE TO TRANSFORM THEIR LIVES

For years, Simon had issues with his digestive system: nausea, bloating, gas. He also struggled with high blood sugar to the point where his doctor told him he was at risk for diabetes. Simon had

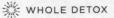

a high-pressure job as a day trader, which he enjoyed but often found overwhelming. Once he'd had a doctor's appointment right after returning from vacation, and he was amazed to discover that his blood sugar reading was much closer to normal. For him, high blood sugar was an issue of both stress and diet: while he was working, he tended to snack constantly on starchy, sugary foods—donuts, bagels, muffins, cookies—simply because that was what was available in the break room at work.

Simon began switching to slow-burning, high-fiber carbohydrates—quinoa, brown rice, lentils, garbanzo beans—which provided him with a steadier, healthier source of fuel. He also began doing some vigorous exercise after work to "blow off steam." Finally, he committed to doing something genuinely fun for at least part of every weekend—some activity that he enjoyed so much, he was able to forget about work. Within a few months, his digestive symptoms were gone, he had lost a few pounds, and his blood sugar was consistently at a healthy level.

Jillian was overworked and fatigued. Her job as an IT executive often left her feeling depleted, and on weekends, she collapsed on her bed in exhaustion. Slowly but surely, she began to develop symptoms: Her skin broke out. She gained weight. She had trouble sleeping. She started to struggle with depression. Jillian needed help.

Inspired by her experience of Whole Detox, she eventually decided to take some downtime: a week's vacation at a women's writing retreat on the Oregon coast. The chance to walk in the woods, mull over her thoughts, and simply enjoy the quiet was a revelation to her. When she returned, she realized she wanted more balance in her life—"more of life and less of work," she told me. She decided to leave her current high-powered job for one that was less taxing and began to live a healthier, more balanced life. Within a few weeks, her symptoms were virtually gone, and she looked more radiant than she had in years.

Peter had suffered from GERD for the past decade. As we explored his history, he realized that his symptoms had begun just after he had started working a double shift as a cab driver. "I need those extra hours to support my family," he told me. However, the acid reflux had become so bad that he often had to pause while driving, getting out of the car to breathe deeply; otherwise, he doubled up in pain.

My "prescription" for Peter was deceptively simple: make some time on Saturday mornings to take guitar lessons, which he'd told me he'd always wanted to do. Within a few weeks, he was writing songs, expressing his emotions in ways he couldn't do before. Although he still leads a high-pressure life, that weekend music break was a huge relief, and soon, his GERD disappeared.

BURNING FUEL

Does food ignite your energy or does it burn up your inner power? Either way, food is closely linked to the FIRE through the digestive system. Or, put another way, the FIRE is represented in the body through the act of transformation: your digestive tract transforms your food into energy, and your organs transform the plants and animals you consume into you.

The digestive transformation begins in your stomach, but your liver, gallbladder, small intestine, and pancreas are all part of each eating event. Your liver produces bile, an acrid, yellow-colored substance that helps you absorb fat. Your gallbladder stores the bile. Your pancreas helps to break down and assimilate sugar (glucose) through the activities of enzymes and insulin, respectively. And your small intestine transfers nutrients from the digested food into the bloodstream, where it nourishes every single one of your cells. All of these organs are therefore part of the third system of health, helping to create the transformative power of the FIRE.

Although protein can give our bodies a needed boost, the fuel that gets us through the day is glucose. All fruits, vegetables, grains, and legumes are ultimately broken down into glucose and other sugars. In fact, we are wired for sweetness, which is why even newborn babies will always prefer the sweeter formulas if given the choice. On a primal level, our bodies understand that sweetness equals energy. And because for most of human history we couldn't ever count on getting enough food, we are wired to want more and more and more.

Here is where we run into the contradictory nature of the FIRE, because we crave sweetness, but it isn't always good for us. Sugary sweets are FIRE foods because they are the quickest type of fuel there is. Refined carbohydrates—white flour and the pasta, baked goods, and snacks made from it—can often be sweet. Even when they are not, they burn quickly and create cravings. Fresh, organic corn is a naturally sweet and healthy food (although note that I have you avoid all corn during the Whole Detox program), but the chips and tortillas made from refined corn likewise burn too hot and are not generally healthy (not to mention that corn is predominantly genetically modified). And of course, one of the least healthy foods on the planet is the sweetener made from corn—high-fructose corn syrup—which is added to sodas and many processed foods, even the ones you wouldn't necessarily expect to be sweet, like soups and condiments. This overload of sweetness dulls our appreciation for it, so we need ever larger portions of sweet foods to be satisfied.

The color of the FIRE is yellow, and many of these unhealthy choices are yellow foods, but I don't want you eating them. Nor do I want you eating quick-burning fast foods—such unhealthy fuel for your inner FIRE! Significantly, fast and processed foods are often the cuisine of choice for people with too much FIRE, because they offer quick bursts of energy and ongoing support for a lifestyle in which you work overly long hours and neglect the rest of your life. Just listen to our language: "fried" foods that make you feel fried; "fast" foods that make you feel rushed. Grabbing food on the run or gobbling it down at your desk creates major digestive problems and pushes your stress levels through the roof. I can't tell you how much healthier it is to slow down, eat with pleasure, and enjoy your meals in a relaxed atmosphere.

Applying fire to food transforms it from raw to cooked, and this, too, is a double-edged sword. Sometimes slow-cooked food is easier to digest than raw, and nutrients often become more bioavailable when a food is cooked. But when you cook a food too long, the burnt, brown, or crisp part contains compounds known as advanced glycation end products, or AGEs. These fiery foods are aptly named, because AGEs speed up the aging process faster than any other compound in food I can think of. How do they do it? By creating inflammation—that is, they set your body on fire.

By contrast, a modest amount of heat can help break down some foods and make them easier to digest. Cooking also makes some valuable nutrients more bioavailable.

What's your happy medium? Eat some raw foods and some cooked. You will see in the Whole Detox program that I incorporate raw smoothies with a cooked dinner, and the lunch is half raw and half cooked. My guidance is when you need to cook, cook slowly, over low heat, and don't cook your foods to the point when they turn medium or dark brown, as in grilling, frying, toasting, or baking. Moderate heat will keep you warm, but high heat will only AGE you. So please avoid browned, crusty, and crispy foods. Inundated with AGEs and yellow foods, we risk premature aging, obesity, diabetes, and metabolic syndrome—all of which have become epidemic among people who eat a standard Western diet.

I do want you eating some yellow foods, the healthy variety: yellow summer squash, yellow bell peppers, wax beans, Asian pears, lemons, pineapple, and bananas. Yellow plant compounds include lutein and zeaxanthin, two carotenoids that are needed for healthy eye function. And lemons contain compounds like bioflavonoids, which support your liver through all phases of detox.

I also think it's good to eat slow-burning carbohydrates on occasion: quinoa, brown rice, and other whole grains. These FIRE foods offer you long-burning fuel whose flame reaches every part of you. Some of you prefer no grains whatsoever, which is fine; however, I have found that some people actually need this sustainable and high-fiber fuel source. Copious studies support the inclusion of whole grains in a mixed diet. The goal is not to let them have "power" over you but to make thoughtful choices about when to include them for your energy.

Another type of healthy FIRE nutrient is the team of B vitamins that are found in many of those slow-burning carbohydrates. Please note that when you supplement with B vitamins, your urine might turn yellow.

B vitamins also help extract energy from your food. They are crucial in glycolysis, the conversion of glucose into energy in your body, as well as for the Krebs cycle, breaking down sugars, amino acids, and fatty acids. Meanwhile, B vitamins help you relax and de-stress so you can maintain a healthy work–life balance.

HEALTHY YELLOW FOODS

- Complex, unrefined carbohydrates, such as quinoa, millet, amaranth, sorghum, and other whole grains
- Soluble fibers—dietary fibers that will support your digestion and give your pancreas some relief by slowing down the release of sugar—found in oat bran, nuts, seeds, beans, lentils, peas, and some fruits and vegetables
- Ginger, a soothing yellow spice that can ease digestive problems like stomach upset and nausea
- Lemon juice and zest to spark healthy detox pathways in the liver and assist with alkalinization of an over-acidic, fiery eating pattern
- Herbs and spices, used in cooking, that add some "heat" to a dish and stimulate digestion, such as chili pepper, paprika, black pepper, cardamom, horseradish, cinnamon, garlic, and ginger
- B vitamins, to help relax and balance stress, and which can be found in many different foods, such as fruits, vegetables, whole grains, and legumes

YELLOW FOODS AND YOUR FIRE

Some FIRE foods are healthy; some are less so. Once you know the range of FIRE foods—many of which are yellow—you can make the wisest choices to fuel your inner flame. Here's a rundown of the main fiery yellow foods with my best recommendations for what to eat and how to eat it.

Carbohydrates

Notice how many carbohydrates you eat at each meal and over the course of a day. To empower yourself with the energy you need, you have to keep checking in with your fuel gauge, balancing the different carbohydrates in your diet. One day you might need oatmeal and lentils; the next day you might crave quinoa and black beans. One day you might carbo-load; the next day you might be completely uninterested in starchy foods. Learn how to tune in to your FIRE to know what type of fuel it needs.

PROCESSED CARBOHYDRATES

We typically grab these foods when we are burnt out and don't have the energy to cook. Ironically, they actually drain our inner FIRE, producing a quick energy rush followed inevitably by a crash. Processed carbohydrates also deplete our bodies of the valuable B vitamins and other nutrients we need for proper digestion and metabolism. It is best for you to let go of these foods as much as you can. Don't let them take your FIRE!

WHEN YOU NEED SOME SWEETNESS

A good general rule is to stick as closely as possible to a sweetener's natural form. Unhealthy, overly processed choices:

- Artificial or synthetic sweeteners
- Brown sugar
- Evaporated cane juice
- Granulated or powdered sugar of any type or color
- White sugar

Natural choices that are healthy in small doses and in combinations with other foods to blunt their glycemic effects:

- Applesauce
- Bananas
- Blackstrap molasses
- Honey, preferably raw and organic
- Juice concentrate
- Maple syrup
- Medjool dates

Try to combine a sweet food with some protein. That combination will modulate your blood sugar response, preventing those deadly spikes and crashes that set you up for cravings, constant hunger, weight gain, and diabetes.

SUGARY SWEETS

I'm sure you've heard this before, but let me say it one more time: sugar is ungodly toxic. It shuts down your detox pathways rather than revving them. It's tough to detox from sugar, but you can do it—your willpower is fiery! And if you can detox from sugar, you can detox from anything!

Now, how did we end up craving sugar in the first place? Through the years, I've observed that people gravitate toward sugar when they feel depleted and need some sweetness. So I would say that craving sugar could be a sign that you need some more joy in your life. If sugar truly made you joyous, I'd have a hard time telling you to avoid it, but the problem is that it's a quick-burning joy that disappears almost as soon as it shows up—again, think of the way a fire flares up quickly to consume a few sheets of paper or a handful of leaves. And the crash after the flare-up leaves you feeling worse than before.

Enough is enough. Finito. No more toxic sugar. There. I said it.

AVOID ARTIFICIAL SWEETENERS

The naming games give it all away: How can we expect anything artificial to spark our natural inner FIRE?

In fact, artificial sweeteners are ugly, toxic chemicals that your body doesn't recognize and therefore can't respond to. As a result, these chemical concoctions generate metabolic changes, disrupt the friendly bacteria in our gut, and might even create *more* weight gain than eating sugar. (But please don't eat sugar either!)

One of my least favorite artificial sweeteners is, ironically, packaged in *yellow:* sucralose. Each molecule is loaded up with three chlorine atoms, and when you recall that chlorine is used to disinfect swimming pools, you can imagine how little you want it in your body. But, honestly, the other artificial sweeteners aren't much better. Just avoid them.

COMPLEX CARBOHYDRATES

Ahhhhh, what a relief to leave toxic foods behind and focus on those that truly nourish our inner FIRE. I know a lot of books out there warn you against carbohydrates, but I don't want you to jump on that bandwagon, because legumes, gluten-free grains, and starchy vegetables are a powerful source of energy that keep your blood sugar steady, in addition to providing you with healthy phytonutrients and fiber.

All carbohydrates contain long chains of sugars. When carbohydrates are refined, these sugars hit your bloodstream too quickly, creating those spikes and crashes. But when carbohydrates are complex (unrefined), they also contain fiber, which turns a fast-burning carbohydrate into a slow-burning one. They also contain many other detoxifying phytonutrients, including lignans, lignins, ferulic acid, and many others. So please don't eliminate carbohydrates from your diet unless under specific guidance by your health-care practitioner—just choose the right ones in the right amounts.

CHOOSE COMPLEX CARBOHYDRATES FOR A STEADY SOURCE OF FUEL

Legumes
- Beans (adzuki, black, chickpea/garbanzo, fava, mung, pinto, white [cannellini, Great Northern, navy], and others)
- Lentils (green, orange, orange/red, yellow)
- Peas (black-eyed, green, snap, snow, split)

Gluten-Free Grains
- Amaranth
- Gluten-free oats
- Millet
- Quinoa (black, red, white)
- Rice (brown, purple/black, red)

Nuts and Nut Butters
- Almonds
- Brazil nuts
- Cashews
- Macadamia nuts
- Pecans
- Walnuts

Seeds and Seed Butters

- Chia seeds
- Flax seeds
- Hemp seeds
- Pumpkin seeds
- Sesame seeds and tahini
- Sunflower seeds

Starchy Vegetables

- Parsnips
- Potatoes (purple, red, yellow fingerling)
- Squash
- Sweet potatoes
- Turnips
- Yams

Low-Glycemic Fruits

"Glycemic" refers to how sugar is released from a food. A low-glycemic fruit releases less sugar within a set time period into your bloodstream than a medium- or high-glycemic fruit. Here are a few examples of low-glycemic fruits suitable for Whole Detox:

- Apples
- Berries
- Cherries
- Grapefruit
- Kiwi fruits
- Nectarines
- Pears

Grains, Gluten, and Digestion

Over the past few decades, an increasing number of people have been having trouble digesting grains and legumes, particularly those that include gluten, a group of proteins found in wheat, rye, barley, and some other grains. Because gluten is used in most processed foods and is added to make many bread products fluffier and lighter, we've all been massively overexposed to it.

The number of gluten-related digestive problems has skyrocketed. The most severe form of gluten problems is celiac disease, which only about 1 percent of the population has. However, it is thought that a much higher percentage have gluten intolerance (referred to as nonceliac gluten sensitivity, or NCGS), a less intense but still problematic response that can generate a number of symptoms, including headaches, acne, indigestion, fatigue, weight gain, and vulnerability to autoimmune conditions. I have it myself, so I know it well. For years, I had pain, swelling, and redness around my finger joints. I consulted with a health practitioner, who thought it was the soap I was using to wash my hands or a lotion I put on my skin, but I knew that couldn't be right. It was truly systemic, and when I removed gluten from my diet, the joint pain and swelling went completely away! I'm proud to say that I am as gluten-free as I possibly can be to this day.

There are many different theories about why gluten intolerance is on the rise. Some of the problems with gluten and with other grains and legumes might be due to the rise of industrial agriculture. The toxic burden in our environment is probably diminishing our digestive and immune functions as well. Consequently, gluten, grains, and legumes have gotten a bad rap, since many people have trouble digesting them or tolerating their effects.

This is a real shame, because whole grains and legumes impart some wonderful phytonutrients and can be high in B vitamins, fueling the metabolic cycles in your body. If digestion is an issue for you, I suggest that you avoid or minimize your consumption of gluten. You can also sprout legumes, which makes them easier to digest. If you use canned beans (not ideal, but I know this is most practical), make sure you buy organic, bisphenol-free brands and drain and rinse them to remove the nondigestible carbohydrates.

COLORFUL GRAINS

Did you know that grains come in many colors? The greater variety you sample, the more different types of carbohydrates, fiber, and phytonutrients you consume. Let your body "taste" the rainbow!

Quinoa: black, red, white

Rice: black (also called purple), black Thai, brown basmati, long-grain brown, short-grain brown, wild

Warming Spices

Flavorings can add a hint of fire to your meal while igniting a healthy digestion. We each have a different tolerance for "hot" foods, so tune in to your
own fire as you choose your spices:

- Black pepper
- Cardamom
- Chili pepper
- Cinnamon
- Garlic
- Ginger
- Horseradish
- Paprika
- Turmeric

Beverages

As I mentioned in the previous chapter, I want you to stay hydrated. But I
don't want you to drink too much during a meal because the liquid can
dilute your stomach acid and cause your stomach to work harder. Iced beverages can also have a chilling effect on the flames of digestion.

If you're drinking a caloric beverage—soda, milk, juice, wine—you're
increasing the amount of energy you consume. You might want to moderate
energy consumption throughout the day by choosing water or herbal tea.

If you're concerned about excess weight or overeating, use fluids to
your advantage: drink 16 ounces of water thirty minutes before a meal
to reduce your food intake—as much as 13 percent, according to some
research. Over time, this practice can lead to greater weight loss when combined with a lower-calorie diet.

TIMING IS EVERYTHING

According to Ayurvedic tradition, noontime is when our "metabolic fire" burns
brightest. We can harness that energy by eating our largest meal at noon.
Breakfast and dinner should be moderate meals because your energy is just
revving up or winding down. Temper your eating accordingly during and even

after your Whole Detox. Follow another traditional principle of detox by eating more cooling foods in warmer weather and warmer, cooked foods in cooler temperatures.

SUPPORT WORK-LIFE BALANCE WITH MIND-BODY MEDICINE

As you learned in the ROOT chapter, stress is one of the major culprits behind chronic disease. Stress at work can easily overwhelm our lives, leading to fiery confrontations with friends, family, or colleagues. When we feel our inner flames burn too hot, we might become inflamed or have redness, pain, or swelling.

That's why keeping stress in check is essential for good health. And mind–body medicine is one of the best ways I know to bring some cool, soothing relief to a hot head and a flaming heart. Such techniques as hypnosis, guided imagery, biofeedback, progressive muscle relaxation, yoga, meditation, and tai chi have been found to be helpful for reducing chronic diseases and symptoms like depression, insomnia, anxiety, irritable bowel syndrome, nausea, and pain, and for managing diabetes and hypertension.

You can also create your own mind–body medicine. Choose one meal a week to eat mindfully—slowly, joyously, savoring every bite. Take a long, slow walk in a beautiful environment. Sit peacefully in an indoor or outdoor space that soothes your jangled nerves and transforms your raging fire into a quiet glow. I've heard it from my patients time and time again: one of the most powerful changes they ever made was to take up meditation, even if it was just finding five minutes each day to sit in peace and stillness.

SUPPORT YOUR FIRE WHILE YOU EAT

It's not just *what* we eat, but *how* we eat that adds to our health. In days seven through nine of your twenty-one-day program, you'll learn how to keep your FIRE in check. Since this is the system that can most easily go out of balance, the following tips will help you maintain your own internal Zen mode even if the outer world seems chaotic and frenzied:

- *Breathe into your center.* Before your first bite of food, take a deep breath into your solar plexus. Engaging your relaxation response will help you better digest your food. I find deep breathing easiest when I am sitting comfortably in a chair with my spine erect, my shoulders back, and my hands in my lap. Then I take three or four deep breaths to center myself into my inner power before beginning to eat.

- *Get in touch with your hunger gauge.* Often we lose sight of our innate sense of physical hunger and our bodies' physical cues to eat. The demands of a busy life may lead us to forget to eat, or to undereat or overeat without realizing it. Staying in touch with your internal eating rhythms—and eating regularly—helps you keep your internal power rather than giving it over to irregular eating times and over- or undereating. Sometimes this takes a bit of retraining! Many of us "think" our way into hunger, or assess it intellectually, rather than connecting to the power of our digestive system as the ultimate gauge. Try rating your hunger before and after eating to tap into how well you are maintaining your fuel reserves. If you find yourself "stuffed" after a meal, you may have inundated your energy input, placing an additional burden on your digestive system to process. Aim for about 80 percent fullness, or a point at which you are not stuffed, but also no longer hungry. Aim for the level at which you are able to take a light walk after eating.

- *Know your fuel.* Eating is meant to energize you rather than deplete your reserves. Some foods give you the punch of power you need, while others seem to drain you of your power. Do you find yourself eating foods that you *know* might "run you down"? When you do, you risk unbalancing your FIRE. Sugar is one such food, and added sugars are ubiquitous in the food supply, even in such unexpected places as salad dressings, ketchups, and sauces. Although they provide an initial burst of energy, in the long run, they will rob you of your energy through the roller coaster of blood sugar spikes and crashes. Stay on an even keel by balancing your sugar intake with dietary fiber and avoid artificial sweeteners, which can set you up for additional cravings and metabolic imbalance.

- *Schedule regular eating times.* Many of my patients find it helpful to create a regular eating schedule of small meals four to six times a day. This might be a good way to retrain yourself to get in touch with your eating rhythm: studies have shown that eating more frequent meals throughout the day (compared to a few large meals) helps us to maintain our blood sugar, and, therefore, provides more energy. However, your eating balance needs to be personalized to your needs: you might need to nibble and graze, or you might need a few large meals.

DETOXING YOUR FIRE: WHAT TO CHOOSE
- Complex carbohydrates
- Soluble fibers
- Yellow foods, such as yellow vegetables, whole grains, ginger, lemon, legumes
- Foods that give you sustained energy over time
- Work–life balance
- A healthy separation from work

DETOXING YOUR FIRE: WHAT TO AVOID
- Processed, highly refined carbohydrates
- Fast and convenient foods
- Foods that are tough to digest and assimilate
- Foods that create excessive bloating, discomfort, distention, or gas
- Eating more at one time than you can digest
- Foods high in sugar or those that unbalance your blood sugar
- Artificial sweeteners of *all* types
- Overcooked foods high in AGEs
- Situations where you feel like you are giving more energy than you are receiving in return
- Feeling that you have to "do it all," so you end up feeling depleted
- Focusing more on the goal than on the journey
- Workaholism—feeling so obsessed with work you can never let it go
- Perfectionism—focusing on trying to get every detail perfect rather than seeing the big picture

TEND YOUR FIRE

Each of the systems of health is a very personal affair—a reflection of your values, personality, genetics, and vision of life. Nowhere is this individuality more apparent than when you consider your relationship to the third system of health, the location of the ego and personal ambition.

Let's go back to my patient Mollie, whom I was telling you about earlier in the chapter. On her first visit, she was slumped in her chair and let out a huge, exhausted sigh.

"I feel totally burnt out," she told me. "I'm just fried. I feel like I'm just going through the motions—no fire, no spark."

I was fascinated by her language, because it so beautifully captured the paradox of the FIRE: too much, and you feel "burnt to a crisp"; not enough, and you lack that essential spark of passion and inspiration.

I began working with Mollie by exploring all the different ways that the FIRE burned in her life. Here's the list she came up with:

- Fiery inspiration sheds light on my goals.
- Energy fuels me and keeps me going.
- When I do too much, I burn out.
- When I have too much to process—information overload, over-thinking, stress, chaos—I feel like my flame is choked and my fire goes out.
- When I'm doing work I really love, I feel like I'm burning with an eternal flame.
- When I've been on overload and I take a break—long enough to feel really refreshed—I feel like a phoenix rising from the ashes!

I love the range of Mollie's images because the FIRE can be so empowering and joyous when it's in balance, and so toxic when we have either too much or too little. It can be hard to forge your own authentic relationship to your FIRE because of all the conflicting cultural and familial messages. Men are supposed to be ambitious; women are supposed to be less interested in worldly achievement than in tending to a home and family. All of us are supposed to work 24/7, endlessly on demand to bosses, clients, colleagues, and social media. Yet many films, TV shows, and popular songs demonize the overly ambitious character, presenting work not as a source of joy and inspiration but as something that interferes with the "true" happiness of love and a fulfilling personal life.

I know many people who find extraordinary inspiration and joy in devoting themselves to their work—indeed, I am one of them! Pretty much any time I'm awake, I'm thinking about the full spectrum of Whole Detox: wondering about the different colors in the spectrum, studying new research about food and light, endlessly fascinated as to what new things I can learn and what new ways I can help my patients, students, and readers. Even my recreation is color based: I paint in deep, saturated shades that make color real and palpable to me. This immersion in my working life isn't a cause of burnout to me, but rather a deep wellspring of joy.

My husband, by contrast, loves his work as an acupuncturist, but when the working day is over, he's delighted to let it go. He comes home and plays music, watches a movie, prepares a delicious dinner. He likes a variety of interests and tasks; unlike me, he isn't drawn to unify and deepen a single, all-absorbing focus.

I believe that both my husband and I have a healthy relationship to the FIRE, but look how differently each of us expresses it! What I hope for you, in every system of Whole Detox, is that you will get to know your FIRE, your ROOT, your FLOW, so you can nourish your entire being.

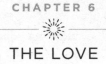

CHAPTER 6

THE LOVE

Love is the total absence of fear. Love asks no questions. Its natural state is one of extension and expansion, not comparison and measurement.

—GERALD JAMPOLSKY

UNDERSTANDING THE LOVE	
Anatomy	Heart, thymus, cardiovascular system, respiratory system
Functions	Circulation, oxygenation
Living	Compassion, expansiveness, loyalty, service
Eating	Leafy vegetables; raw, living greens; green foods

THE SCIENCE OF THE LOVE

The fourth system of health, the LOVE, is based in the heart and the lungs. The heart is an especially fascinating organ about which current medical opinion is evolving rapidly. For many years, conventional medicine considered the heart as little more than a pump—a mechanical device rather than a dynamic organ. Of course, even as a pump, the heart is a pretty amazing instrument. Every day it moves thousands of liters of blood through every inch of your body, disseminating the life force to your lungs, muscles, bones, eyes, ears, and brain, supplying every one of your cells with life-giving blood.

Recently, however, cutting-edge research has brought us to a more advanced view, seeing the heart not just as a pump but as a complex participant in the neuroendocrine system, producing hormones that activate the body in a variety of ways. Indeed, a group of scientists at the University of Ottawa have advanced a new specialty: cardiovascular endocrinology, the study of the biochemical effects of the heart. If the heart is a core player in the endocrine system, that means it affects thought, perception, and emotion as well as providing our cells with blood.

Recent research has also taught us that the heart is related to our emotions. All those metaphors about "let your heart guide you," "a heartfelt emotion," and "being heartbroken" have an actual physical component. When you are stressed or distressed, your heart beats faster, your blood pressure rises, and stress hormones inflame your system, putting you at risk of heart disease, stroke, and other cardiovascular ailments, which we now know are sparked and fueled by inflammation. When you are calm and full of joy, your heart beats at a healthy rhythm and your blood courses through your arteries at a healthy pressure.

Grief, Loss, and Your Heart

Grief, too, affects the heart. When someone is overcome with grief, their heart might even stop beating; researchers have documented cases of loss or rejection producing literal ailments of the heart. Just a glance at some press releases on recent research yields a host of evocative titles: "In Young Women, Depression Can Mean Literal Heartbreak," "Literal Heartbreak: The Cardiovascular Impact of Rejection," and "Why a Broken Heart Literally Hurts."

Other research shows that the loss of a beloved spouse can harm the heart of an elderly person. A study of more than ninety-five thousand Finns found that widowed men over sixty-five were at greater risk for ischemic heart disease. Puerto Rican researchers also concluded, "From clinical experience, we observed that the psychological category 'experience of loss' was associated with the onset and development of coronary heart disease." Research results supported this clinical observation.

Finally, a suggestive body of research has found numerous associations between bereavement and heart disease—a medical explanation of the bro-

ken heart. Bereaved spouses are at greater risk for heart disease. Even childhood losses can affect adult cardiovascular function, according to a study
conducted at Duke University's Psychiatry and Behavioral Sciences department.

The Cardiovascular Benefits of Love and Compassion

Love as well as grief can affect the heart. One study found that training
women to have compassion for themselves modulates heart rate variability (HRV) as well as reduces anxiety and evokes a cardiac parasympathetic
response—that is, a relaxation response in the heart. In other words, having
compassion for yourself literally eases your heart.

Likewise, in 2015, a group of researchers tested the effect of a loving-
kindness meditation on nitric oxide, a compound affecting blood pressure
and heart health. The results suggested that the relaxing effects of meditation may well be the result of biochemical changes related to nitric oxide.

Heart and Lungs

Of course, we can't view the heart in isolation from the lungs; our blood
must be oxygenated as it circulates throughout our body. If the lungs don't
draw in enough air, the circulatory system is affected: red blood cells get
less oxygenation and we end up having less energy. Most people breathe
shallowly, not having the full benefit of expanding the lungs wide and open
to release old toxins. Keep in mind that you can detox simply by taking a
deep breath—it's free and fuels both your heart and lungs, supporting the
two primary functions needed for survival.

Just as the heart and blood have a literal and a metaphoric power, so
does the air we breathe. Air, after all, is the staple of our life force. Breathing
deeply calms us; shallow, rapid breathing can make us anxious. Put more
scientifically, deep breathing activates the parasympathetic nervous system
(responsible for the relaxation response), while shallow, rapid breathing
activates the sympathetic nervous system (responsible for the fight-or-flight
reaction, or the stress response).

When we expand our lungs, our chest expands too, and as it relaxes, so
does our heart. And when our body expands in that fashion, we feel more
open to love, compassion, and service, extending outward to care for others

as well as inward to care for ourselves. As we consider the fourth system of health, we'll be looking at both the physical and the emotional sides of your loving heart and your expansive lungs.

THE POWER OF GREEN

You might have thought that red would be associated with the heart; however, green is the color of the fourth system of health. Researchers have discovered some fascinating links associating this color with the heart. For example, an Austrian experiment found that exposing people to green fluorescent light seemed to have a soothing effect on their hearts, affecting heart rate variability (HRV). People who endure continual worry and anxiety seem to have decreased HRV, which is also associated with a number of disorders, including congestive heart failure and depression. If exposure to green light increases HRV, we can imagine that has heart-protective effects and might help to heal grief—precisely the associations suggested by the fourth system of health.

To bring more of the LOVE into *your* life, take a walk in the woods or on some green grass. Breathe in the loving breath of nature and revel in the expansiveness of greenery.

If the weather is against you or if the nearest green space is too far away, bring the green to you in the form of plants at home or at work. Even a small representative of something green—living, growing, sprouting—can bring the expansiveness of love and compassion into an everyday world that may feel like it's collapsing down on you. Consider an herb garden in your kitchen window or a potted fern on your desk—anything to which you can direct love and feel love coming back in return.

Plants and nature not your thing? Go the other way with some green money. Spend something on self-care in the form of a massage, a funny movie, a bottle of scented lotion—something that makes you open up and remember just how wonderful you are.

GET TO KNOW YOUR LOVE

Love is perhaps the greatest nourishment that exists. Human beings thrive on it. We feed ourselves with heart symbols plastered on T-shirts, bumper stickers, books, and cards. As Mother Teresa said, "The hunger for love is much more difficult to remove than the hunger for bread."

Sometimes we use food to show love. We prepare a beautiful dinner for a loved one. Or we invite someone we love to eat with us. One of the oldest human traditions is "breaking bread" with family, community, and even with strangers whom we choose to welcome, while we refuse to eat with enemies and people we don't trust.

We're used to thinking of love as a relationship between two people. Love, however, starts with the self, and that includes the way we feed ourselves. By eating healing meals, we express love for our bodies. When we love ourselves, we know, intuitively, what kind of food our bodies need—we "follow our hearts" in choosing what to eat. When self-love is starved, or blocked, it's harder to choose the right foods or to stop eating when we've had enough.

Focusing on the fourth system of health can be a challenge for many of us, especially when we confuse self-care with selfishness. Getting the nutritional support for our fourth system can be overlooked as well, since many of us don't recognize the crucial importance of loving green foods and minerals for both heart health and emotional health.

If we move from the physical nature of the heart to its metaphorical symbolism of love, we must then consider the nature of love itself. I like M. Scott Peck's definition, from *The Road Less Traveled*: "The will to extend one's self for the purpose of nurturing one's own or another's spiritual growth." If that's our definition, we can see at a glance why love must always include self-love. How can we become capable of nurturing another's growth if we neglect our own?

As we have seen, conventional medicine associates the heart and lungs because of the role of the lungs in oxygenating the blood and supporting the heart. In TCM, the heart is the source of love, while the lungs are the seat of grief.

At first glance, this might seem odd: How could love and grief be related? And indeed, in some ways, they are polar opposites. Love makes us feel expansive, caring, and larger than we were before. Grief can make us feel constricted, wounded, shrunken, or hunched over in pain. Love moves us to care, for others and ourselves. Grief can lead us to frozen indifference, stony numbness, a refusal to care lest we get hurt again.

And yet any time we love, we open ourselves to the grief and pain of loss, just as any time we experience grief fully, rather than resisting it, we allow that painful emotion to pass through us, leaving us open and ready for love. Hence, the heart (love) and the lungs (grief) work together as yin and yang, sunlight and shadow, exhalation and inhalation, diastolic (the heart expanding outward) and systolic (the heart contracting inward). If we see love and grief as two aspects of the same journey, we may become more able to both honor our grief and let it go, so we can expand into love once more. This is why I believe so deeply in the power of the heart. The heart is the inner fulcrum, or the sovereign organ, that brings together our earthly self and all the contraptions of survival, emotion, and power, with our higher will, intuition, and soul. Those who have truly tapped into their wellspring of self-love will let their passions be their guiding principle for decision making. In other words, they will follow their heart, connecting in the highest way to related qualities of forgiveness, gratitude, love, and service.

BALANCE YOUR LOVE

You might think, *The more love, the better*, and if you mean the experience of love, you would be right. When it comes to the topic of love within our Seven Systems of Full-Spectrum Health, however, the LOVE can most definitely be out of balance, just like any of the other systems.

A person with a healthy LOVE
- is full of passion for issues that are close to their heart;
- can love in a balanced way of caring, but not feel overly committed;
- is a natural "healer" type of person;
- is empathic and tuned in to others' feelings, but doesn't get dragged into them;

- has emotional wisdom;
- knows how to balance the head and the heart;
- is generous, but not to the point of draining themselves;
- has an open heart with healthy boundaries;
- gives and receives in equal measure;
- has normal breathing;
- has hands that are slightly warm, not cold;
- has normal blood pressure and overall good heart health;
- is open to sharing their meals and enjoys family-style eating; and
- loves eating vegetables and engages in plant-based eating.

A person with an underactive LOVE
- has difficulty forgiving themselves and others;
- has the feeling that their heart is shut down due to hurt and trauma, and can't be healed;
- tends to dwell on past events;
- might lack passion;
- tends to focus on their suffering and pain;
- is often not in touch with others' feelings since they tend to be overwhelmed by their own;
- might be perceived as cold or uncaring;
- might hold back love because of painful feelings;
- has a head that rules their heart;
- has shut people out of their life;
- might have become stingy, jealous, and bitter;
- doesn't like to be touched;
- tends to take more than they give;
- has trouble taking care of themselves;
- feels paralyzed by deep past hurts;
- breathes heavily and erratically, and might have asthma or sleep apnea (their breathing stops or is interrupted during sleep);
- has cold hands and a stagnant circulation;
- might have low blood pressure;
- might have a low heart rate;
- might have blockage and/or calcification in their arteries;

- prefers not to share;
- avoids vegetables;
- rarely eats or likes eating leafy greens and salads; or
- might have become numb because of a series of disappointing, painful events in childhood or because of a childhood lack of love.

A person with an overactive LOVE
- is often a martyr type or feels they have to sacrifice themselves;
- might feel overly hurt at the slightest sense of pain inflicted toward others and may even feel their pain for them;
- is a people pleaser;
- seeks others' approval for their sense of self-love;
- overextends themselves repeatedly;
- neglects their self-care;
- might be frustrated or angry about not being nurtured but has trouble asking for nurturing;
- might care more about others' feelings than their own, which might create bitterness;
- is often anxious, especially when it comes to ensuring that others are content;
- tends to extend care outward, rather than inward;
- might make dinner for everyone else and leave themselves out or eat standing up;
- might be very touchy-feely and likes to give hugs;
- is extremely loyal, but might resent it when they perceive others aren't equally loyal;
- might be overly devoted to a cause to the extent they neglect their own needs;
- is effusive with passion;
- has a heart that rules their head and might not use logic;
- breathes quickly and shallowly, and is subject to hyperventilation;
- might have high blood pressure;
- might have warm hands or red palms;
- might flush in the face or chest area easily;

- might have a high heart rate and abnormally fast heart rhythm, and might be subject to anxiety and heart palpitations;
- might have a personal history of breast cancer or of cysts or lumps in the breasts;
- expresses love by making food for others, but can become offended if the food is not eaten; or
- tends to eat lots of green leafy salads or vegetables and not be as balanced in getting quality protein.

PRACTICE SELF-COMPASSION:
HOW THE LOVE DETOX WORKED FOR HALEY

Haley was a woman in her early fifties who described herself to me as "brokenhearted." She had just ended a long, painful relationship with a married man, a relationship that she told me had been sometimes loving but which often had left her feeling "starved" and "heartsick."

She told me that as her relationship was ending, she found herself weeping frequently. She also felt anxious, waking up in the middle of the night with her heart racing. During the day, she sometimes got heart palpitations, "until it feels like my heart is jumping out of my chest."

Haley had always been a somewhat anxious person, but when these panic attacks struck, she felt as though nothing could ever console or calm her. "I feel that I'm the only one who will ever be there to take care of me," is how she put it, "and what I can offer to myself is just not enough."

Haley and I agreed that our work would begin by looking at the issues of self-nourishment and self-love. She seemed to have a lot of compassion for others and I wanted her to extend some of that compassion to herself. These issues are often viewed as psychological, but I see them as nutritional also. According to the fourth system of health, plant foods are LOVE foods, and I thought that by eating more green vegetables, Haley could support the process of healing her heart. I also thought that magnesium—used for establishing a healthy, regular, heart rhythm—would ease the palpitations and anxiety.

Haley was skeptical that simple changes in diet and a few supplements could shift her outlook, but she agreed to give my suggestions a try. To her amazement, the green foods and magnesium did indeed make a difference, and within a few weeks, she felt much calmer and more optimistic.

I also taught her some mindful breathing techniques that I believed could ease her pain and soothe her anxiety. I explained that she could focus on her breathing when she felt anxious but also when she felt alone and uncared for. Because both the lungs and the heart belong to the fourth system of health, breathing deeply and mindfully is good for the heart, physically and metaphorically. Slowing the breath allows the physical heart to find its healthy rhythm, while connecting to the breath enables us to transform the constricting emotions of grief and despair into the expansive feelings of love and compassion.

Fortified by these physical approaches, Haley was ready to take a more emotional journey, exploring all the ways in which she nurtured others before she took care of herself. Like many people—and particularly like many women—Haley had been brought up to believe that self-care was selfish, that a good person put others first. Longing for love and nurturing, she had generously cared for the other people in her life, but she felt guilty, anxious, and ill at ease whenever she tried to care for herself. At the same time, she admitted, she frequently felt frustrated and even bitter at the lack of balance in her relationships. "I would like more of a two-way street," she told me. "But the care seems to go only one way."

Over time, she came to see that if she always put others first, she was likely to find that other people were only too happy to receive without giving back. If she wanted more balance in her relationships—both at home and at work—she needed to tip the balance herself by finding ways to turn her love inward as well as outward.

When I reminded her of M. Scott Peck's definition of love, she readily agreed that she felt love for her ex-partner, for her two sisters, even for some of the coworkers at her job. She wanted what was truly best for them and was committed to helping them get it. But when I asked her how this related to her—what she had done lately to ensure her own growth into the best possible version of herself—she was at a loss. "I don't think of having a duty or obligation to *myself*," she said finally, "but I guess I do."

"I'm struck that you use the words 'duty' and 'obligation,'" I replied. "Is that how you think of love toward others?"

Haley took a surprised breath. "No," she said slowly. "I give to others because I want to, because I feel the rightness of it."

"Then why can't you give to yourself in the same way?" I asked.

Haley felt uncomfortable with the idea of giving to herself, but she could see how loving and caring for herself might be what she needed right now. She could also see how self-love and self-care might help to dissolve some of the bitterness and frustration she felt over "always giving to others and never really having them give back to me." Together we made a list of five things she could do in the coming week to turn her love and generosity inward:

- Get a massage at a local spa, and take a walk in the botanical gardens afterward.
- Clean up her home office, bringing in some flowers and an inspiring poster, so her personal workspace felt like a lovely, healing, serene place.
- Go to a funny movie she'd never quite made time to see, which starred two of her favorite actors and seemed like it would be a fun night out.
- Make sure to use a nontoxic, rose-based moisturizer twice a day, so her skin felt cared for.
- Spend five minutes at the end of every day breathing deeply and allowing herself to review what was good about herself and what was right about her life rather than always focusing on where she and her expectations had fallen short.

Haley was surprised at how difficult these seemingly pleasurable activities were to perform. I asked her how hard it would have been had they been for someone else—had she been booking a massage, setting up a movie date, or buying moisturizer for her ex-partner, one of her sisters, or a close friend. She agreed, "Nothing could stop me," if her care had been directed at somebody else. I urged her to extend that same commitment to herself as the best possible way to heal her LOVE.

FOREST DETOX

The power of green takes on a new dimension with "forest bathing"—time spent walking or sitting in a forest environment. In another example of how fourth-system elements come together, time in the greenery has significant implications for heart health and hypertension.

This therapeutic technique originated in Japan, where it is known as *shinrin-yoku*, or "taking in the forest atmosphere" or "forest bathing." Recent research has ratified the cardiovascular benefits of this green practice. In the words of one research team,

> The results show that forest environments promote lower concentrations of cortisol, lower pulse rate, lower blood pressure, greater parasympathetic nerve activity, and lower sympathetic nerve activity than do city environments. These results will contribute to the development of a research field dedicated to forest medicine, which may be used as a strategy for preventive medicine.

GREEN FOODS AND YOUR LOVE

Just as the heart brings together our physical and emotional selves, vegetables unite the rootedness of the earth and the literal and symbolic blossoming into an expansive space. Green foods are particularly nurturing—luckily, nature has provided us with a lot of them! In fact, green is the color most predominant in nature, offering us many chances to heal.

I associate the color green with the elements of healing and expansion. Just as the leaves on a tree open naturally, green represents an unfolding of love, service, and gratitude from within.

Within food, green indicates the presence of chlorophyll, king of the antioxidants. High-chlorophyll foods, such as spirulina, wheatgrass, alfalfa grass, barley grass, and chlorella, cleanse the blood and promote good circulation. Chlorophyll can also help bind heterocyclic amines—the carcinogens that develop when meat is cooked. I highly recommend pairing meat with green foods rich in chlorophyll because of the ways chlorophyll can bind carcinogens.

Besides chlorophyll, vegetables—green and otherwise—supply our body with several thousand varieties of phytonutrients, plant compounds that impart color and special functions to a plant:

- red, orange, and yellow carotenoids and xanthophylls
- yellow-green chlorophyll, catechins, isoflavones, lutein, and zea-xanthin
- blue-purple anthocyanidins, hydroxystilbenes, and phenols
- tan-white allicin, lignans, lignins, and tannins

Other vitamins and minerals can also support your LOVE:
- *Magnesium, potassium,* and *calcium* keep heart rhythms regular and reduce anxiety.
- B *vitamins,* especially *folate* (B9) and *cobalamin* (B12) maintain healthy blood flow and lower homocysteine, a compound associated with blood clots, heart attacks, and strokes.
- *Phytosterols,* a class of compounds in plant foods, help to reduce levels of "bad" (LDL) cholesterol, keeping the cardiovascular system healthy.
- *Phytoestrogens*—isoflavones, coumestans, stilbenes, and lignans—support your heart, balance your estrogen, calm your mood, and promote your health.

I never cease to be amazed by the impact of leafy green foods and green supplements upon a cardiovascular condition. For example, my patient Samuel was told by his cardiologist that he had a 70 percent blockage in his carotid artery, a condition usually requiring an intervention to open up the artery. Unwilling to engage in such a drastic procedure, Samuel was in desperate hope of a dietary solution. At my suggestion, he began eating leafy green salads every day for lunch and exercising on a daily basis, along with stopping his smoking habit, and within months, his blockage was nearly gone.

Likewise, Luke had been struggling for years with high blood pressure, for which he was taking several medications by the time he came to me. His wife—a longtime patient of mine—begged him to come see me, and finally, frustrated with his medications' many side effects, he agreed. I convinced him to start eating more green vegetables—broccoli, Brussels sprouts, kale, collard greens, spinach, chard, and escarole. He had always hated vegetables, but his wife found a number of creative and healthy ways to cook these greens: lightly sautéed with garlic, steamed in coconut milk, garnished with pine nuts and currants. Within two months, to his doctor's astonishment, Luke was able to significantly reduce his medications, and after six more weeks, he was off his meds entirely.

As I said, green foods—the LOVE foods—are some of the most potent medicines I know. So come with me on a tour of these healing foods to support your heart, lungs, and sense of LOVE.

PHYTOSTEROL CONTENT IN SELECT FOODS*

Food	Serving size	Phytosterols (milligrams)
Sunflower seed kernels, dried	½ cup	374
Rice bran oil	1 tablespoon	162
Sesame oil	1 tablespoon	118
Sesame seeds, whole	1 tablespoon	64
Avocado	½	57
Almonds	1 ounce	39
Sunflower seed butter	1 tablespoon	33
Asparagus, raw	1 cup	32
Olive oil	1 tablespoon	22
Pickles, sour	1 cup	22
Lettuce, green-leaf	1 cup	14
Sunflower seed oil	1 tablespoon	14

*It is thought that the diets of early humans contained an average of 1,000 milligrams of phytosterols per day because of the high intake of plant foods.

IF YOU ARE TAKING BLOOD THINNERS

If your health-care provider has prescribed you warfarin, Coumadin, or any other blood-thinning drug, talk with them about your intake of leafy green vegetables. As we have seen, vitamin K helps prevent blood clots—a potentially dangerous effect if you're taking a blood thinner—and you might need to avoid many green vegetables while you're on that medication.

If that is your situation, consider buying some liquid chlorophyll from a health-food store, and put ¼ teaspoon into an 8-ounce glass of water. Sip it throughout the day to get the benefits of this detoxifying plant compound. Chlorophyllin, a stabilized form of chlorophyll, is another substance that will bind toxins in the body coming in from foods like grilled meats. My patients have even told me that taking chlorophyll improved their body odor after a while—perhaps because the chlorophyllin binds the toxins that can create an unpleasant smell.

Phytonutrients

Phytonutrients are biochemical compounds found in plants—literally, since the word *phyton* means "plant" in Greek. They support the plant's health in various ways, and they support our health too.

Compared to everything else we consume, phytonutrients are a mere drop in the nutritional bucket. On average, you probably eat about 200 daily grams of carbohydrates, about 100 daily grams of protein, and more than 50 daily grams of fat. Yet even if you've loaded up your plate with fruits and vegetables, your daily phytonutrient consumption probably totals less than 1.5 grams—less than 1 small teaspoon each day.

Welcome to the power of the tiny, because this small, seemingly inconsequential amount can bring about significant changes in your metabolism. Welcome, too, to the power of diversity: a 2006 research study shows that you get far better health results eating small amounts of several different phytonutrients than large amounts of just a few. Combining plant compounds seems to maximize their synergy, with each expanding the power of the others. I think this is a wonderful symbolic image of service: giving to others makes you stronger, but you also need others to give to you.

You've probably heard that our goal should be nine to thirteen servings of fruits and vegetables each day—and, preferably, these are widely varied servings, covering the full spectrum of colors and the broadest possible range of phytonutrients. Unfortunately, the average American barely makes it to 3.6. I have to believe that the "phytonutrient gap"—the deficiency in rainbow compounds—is at least partly responsible for the skyrocketing rate of heart disease in the United States, which has become the number one killer of people in industrialized countries, with Canada, Europe, and Australia also high on the list. When I think of Samuel and Luke, whose vegetable consumption made their heart problems disappear, I wish I could convince every person to reach for the vegetables.

I'm so happy I could at least help my father, who for years struggled with a heart condition and high blood pressure. He now proudly touts his green smoothie every day as his mainstay, and indeed, Whole Detox has improved his blood pressure considerably and even allowed him to reduce his medications. What a relief!

So reach for those greens and enjoy your morning smoothie. If my father can do it, I know you can too.

Phytodetoxification

This intriguing new term has just made its way into the scientific literature, although my nutritionist colleagues and I have been familiar with the concept for quite a while. It describes the ability of plants to detoxify organisms like human beings—to help bind industrial chemicals, heavy metals, and endocrine disrupters so they cannot damage our bodies. As you can see, we need plants desperately. We simply can't do without them if we expect to stay clean in a toxic world.

Plants don't simply rid your body of toxins, however. They also open your heart and your circulation with their chlorophyll and vitamin K. As if that weren't enough, plants help us better connect to nature. If you've ever grown your own herbs in your kitchen windowsill or maintained a garden of any kind, you have experienced the love that results as you shower your beloved plants with the care and nourishment they require to survive, thrive, and nourish you right back.

Although I've met many nutritionists who would fight over meat, dairy, and even fish, I've never met a health expert who says we should not eat plants. Plants just make people . . . happy!

So when it comes to taking care of yourself, focus on plants of all types. Grow some, eat lots, and let them teach you about giving yourself more love, in all its forms. After all, no matter what diet we follow—Paleo, vegan, or flexitarian—we are all eating plants. Truly, plants are the great unifier!

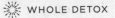

Phytoestrogens

As the name suggests, "phytoestrogens" are the plant form of estrogen, but they are from one hundred to one thousand times weaker than the estrogen in the body. Phytoestrogens can be healing for your heart by assisting with an open circulation, and they provide a way to smooth out hormonal fluxes, especially for women approaching perimenopause and menopause, when the body's own estrogens are in decline.

A common source of phytoestrogens is soy, which has the potential to be a healthy food when not genetically modified. You won't find any soy in your twenty-one-day program, because many people have an allergic response to it. However, if your health-care provider hasn't cautioned you against eating it based on your physiology, you can do your heart a favor by enjoying a moderate amount of fermented, organic, non-GMO soy products in the form of miso or nattō.

Another phytoestrogen that is even more potent than soy is flaxseed. Studies suggest that getting more flaxseed in your diet might improve your heart health by reducing cholesterol and other blood lipids, in addition to potentially being protective against some hormonal cancers.

GOOD SOURCES OF PHYTOESTROGENS

Food	Phytoestrogens (μg/100g)
Flaxseed	379,380.0
Soybeans	103,920.0
Tofu	27,150.1
Soy yogurt	10,275.0
Sesame seeds	8008.1
Flax bread	7540.0
Multigrain bread	4798.7
Soy milk	2957.2
Hummus	993.0
Garlic	603.6
Mung bean sprouts	495.1
Dried apricots	444.5
Alfalfa sprouts	441.4

Dried dates	329.5
Sunflower seeds	216.0
Chestnuts	210.2
Olive oil	180.7
Almonds	131.1
Green beans	105.8
Peanuts	34.5
Onions	32.0
Blueberries	17.5

Note: If you have a hormone-sensitive cancer or are taking drugs for hormonal issues, check with your health-care professional about your intake of high-phytoestrogenic foods.

Heart-Healthy Crucifers

The word "crucifer" means "cross," which refers to the cross pattern you can see in the arrangement of the four petals of these plants' flowers. Crucifers include broccoli, cauliflower, collard greens, mustard greens, cabbage, bok choy, arugula, and Brussels sprouts, all of which support your heart as well as offer your entire body antioxidant protection against toxins and inflammation. In a large study conducted with Chinese adults over more than ten years, scientists discovered that eating more vegetables—and especially more cruciferous vegetables—led to improved heart health and increased longevity. Crucifers might also have an anticlotting effect that can keep blood flowing smoothly and help to prevent stroke.

That stinky smell shared by crucifers means they contain sulfur, an essential compound for guarding the body against toxins. Sulfur-containing compounds, such as the sulforaphanes found in broccoli and cauliflower, help to detox the body, supporting the work of the intestines and liver in ridding the body of contaminants. If you want to get the maximum detox, antioxidant, and anti-cancer benefit from your crucifers, chop them up with some garlic and onion and then let the raw vegetables sit for about five minutes before cooking. This short period of time gives "plant actives"—the bioactive compounds that protect against illness—a chance to form.

Sprouts and Leafy Greens

The raw, living, active components of young sprouts (broccoli, alfalfa, or mung) and leafy greens (romaine, red leaf, butterhead, escarole, and arugula) provide us with the vital, healing nutrients that move us into expansion. These foods offer our body substances that assist with the circulation of blood throughout the vascular system as well as provide us with protective compounds, such as indoles and chlorophyll. If you are following a low-oxalate diet due to kidney or gallbladder issues, remember that several green leafy vegetables contain oxalates:

- Beet greens
- Beet root
- Collard greens
- Kale
- Okra
- Parsley
- Spinach
- Swiss chard

Heavy metal accumulation in the body, such as lead, cadmium, and mercury, has been connected to high blood pressure and cardiovascular disease. Chlorella and, to a lesser extent, cilantro may be helpful in binding heavy metals, as has been shown in animal studies.

MAKE YOUR OWN SPROUTS—IT'S EASY!

You can make your own sprouts using a widemouthed glass jar and screened lid. Most health food stores will sell you seeds: alfalfa, broccoli, garbanzo bean, lentil, mung bean, mustard, radish, red clover, and sunflower. Make sure you wash your sprouts extraordinarily well, because dirty sprouts have been implicated in foodborne illness outbreaks. Also, if you have an autoimmune condition, avoid alfalfa sprouts, which contain a compound called canavanine that might cause inflammatory flare-ups in sensitive individuals.

Microgreens

Microgreens—the edible seedlings of vegetables and herbs—are some of the most nutrient-dense foods I know. Sprouts and microgreens are different: sprouts germinate in water, usually within forty-eight hours, and form roots, stems, and undeveloped leaves, whereas microgreens need soil and sunlight, and take about seven days to grow before they are ready to eat.

The tiny leaves of microgreens are usually very pungent in taste and have vibrant hues. They can be served as a main salad or as a garnish on a salad or sandwich. In an analysis of twenty-five microgreens, those that scored highest in vitamins and phytonutrients (vitamin C, tocopherols, carotenoids, phylloquinone) were red cabbage, cilantro, garnet amaranth, and green daikon radish.

GETTING THE MOST FROM YOUR GREEN TEA

Green tea is another heart-healthy food rich in antioxidants. What I recommend during the Whole Detox program is decaffeinated green tea. Steep green tea for eight to ten minutes to maximize the release of the anti-cancer compound epigallocatechin gallate (EGCG). Black pepper helps EGCG linger in your body, so try pairing some green tea with a dish that contains freshly ground pepper, like soup or a salad. One of my nutritionist friends doesn't like the taste of green tea, but she knows how good it is for her, so she uses it as the base for her morning smoothie—a great way to hide the tea but get the benefit!

Whenever you can, choose water with minerals for your tea, rather than distilled water. The minerals in water bring out the tea's flavor a bit more, and it's actually healthier.

SUPPORT YOUR LOVE WHILE YOU EAT

As we have seen, there are so many ways in which plant foods add to the quality of your health. In days ten through twelve of your twenty-one-day program, you'll learn what you need to do to support your LOVE. Meanwhile, here are some quick tips on how to expand your LOVE into your everyday meals:

- Before starting to eat, take a couple of seconds to move from your busy head into your beautiful heart. You can easily do this by thinking of a time when you felt loved. Let your heart go to that feeling of being filled with love. Imagine that this feeling infuses your food. Sit in that loving space for twenty to thirty seconds.

- Have a heart image visible in your space. Eat from heart-shaped bowls, and put heart stickers on your refrigerator, blender, kitchen cabinets, and drinking containers, to keep the spirit of love alive in the places where you cook and eat.
- Give thanks for your meals: to the person who prepared it (even if it's yourself, which is one step closer to self-love!) and to the animals and plants that gave their lives so you would be nourished. Research suggests that gratitude has lasting health effects. Think of how it might help you to appreciate the meal and even digest it better.
- Share meals with others whom you love. Eating is the ultimate unifying experience—we all need to eat as human beings, so what better way to "feel the love" than to eat together.
- Sing while preparing food; invite the element of air to honor your lungs, which work so closely with your heart to oxygenate the blood.

DETOXING YOUR LOVE: WHAT TO CHOOSE
- Cool, leafy, raw greens that can soothe and open the heart with vasodilators, agents that promote the expansion of blood vessels
- Taking good care of yourself
- Giving yourself time to love yourself, through "me time" or other healing practices
- Breathing deeply
- Being in nature, especially the forest ("forest bathing")

DETOXING YOUR LOVE: WHAT TO AVOID
- Foods that clog the arteries: meat and poultry, which contain too much toxic animal fat
- Foods that cause vasoconstriction or high blood pressure: excessively salty foods
- Foods that cause breathing difficulties due to an allergic reaction
- Life events or situations that cause high blood pressure
- People-pleasing behavior
- Being the martyr or feeling that you have to rescue people

EXPAND INTO YOUR LOVE

As you look over the lists portraying a healthy LOVE, an overactive LOVE, and an underactive LOVE (see pages 137–140), you can see how complex the relationship is between love and grief, and how challenging it can be to keep your heart open, but not too open. The LOVE opens us to connection and intimacy, but it can also make us more vulnerable to abuse and neglect. Compassion and service to others can enrich and deepen our lives, but they can also lead us to neglect the crucial work of self-compassion and care for ourselves. Grief and loss can cause us to harden our hearts, but they can also be the inspiration that softens our hearts and makes us appreciate the loved ones who remain.

This is why I see Whole Detox as such a personal journey, and as a never-ending one. Your vision of a balanced LOVE is likely to evolve over time, appearing very different to you with every passing decade. The first step on this journey is awareness, so you can identify and overcome every barrier that keeps your LOVE from flourishing as you deserve.

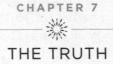

CHAPTER 7

THE TRUTH

That inner voice has both gentleness and clarity. So to get to authenticity, you really keep going down to the bone, to the honesty, and the inevitability of something.

—MEREDITH MONK

UNDERSTANDING THE TRUTH	
Anatomy	Thyroid gland, ears, nose, mouth, throat
Functions	Speaking, chewing, hearing, smelling
Living	Speaking one's truth, choice, decisions
Eating	Mindful eating, varied flavors, moist and liquid foods, sea plants

THE SCIENCE OF THE TRUTH

If you move up from the heart and the fourth system of health, you reach the base of the throat: home of the voice box, the thyroid gland, and the fifth system of health, the TRUTH. This system also encompasses the ears, nose, and mouth, so it oversees hearing, smelling, and your sense of taste.

The thyroid is an incredibly important gland whose impact is often underestimated in conventional medicine. Through its effects on your metabolism, your thyroid gland helps to regulate your weight as well as regulating your mood, mental sharpness, and overall well-being. Even a slightly underperforming thyroid can produce significant symptoms, including

depression, fatigue, listlessness, brain fog, and weight that seems impossible
to lose, while an overactive thyroid can cause rapid and erratic weight loss
as well as anxiety, sleeplessness, and a racing heart.

Underactive thyroid is a widespread problem in the United States, especially for women over forty. However, conventional tests for thyroid tend to
target only the most serious problems and miss many of the smaller ones.
That's why giving your thyroid the comprehensive support it needs is so crucial for Whole Detox. Many of my patients are amazed at how much clearer,
sharper, calmer, and happier they feel once they start detoxing the fifth system,
and many also find that it suddenly becomes surprisingly easy to lose weight.

Taste, Variety, and Your Health

Weight loss may be helped by a healthier thyroid, and it may also be related
to an enhanced sensory experience of food. Yes, you heard that right: smell,
taste, and texture can make a huge difference in how your body responds. If
you eat monotonously, your body will crave variety, leading you to overeat,
in search of the food or taste you didn't get. I've also seen patients who
avoid sugar suddenly become obsessed with sweetness, finding it nearly
impossible to resist their sugar cravings.

Conventional medicine tends to ignore taste, but cutting-edge research
has discovered what I and my colleagues always knew: taste is pivotal to
food, weight, metabolism, and appetite, and we neglect it at our peril. In
fact, research suggests that our taste is impacted by our emotional state.
Researchers at Cornell University assessed taste and emotions of 550 people
who attended hockey games. There were a total of eight games, four wins,
three losses, and one tie. Findings revealed that positive emotions during the
winning games correlated with enhanced sweet and diminished sour inten-
sities while negative emotions lead to heightened sour and decreased sweet
tastes. In other words, when life is "sweet," you taste things sweeter, and,
when life is "sour," you taste them that way, too. It's a novel concept in nutrition to say that how we taste says something about our lives! Recent studies
have identified taste receptors in our intestines, airways, brain, and even in
the testes and sperm. Bitter taste receptors seem to play a unique role in our
gut function, metabolism, thyroid function, and body weight—so begin to
fight weight gain and indigestion by steaming up some bitter leafy greens!

You'll also want to examine food type, and here, too, your body seeks balance. For example, if you consume a high-protein breakfast, you're likely to find yourself craving carbohydrates for lunch. And if you tell yourself, "I'm never eating carbs again," the cravings might become overwhelming. This wish for balance isn't caused by a sweet tooth or lack of willpower; it's fundamental to human biology, confirmed by research showing that sweetness is an inherent taste that attracts us from birth.

The solution? Make sure that you sample the whole spectrum of tastes every day and, ideally, at every meal. Get some sweetness from carrots, sweet potatoes, pears, and berries. Savor the sourness of citrus fruits and tart green apple. Enjoy the bitterness of greens and eggplant. Take in the wonderful taste of sea salt or pink Himalayan salt sprinkled on your stir-fry. Pique your taste buds with savory (umami) seaweed, tamari, and miso (organic only, please!). This variety of tastes will awaken your mouth, nose, and throat to the stimulating scents and flavors, spurring your thyroid to optimal function and revving up your metabolism. Just by stimulating your olfactory sense through the smells of food, you begin the digestive process.

I also urge my patients to add modest amounts of natural sweetness into their diets with sweet fruits (dates, figs, raisins, prunes) and natural sweeteners (raw honey, molasses, maple syrup). When I traveled to other countries, like Taiwan and Nepal, I noticed that small amounts of savory and sweet sauces, pickled foods, and other delicacies are part of almost every meal, which reflects the principles of traditional medicine.

A Full Voice for a Whole Self

We use our mouths to consume food, but we also use them to speak. Accordingly, life issues for the fifth system include authenticity, choice, and finding your voice. If you can tell the world your truest thoughts—if you can share your most genuine and authentic self—you have taken a huge step to support your TRUTH.

Some fascinating research suggests that we ignore our personal truth at our peril. In 2014, a group of German scientists published a study with the intriguing title "Lying and the Subsequent Desire for Toothpaste." They were curious about the relationship between a person's sense of doing something wrong and his or her wish to be cleansed, which they called the Macbeth effect, after the famous scene in Shakespeare's *Macbeth* in which a murderous queen dreams over and over that she cannot wash the blood from her hands. The scientists asked a group of subjects to commit either a moral or an immoral act—that is, either to tell the truth or to lie. Then the subjects had to rate the desirability of various products. Lo and behold, the people who lied gave higher ratings to cleaning products while a functional MRI revealed increased activity in the sensorimotor areas of the brain—the parts of the brain that experience taste and smell. "The results demonstrate neurobiological evidence for an embodiment of the moral-purity meta-phor," the scientists wrote. "Thus, abstract thoughts about morality can be grounded in sensory experiences." Or, put another way, the fifth system of health brings together our sensory experience of smell and taste with our inner sense of truth and authenticity.

We also use our mouths for singing, and a growing body of evidence suggests that singing benefits our immune system by lowering stress and reducing inflammation. A 2004 study in the *Journal of Behavioral Medicine* found that people who listened to choral music responded with a drop in secre-tory immunoglobulin, a common marker of inflammation, as well as in the stress hormone, cortisol. However, *singing* choral music had even more beneficial effects. Finding our voice, it seems, is good for our health as well as our happiness, since subjects reported increased well-being after just one sixty-minute rehearsal. "These results suggest that choir singing positively influences both emotional affect and immune competence," the German researchers concluded.

A Swedish team came up with similar findings in a 2003 study entitled "Does Singing Promote Well-Being?" In this experiment, amateur and pro-fessional singers were given a singing lesson while scientists used an elec-trocardiogram (ECG) to record their cardiovascular activity. The researchers also analyzed subjects' blood, looking for biochemicals that indicate stress (primarily cortisol) and inflammation as well as measuring HRV.

As might be expected, the professionals revealed increased "arousal" during the lesson; that is, they were more worked up, anxious, and excited. To them, singing was serious business, and their test results reflected that tone. However, the amateurs found the lessons an occasion for "increasing joy and elatedness." Unlike the professionals, they weren't worried about their results, so they simply relaxed and enjoyed the experience of using their voices. As the researchers put it, "The amateurs used the singing lessons as a means of self-actualization and self-expression as a way to release emotional tensions." Both amateurs and professionals felt more "energetic and relaxed" after the lesson, however, suggesting that tapping into the power of the fifth system of health is good for immune function and stress.

Finally, a 2010 Hong Kong study divided people aged sixty-five through ninety into two groups. One group was given thirty minutes a week to rest; the other spent the same amount of time listening to music. Researchers found that quality of life improved significantly among the music listeners compared to the control group.

The Hong Kong study tested only listening—and indeed, the ears are part of the fifth system—but I have to wonder what might have happened if, like the German subjects, the Chinese participants had also been given the chance to sing. A 2015 study of 258 older English adults answered this question. They found that community group singing favorably affected quality of life in these seniors: they had less anxiety and depression. My takeaway from the research is that it is healthy to be listening and vocalizing.

I have wondered whether these messages shut down not only one's unique voice but perhaps thyroid activity too. I have seen associations between women with hypothyroidism (low thyroid activity) and an inability to speak freely. Maybe this is just coincidence, but I find it fascinating to watch patterns of how what we say (or, in this case, don't say) translates into bodily symptoms and complaints.

THE POWER OF AQUAMARINE

Aquamarine is the color of the TRUTH, and we nourish our mouth, throat, and thyroid with sea vegetables that come out of shining blue-green oceans— foods that connect us to the ocean just as root vegetables connect us to the earth. The iodine on which our thyroid depends comes from such sea plants as nori, dulse, arame, and kelp. These foods are also rich in selenium and zinc, deficiencies of which are a common cause of thyroid problems.

To tap into the power of aquamarine, turn your head and look up at the sky or out at the expanse of the ocean, allowing that vast blue perspective to help you gain *your* perspective. If you don't have access to a broad vista, keep a blue stone—turquoise or lapis lazuli—on your desk or bedside table. Quiet your mind, gaze at the blue, and allow the right decision to emerge.

You can also lubricate your throat with warm, soothing tea or soup sipped from an aquamarine mug. Drink in the color along with the heat and the nourishment.

Finally, when you want to focus on the power of your voice, slip on an aquamarine scarf, tie, or necklace. Bring that color to your TRUTH center and amplify the force of your personal truth.

GET TO KNOW YOUR TRUTH

One of our gifts as humans is to express our personal truths through words. Our throat is a meeting place for the passions of our heart as well as for the thoughts and insights of our mind.

Julian is an accomplished musician, a classical flautist who also teaches a select number of students. He sent me the following e-mail after doing some work on his TRUTH:

> I'd like to share an increase in my awareness while playing my flute yesterday. I have a few students, and during lessons yesterday I felt there was an unusual ease of playing. My throat was relaxed, I was able to play technical passages easily. I think your approach has freed my creativity in that I was very excited how quickly and clearly I could play and how resonant my sound was. It was so refreshing that I practiced an hour after I finished teaching. It was rejuvenating and I felt free.

Julian's message speaks to the close connection between our bodies and the whole of our lives. Set free to express his own particular artistic truth, Julian was able to reach a new level of physical performance. Just as Padma's thyroid issues and her ability to speak her truth were interrelated, so was Julian's creativity profoundly affected by his physical self—and vice versa.

BALANCE YOUR TRUTH

Balancing your TRUTH means finding a healthy relationship between speaking and listening; accepting your uniqueness and becoming obsessed with it; and holding fast to your inner truth and remaining open to the truths of others. Here are some factors to keep in mind as you think about balancing your TRUTH:

A person with a healthy TRUTH
- is true to themselves;
- accepts their uniqueness;
- feels free;
- lives a life that seems to fit who they are;
- feels comfortable speaking what is on their mind in whatever way is most effective for the situation;
- speaks and listens to others in equal measure;
- has a strong voice and sense of presence when speaking their truth;
- expresses themselves well in many ways, not just verbally;
- makes prompt decisions, but not hasty ones;
- doesn't violate the freedom of others;
- is comfortable speaking, even publicly, but doesn't necessarily seek out attention by speaking loudly or shying away;
- has healthy mouth, gums, teeth, neck, and nasal passages and normal throat moisture and mucous;
- eats the amount of food their body requires with an average appetite;
- is generally able to make time for regular meals away from other activities and focuses on enjoying the scents, tastes, and textures of each meal;
- makes time to eat with awareness, without engaging in other activities or becoming distracted by visual cues or noises; and
- eats moist fruits and drinks soups, sauces, and juices on a regular basis.

A person with an underactive TRUTH
- is often soft-spoken and feels uncomfortable exposing who they are, a shy person who doesn't like to speak up;

- is often embarrassed about speaking their views and might even cover up their true opinions;
- might gossip, start rumors, blackmail, or lie;
- speaks slowly, perhaps with a stutter or pausing to search for words;
- makes decisions slowly and might even be paralyzed by making decisions;
- often lets others make decisions for them;
- after a decision is made, often feels they have made the wrong choice;
- likes to fit in with everyone else;
- might project a sense of inferiority or exaggerated humility;
- embraces a "victim" mentality, feeling shackled and imprisoned by what they are told to be because it doesn't fit who they are, yet they are reluctant to speak up;
- prefers to process their thoughts and emotions through writing rather than speaking;
- has a phobia about public speaking;
- might have dry lips, mouth, throat, or nose;
- might be subject to bouts of laryngitis;
- might have a neck sore to the touch;
- might have lost teeth;
- might have jaw soreness or TMJ (temporomandibular joint);
- has a slow metabolism, low thyroid activity, and perhaps even hypothyroidism;
- might have a small mouth proportionate to their face and brittle, small teeth that tend to break easily, with lots of spacing in between;
- might have hearing loss;
- might feel they are vulnerable and likes to wear turtlenecks and scarves to protect their neck;
- might have a soft voice;
- might feel like they have a lump in their throat ("plum pit" in TCM);
- sometimes has an issue with swallowing or tasting;
- has a weak appetite and might not eat enough food;
- eats slowly in long, drawn-out meals;
- might experience challenges in their ability to communicate

with others in an authentic way, often with respect to their food choices and/or how they eat;

- might keep secrets when it comes to health and eating, such as eating snack foods in private;
- might not get enough liquids or "water foods," whether fruits, soups, sauces, or juices; or
- might have lost their sense of taste or have impaired taste.

A person with an overactive TRUTH

- is vocal and outspoken;
- might use foul language consistently;
- would rather talk than listen, and would rather be the object of attention;
- doesn't necessarily know what is true for them, and may be using excessive chatter as distraction from what is true;
- makes decisions quickly;
- sees themselves as special and different from everyone else;
- might project a sense of grandiosity or superiority;
- values their freedom and may have strong resistance to authority;
- might be so concerned with their own point of view that they violate others' sense of freedom or overstep their bounds;
- processes thoughts and emotions verbally;
- tends to overload the senses by doing too many things at once, such as always playing music in the background or talking on the phone while watching TV;
- might speak too fast;
- might have inflammation surrounding the mouth, gums, teeth, jaw, neck, or nasal passages;
- is prone to sore throats;
- might have shooting neck pain;
- has a fast metabolism and perhaps excess thyroid activity or hyperthyroidism;
- might have acute hearing or even ringing in the ears (tinnitus);
- is prone to vertigo;
- might have a high-pitched voice;

- has a strong appetite and might eat excessively without gaining weight;
- eats in a hurry and frequently on the run and/or while doing other things, such as listening to the radio, talking with others, watching television, driving, or working;
- might be eating constantly;
- might get hiccups after eating;
- might be overly drawn to fruits, soups, sauces, juices, and might even prefer to drink their meals rather than chew them because it's faster and more efficient; or
- always has something in their mouth, such as food, a pen, gum, mints, or candy.

LEARN TO SPEAK YOUR TRUTH:
HOW THE TRUTH DETOX WORKED FOR IRIS

Over the years of dealing with my own health and that of others, I have seen again and again how important it is to be true to ourselves in all arenas of our lives, including foods, eating, and our health. If we can't say no to the demands of others, we might also find it hard to say no to the foods that don't really serve us. The throat is a place of self-expression, but it's also the gateway for food to enter our body. When we come from a place of healthy expression, speaking clearly and truthfully, and eating mindfully, we can more easily choose the foods that our body truly wants and needs.

This was a challenge for my patient Iris, a faithful churchgoer who struggled every Sunday with the donuts, pastries, and brownies served as part of the after-service coffee hour. If one of Iris's friends offered a home-made cookie or "just a taste of my favorite cake," Iris felt unable to say no, even though she knew that sugary foods gave her migraines. Somehow, she just couldn't speak up for herself, preferring the agony of a day-long head-ache to the prospect of speaking the truth.

When she came to me for help, we quickly identified sugar as one of her food triggers, but then I realized she already knew that. Unlike some of my patients, she had long ago figured out which foods were good for her and which were not. The problem wasn't *knowing* her truth but *speaking* it.

Iris had other symptoms that led me to think her fifth system needed some support. She suffered from a dry throat, especially in the evenings. She had subclinical hypothyroidism—an underperformance of her thyroid gland—which didn't show up on conventional medical tests but revealed itself in a multitude of symptoms: fatigue, brittle nails, constipation, always feeling cold, brain fog, and an extra fifteen pounds that just wouldn't go away. She also suffered from TMJ, a pain in the jaw that comes from clenching the mouth shut and grinding the teeth. She told me that for years she had worn a mouth guard while she slept, but the soreness had persisted.

I was struck by the image of a clenched jaw, as though Iris was biting down on her words and refusing to release them. Indeed, as we talked, I noticed how reluctant she was to use her voice. She spoke so softly that I could barely hear her, and she frequently apologized, corrected herself ("Maybe that isn't true . . ."), and offered to defer to me ("I mean, I don't know. What do you think?").

She clearly needed support for all of her fifth system. For her chronically dry throat, I suggested a soothing cup of licorice tea after dinner. To address the hypothyroidism, I recommended she cut out gluten, a protein found in many grains, including wheat, rye, and barley. Gluten is often responsible for "molecular mimicry," a process whereby the immune system confuses gluten molecules with the molecules of your thyroid gland. A sensitive immune system releases "killer chemicals" to zap the gluten molecules, but the mimicry causes them to attack thyroid tissue as well. Cutting out the gluten resolves this process and allows the thyroid gland to operate more effectively.

For further thyroid support, I suggested she get more iodine and potassium into her diet by eating the sea vegetables that are part of the fifth system: dulse, hijiki, and nori. I urged her to choose warm, soothing foods that would feel comforting and nourishing in her mouth and throat.

I also gently asked her about her soft voice and her fear of public speaking. She told me that as a child, whenever she expressed an opinion, someone in her loud, raucous family would tease her, often to the point of ridicule. If she objected, she would invariably be told, "Stop being so sensitive" or "You don't know what you're talking about!" Iris had learned that it was easier to suppress her truth—her opinions and her feelings. She had carried this suppression into her adult life.

As she recounted these experiences, her voice got a bit stronger and I heard the beginnings of anger. "How did you feel about all that teasing?" I asked her.

"I hated it!" she burst out—and then looked surprised. I wondered if this bottled-up anger was behind her painfully clenched jaw.

Over the weeks I worked with Iris, her throat discomfort vanished, her jaw pain subsided, and her excess weight began to come off. A combination of emotional support for speaking her truth and nutritional support for her throat and thyroid had helped her detox her fifth system of health.

INTEGRATE THE TRUTH

I like to refer to the fifth system as the seat of integration, where we unite many diverse elements to create something new.

For example, we combine thoughts from our mind and passions from our heart to create expression through our throat. Or when we cook, we bring together fire, metal, and air (on our stovetop) with earth (food) and water (broth) to make a miraculous new entity called a soup. And, once again, you combine these elements in your throat: breathing in the fragrant scents that trigger your taste buds and bringing the vegetables and liquid into your body's cells. The fuel that warmed your soup also becomes part of your body, as does the warm air that radiates from every bite.

MOIST FOODS FOR YOUR TRUTH

Foods for the fifth system support your throat and thyroid. They are often warm, moist, and soothing as well as rich in the minerals and nutrients your thyroid needs. Here are some of the main types of TRUTH-full foods:

Sea Plants

Sea vegetables embody the symbiotic relationship between the elements of water and earth. Many of my patients haven't ever tried sea vegetables when they come to me, and perhaps this is your experience as well. I urge you to go on an "ocean journey," exploring all the different ways you can incorporate sea plants into your diet. Here are a few suggestions to get you started:

- Sprinkle dry dulse flakes on top of a salad.
- Add any sea plant variety to soups, stews, or broths. Nibble on dry dulse as a snack.
- Use a sheet of nori to make yourself a wrap.
- Instead of a salt shaker, keep a seaweed (kelp) shaker on your dinner table.

MEET SOME SEA PLANTS

- *Arame:* This species of kelp is frequently used in Japanese dishes. Its dark-brown strands have a firm texture and a mild, almost sweet flavor. You can add it to a wide variety of dishes, include pilafs, soups, casseroles, and even some baked goods, such as muffins. Arame is rich in a wide variety of minerals, including calcium, iodine, iron, magnesium, and vitamin A.
- *Dulse:* A red algae that grows on the northern coasts of the Atlantic and Pacific, dulse is dried into a texture something like jerky or a fruit roll-up to make a super snack food. When ground into flakes or a powder, it becomes a useful flavor enhancer for meat dishes, chili, soups, chowders, sandwiches, salads, pizza dough, and bread dough. You can also pan-fry dulse into chips, bake it in the oven covered with cheese or salsa, or microwave it briefly and then eat it with butter, as they do in Iceland. Dulse is a great source of iodine.
- *Kombu:* This type of kelp is used to flavor broths, stews, and rice dishes. It's also eaten as a vegetable and a snack, while transparent sheets are used to wrap rice and other foods. You can use kombu to soften beans during cooking and to chemically alter the beans to reduce flatulence. Like most sea vegetables, kombu is a good source of iodine.
- *Nori:* You might know nori as the seaweed used to wrap sushi. You can throw some into your soup and noodle dishes or eat it in the form of a soy-flavored paste. Nori is rich in B12, making it an excellent food for all of us but particularly for vegans, who frequently need to supplement with this vitamin.

I'm always excited to recommend sea plants to my patients, because these tasty vegetables benefit multiple body systems with an abundance of nutrients, including minerals, alkaloid antioxidants, and sulfated polysaccharides. Alkaloids and antioxidants are types of plant compounds that have a wide variety of protective effects. Sulfated polysaccharides are likewise protective against inflammations, bacteria, viruses, microbes, and tumors while supporting immune function and the digestive system. One such compound, fucoidan, appears to have anti-cancer, anti-inflammatory, cholesterol-lowering, and even anti-obesity effects.

Sea plants are especially good for the thyroid gland, supplying such crucial minerals as iodine, selenium, and zinc. While all sea plants are bathed in iodine, the brown sea plants seem to have the highest amounts, especially arame, kelp, kombu, and wakame. However, the mineral content—and particularly the iodine levels—can vary greatly depending on where and when a plant was harvested.

When we look at getting iodine from sea plants, we don't just measure the plant's levels of that mineral; we also look at how bioavailable the iodine might be. This factor varies greatly depending both on the type of seaweed and on your body's iodine level.

Iodine is a crucial mineral. If you have a thyroid condition, especially an overactive thyroid, check with your health-care practitioner before introducing large amounts of sea plants into your diet, because these can be contraindicated for hyperthyroidism.

Another cautionary note: sea plants' proficiency at absorbing minerals means they also tend to absorb heavy metals. This can vary depending on the type of plant and where it was grown—that is, how contaminated the water was. Check the label or ask your supplier whether they have tested their batches for heavy metals. Hijiki has been known to contain higher amounts of arsenic than other types. Choose certified organic options when available.

Finally, some species of sea plants may modify hormone metabolism. In a small case study series, three premenopausal women were given the edible brown kelp *Fucus vesiculosus* (bladderwrack). In response, their menstrual cycles were lengthened by five to fourteen days. One woman saw a drop in estrogen while her progesterone levels increased, often a beneficial effect. The researchers suggested that this may be why estrogen-sensitive cancers are lower in populations like Japan's, in which sea vegetables are part of the everyday diet.

Moist Fruits

Fruits tend to be high in water content, so they are a perfect food to lubricate your throat. Some of my favorites are cantaloupe, watermelon, oranges, kiwi, nectarines, peaches, honeydew melon, and grapes. You can just imagine their moist, soft texture as I name them and feel how soothing they will be when you actually eat them. When your throat is moist and open, you'll find speaking more comfortable, and perhaps you'll be more likely to use your voice.

Make sure to choose fresh whole fruits rather than those that are in toxic cans or have added sugars. Your best bet is to consume whole fruit, including its fiber, rather than fruit juices, which can be very high in sugar. If you would like to choose a fruit juice, select those with no added sweeteners. Change up your fruit and fruit juice choices regularly—make sure you're getting a wide nutritional variety.

WATER + FRUIT = SUPER-HYDRATION

Hydration is crucial to the second system of health, while keeping your throat moist and relaxed is important to the fifth system. Both systems of health are concerned with expression: creativity for the second and verbal expression for the fifth. When we feel in the flow of being creative, our channel of TRUTH can open wide to let it out!

You can use a combination of water and food to enhance hydration. Add sliced cucumber, strawberry, melon, lemon, or orange to give your water a tangy twist. You'll drink more, and the time you spend savoring the subtle flavors will make your taste buds happy.

Soups, Stews, Sauces, and Smoothies . . . Oh My!

Liquid foods keep your throat moist and lubricated, quench your thirst, and load up your body with detoxifying nutrients. I especially like to recommend soups and stews during Whole Detox because true nutritional synergy occurs when you put diverse ingredients together with a little heat: sometimes you get improved bioavailability of nutrients, and often the ingredients just taste better and more interesting in combination, especially on the second day! Preparing soups and stews can also lead to olfactory stimulation, creating pleasant aromas that can affect your appetite. One study conducted in the Netherlands showed that healthy women exposed to a concentrated tomato soup aroma ate 9 percent less of a bland soup base than when they hadn't had such concentrated exposure.

Of course, I would much prefer that you toss ingredients into a large saucepan with water or broth to make that soup rather than get it from a can. A study at Harvard University showed that "consumption of 1 serving of canned soup daily over 5 days was associated with a more than 1000% increase in urinary BPA [bisphenol A]." Get the soup, but lose the bisphenol A coating in the can!

Soups can warm and open up the throat area and create more ease in eating. Spooning in warm soup takes longer than gobbling up your food, which might help you to slow down and savor each moment of your eating experience. Research also suggests that soup is good for weight loss: consuming any type of low-calorie soup before a meal can reduce the amount of food intake by as much as 20 percent.

Sauce can enhance a meal by making a vegetable tastier or pulling a dish together. Sauce can also cue us to release saliva and other digestive fluids and enzymes, promoting smoother digestion. Another benefit is the healthy fat in an oil-based savory sauce enables us to absorb carotenoids and fat-soluble vitamins; you miss a lot of nutritional benefits from vegetables and salads when they are fat-free! A vinaigrette or mustard dressing is always a delicious choice, but my favorite is sesame tahini made with sesame oil, so you'll have the chance to taste quite a bit of this super-creamy sauce in the Whole Detox recipes.

Smoothies and juices made of fresh fruits and vegetables can be another efficient way to consume the nutrients we need. Even my father, who is not the healthiest eater, can get his green smoothie down for breakfast every day. It's a great way to get in a load of nutrients first thing in the morning, which is why the Whole Detox meal plans consist of a smoothie a day.

I suggest you use a fruit and vegetable pulverizer, such as the Nutri-Bullet, Vitamix, or Ninja (my personal favorite) to get the whole food rather than just the juice. Oh, and one more thing: chew your smoothie. That's right! Keep that smoothie in your mouth rather than chugging it down, so the microbes and enzymes in your mouth can begin the process of digesting and utilizing nutrients. Green plants like arugula and spinach contain dietary nitrates that convert into nitric oxide, which allows your blood vessels to open wide. Your saliva helps in the process. So slow down when drinking smoothies!

Herbal Teas

I recently co-authored a scientific review paper on foods that influence detox pathways. You might be surprised to find out that one of most influential detoxers is tea, including black, green, honeybush, chamomile, dandelion, peppermint, and rooibos.

While herbal teas can be medicinal, with potent effects on your body, they can also contain heavy metals. Many people ask me about radiation in some of the green teas coming from Japan. The best rule of thumb, as with everything, is to choose from a varied selection, rotating your teas every three to four days. Choose organic tea leaves, and ask the manufacturer of the tea if they are checking for heavy metals and other contaminants in the finished product.

One of my favorite things to do is add a little bit of raw honey (the best is manuka honey or get a source of local honey) to herbal tea to coat my throat and boost my immune function. I remember when I had a bout of laryngitis some years ago. The tea and manuka honey seemed to make all the difference in getting my voice back, or at least soothing my throat until I could recover!

Foods with a Cultural Flair

With five tastes and five senses to honor as part of the fifth system, it's important to open up our exposure to a variety of foods. I like to have people expand their culinary horizons by engaging in various cultural foods, traditions, and practices around eating. Choosing to eat just one way all the time does not expose you to the full truth of the eating experience—a landscape that can be exploratory and healing. You will see that I have brought along some ethnic recipes within the Whole Detox, sometimes via such spices as tandoori and curry.

Food can often be the gateway to cultural insights. Why is the Mediterranean diet so popular and so healthful? Perhaps it's the food, but it could also be the Mediterranean way of eating: relaxed meals that take place over hours, usually in the company of family and friends.

So find out how people in Thailand eat coconut curry. Discover how Costa Ricans feel about their staple dish of rice and beans. Let your curiosity usher you into a mealtime adventure! It might be as medicinal as the food itself.

SUPPORT YOUR TRUTH WHILE YOU EAT

- Go slow, with slow-food restaurants, slow eating, and especially slow chewing. Eating too quickly can pack on the pounds. Research with children has associated fast eating (more bites per minute) with greater body weight.

- Put your awareness into eating so you get the most from the experience and don't feel like overeating. Studies show that cultivating a daily practice of mindfulness can help to reduce stress, binge eating, and emotional eating.

- Choose truthfully. Check out every choice about food that you are presented with and make sure it resonates with your inner truth.

- Become aware of the truth of your portion sizes. Do you remember that phrase "The eyes are bigger than the stomach"? Cup your hands together so you can get a sense of how big your stomach is, then use your innate awareness to stop eating when you've genuinely had enough. And watch out for those large portions, which cause us to eat 16 to 26 percent more than we would have normally.

- Expand your range of choices: look wider and broader, explore and discover, be adventurous. Shake up your food routine and try some foods you might not normally eat: perhaps Indian, Middle Eastern, European, or Ethiopian.

- Keep a food log to identify food ruts—habits that restrict your self-expression through food.

- Allow yourself to be free of dieting. Research shows that the more we feel restrained in our eating, the more likely we are to feel anxious, depressed, or unsettled.

DETOXING YOUR TRUTH: WHAT TO CHOOSE

- Iodine-rich sea vegetables to support your thyroid and supply you with needed minerals
- Soups, sauces, and juices that will lubricate your throat, as well as fruits that contain a lot of water: melons, grapes, tropical fruits, peaches, and plums
- A wide variety of tastes, which will make your tongue and taste buds sing!
- Humming, singing, or chanting to discover the true contours of your authentic voice
- Greater awareness of your daily habits, including your food choices, schedule, and tasks, in order to make the choices that truly serve your body, your spirit, and your purpose

DETOXING YOUR TRUTH: WHAT TO AVOID

- Environmental and food-based toxins that impair thyroid function, such as those that have chlorine, bromine, and fluorine (chemicals frequently used as pesticides, preservatives, and flame retardants)
- Gulping foods down, making them difficult to swallow and, ultimately, to digest
- Silencing your truth by not speaking up when you feel the need to
- Speaking in a truthful but cruel, insensitive, or uncompassionate way
- Gossiping, lying, swearing, threatening, exaggerating, or becoming cold and unresponsive

SPEAK YOUR TRUTH

Learning how to manifest your inner truth—how to express yourself authentically and make choices that align with who you are—is a lifelong process. There is no one right way to speak your truth, and there is certainly no easy way. Venting your thoughts without a filter is not necessarily the best way to speak your truth, but nor is clenching your jaw and biting down on every word that might possibly displease someone. Remaining in a relationship, a job, or a personal situation that violates your sense of inner truth is not good for your fifth system, but nor is breaking a commitment at a moment's notice or flitting from one "shiny object" to another. Knowing and speaking your truth can be a challenging process, but such an incredibly worthwhile one!

I myself struggled for years with questions about how to manifest my inner truth. As a scientist working in laboratories and academic settings, I wasn't always sure how to bring in the part of me that loved yoga, meditation, and alternative approaches to healing. I certainly never told my scientific colleagues about my abstract, vividly colored paintings! My career continued to progress, but I paid a heavy price. Because I wasn't speaking out of my deepest sense of inner truth, I'd return from a day's work or a scientific conference completely drained of energy, feeling dried up and shriveled, as though I might completely disappear. Perhaps I had more room to be "different" than I thought. Yet my childhood experience of a "health-conscious" mother, who also held strong religious beliefs, made me very anxious about not fitting in.

Then one day I noticed something curious. I nearly always wore either a scarf or a turtleneck, something to cover my neck and throat. I remember once before a TV appearance, I was determined to wear a high-necked sweater. My agent tried to talk me into another outfit, and I just froze with fear.

"Deanna, why can't you wear something that reads better on camera and is more flattering?" she asked me.

"I feel exposed," I told her. And then I started to wonder: What was I hiding?

Now I'm fortunate to have a career in which I can manifest all my inner truth: not just the scientist but also the yogi, the artist, the person who believes that psychology and spirituality are just as central to our health as nutrition and biology. It took me a long time to arrive at this place of truth, but it was so, so worth it. And the turtlenecks are gone, although I still like to wear scarves every once in a while!

How will you manifest your inner truth? What silence might you break? What knowledge will you bring to light? How will you make your voice heard?

Your answers may be slow in coming—or they might be right at the tip of your tongue. Either way, I invite you on your journey to detox your own TRUTH.

CHAPTER 8

THE INSIGHT

There is a universal, intelligent life force that exists within everyone and everything. It resides within each one of us as a deep wisdom, an inner knowing. We can access this wonderful source of knowledge and wisdom through our intuition, an inner sense that tells us what feels right and true for us at any given moment.

—SHAKTI GAWAIN

Intuition and concepts constitute . . . the elements of all our knowledge, so that neither concepts without an intuition in some way corresponding to them, nor intuition without concepts, can yield knowledge.

—IMMANUEL KANT

UNDERSTANDING THE INSIGHT	
Anatomy	Pituitary gland, brain/neurotransmitters, eyes
Functions	Seeing, thinking, intuiting/imagining, sleeping/dreaming
Living	Cognition, visualization, sleep
Eating	Stimulants (caffeine), depressants (wine), mood-altering foods (cocoa-based foods), blue-purple foods

THE SCIENCE OF THE INSIGHT

One of the most mysterious, fascinating organs in the body is the human brain. Scientists, philosophers, and mystics have all puzzled over the workings of this organ, trying to grasp the interconnections between mind and body, matter and spirit, thought and action, biochemistry and intention.

I don't pretend to have solved these age-old mysteries. But I do have an approach to healing, supporting, and sharpening your brain. Use Whole Detox to remove barriers in your sixth system of health, and watch your mood improve, your thinking sharpen, your understanding expand, and your sleep become deep, restful, and restorative.

As you already know from reading chapter 1, your brain is a biochemical marvel. Composed of fat, powered by electricity, and animated by a wide variety of chemical compounds, your brain processes thoughts, feelings, perceptions, and sensations, all while making sure your heart keeps beating, your lungs keep breathing, and your stress and relaxation responses fire off as needed. Oh, and let's not forget the brain's role in regulating digestion, hormonal activity, immune function, and countless other bodily functions. We can view these activities in biochemical and electrical terms, as integral facets of personality and worldview, in spiritual terms, or in some combination of the three. My purpose in this chapter is not to sort out which is which—far from it. I want you to see how important it is to support your brain in all dimensions—through revitalizing foods, vivifying activities, helpful thoughts, and practice in mindfulness—so your brain is in shape to perceive the world clearly, experience the full range of emotions, and make good decisions to advance your life.

A common challenge in supporting the brain, however, is that different disciplines tend to focus on their own areas of expertise—either physical or psychological—without seeing how all of these factors interact. A related challenge is that brain scientists tend to focus on brain chemicals, not realizing the extent to which other biochemicals affect the brain.

For example, a rich new area of study concerns the way insulin influences the physical structure of the brain. Insulin is the hormone that helps you metabolize glucose, or sugar; it's not usually considered a brain chemical. Yet, medical researcher Dr. Suzanne Craft has demonstrated that people with insulin resistance may be prone to more rapid aging in the brain and greater vulnerability to Alzheimer's and dementia. This phenomenon has been referred to as type 3 diabetes.

The brain, after all, is known to use a lot of sugar, which is why you might become ravenously hungry after a long, sedentary session of writing, reading, or thinking hard. But when there's too much insulin in your system, your brain shuts down its insulin intake, putting it at risk of an insulin shortage. We need insulin in our brains to metabolize glucose and to counteract a substance known as amyloid protein. Too little insulin, and the amyloid builds up, the threat of glucotoxicity grows, and inflammation goes wild, putting you at a significantly increased risk of dementia.

The brain has receptors for other hormones too. Estrogen receptors play a role in mood and cognition, which is why your moods go haywire and your brain gets foggy when estrogen levels drop, whether during the menstrual cycle or in menopause. Thyroid receptors help regulate metabolism, mood, and cognition, which is why even subclinical changes in thyroid can make you feel anxious, listless, or depressed (see chapter 7). The list goes on and on, since just about every important biochemical in your body has a role in the health of your brain.

Fortunately, the first five phases of Whole Detox have helped balance and support these hormones. And now, in phase six, we'll focus on the brain itself. Whew! Get ready for clearer thinking, improved mood, and better sleep.

Using the INSIGHT to Create Health

A scientific study by researchers at the HeartMath organization has defined intuition as "a process by which information normally outside the range of conscious awareness is perceived by the body's psychophysiological systems." Intuition is elusive; it appears on its own timetable and by definition resists submitting to our conscious control. The impromptu nature of its appearance makes it hard to test and even harder to measure, though a growing number of neuroscientists and other brain researchers have tried. The result is an exciting set of studies that suggest you can often harness your mind to heal your body.

For example, a 2013 study published in *Pain Research and Management* indicates that when children aged ten to fourteen years are taught the techniques of "mindful attention," they can better cope with pain. Rather than trying to ignore a painful stimulus, children seemed to do better by learning new ways to pay attention to it.

A 2012 article in *Psychology and Health* suggests that guided imagery and relaxation training can improve the lives of patients with inflammatory bowel disease, a painful and distressing condition that typically erodes quality of life. The notion that "brain training" can ease the pain of this condition offers exciting possibilities for managing other chronic conditions.

In fact, studies show that relaxation and guided imagery techniques can be useful for a wide variety of conditions that cannot be easily treated by conventional medical means: the discomfort of pregnancy's last trimester, the pain of giving birth, and the distress of chronic tension headaches, among others. I look forward to seeing further scientific exploration for this rich resource in health care.

THE POWER OF INDIGO

Indigo—the glowing color that comes between blue and violet in the rainbow—is associated with many elements of the INSIGHT: creativity and insight, alertness and improved cognitive function, and better sleep. Here are just a few examples of the power of indigo:

- A 2009 article in *Science* suggests that blue light helps people perform better on creative tasks.
- A 2008 British study found that exposing workers to blue-enriched white light improved self-reported alertness, performance, and sleep quality.
- An Australian experiment discovered that exposure to blue light made experimental subjects less sleepy as they tried to complete prolonged tasks during the night.
- Swiss researchers found that exposure to morning blue light seemed to improve daytime cognitive performance and well-being as well as help to modulate levels of melatonin (the hormone that helps you sleep) and cortisol (the stress hormone that helps you wake up).
- When motorists were exposed to blue light in their cars at night, their driving seemed to improve, according to a 2012 French study.

To access the power of indigo, stare into the vast nighttime sky, so deeply blue that it appears black. Quiet your mind and feel your insight awaken.

Intuition often comes to us through dreams, so consider indigo sheets for your bed or perhaps an indigo towel to wrap yourself in after your nightly bath. Better yet, keep a dream journal with an indigo cover and allow your inner voice to speak to you through its pages.

GET TO KNOW YOUR INSIGHT

The INSIGHT and Intuition

The INSIGHT includes both our physical eyes and the "in-sight" that draws upon our inner vision. Our intuition, often referred to as the "sixth sense," integrates all of our prior experience to produce insights that often seem mysterious and that frequently help us bridge the gap between our tiny individual selves—the microcosm—and the macrocosm of life. If we can harness our intuition effectively, we can use it to guide our lives.

Intuition can come to us directly—through what we see, hear, and feel. It can also come through dreams or via that quiet inner voice that speaks only in stillness. Remarkable as it may seem, nourishing the sixth system of health with balanced amounts of unsweetened cocoa powder, spiced foods, and blue-purple foods can often help us tune in to our cognition and even modulate our moods, which may ultimately open the gateway to our intuition.

Many of the foods that may spark our brain are tiny: spices, a teaspoon of cocoa powder, a few grains of coffee (although note that on your twenty-one-day Whole Detox, you will avoid caffeine). The notion of small substances making a large impact fits well with the concept of intuition: one of its functions is to connect the small to the big, the microcosm to the macrocosm. Have you ever noticed a tiny detail—perhaps the twitch of someone's mouth or an unusual word they used—and thought, *Oh, I get it—she's jealous* or *Now I see what's going on—he's planning to fire half the department?* Just as tiny stimulants and spices can spark your brain, so can seemingly insignificant details inspire your intuition.

Even the most logical, rational scientists have relied upon intuition and other types of knowing; the history of scientific discovery is full of insights born during dream time. Dmitri Mendeleev, the chemist who first organized the periodic table, struggled for hours to arrange the different elements in a logical order and then fell asleep at his desk. When he awoke, he had the solution: organize the elements according to their atomic weight. His INSIGHT had operated via an intuition his conscious mind could not access.

Likewise, August Kekulé could not seem to graph the structure of the benzene atom. Then he dreamed of a snake devouring its own tail, and he awoke to understand that the carbon atoms in benzene are arranged in a series of rings.

Daphne had a similar experience—though in our case, we actively worked to support her INSIGHT through nutrition. A web designer who routinely created beautiful, functional websites supported by elegant systems of computer code, Daphne had been stuck on a particular issue for several days. She had skipped meals, worked late into the night, "overdosed" on milk chocolate, skimped on sleep, and generally depleted her sixth system in a desperate attempt to force a solution. She began to feel as though the more she struggled, the less able she was to solve the problem.

She had worked with me several years prior, so she finally gave me a quick emergency call. I suggested that she lay off all the milk chocolate and start to load up on blue and purple foods—blueberries, blackberries, purple kale, purple cabbage—because I knew that the purple-pigmented proanthocyanins supported the brain's plasticity by reducing inflammation. "Maybe you can open up a new neural pathway that will lead you to your solution," I said, only half joking. Knowing how crucial sleep is to the brain, I also told her to get a good night's sleep.

Reluctantly, she agreed. She continued to address the changes in her diet and routine, and finally, weeks later, she woke up with a new idea that proved to be just what she'd been looking for. "I can't believe I solved the problem in my sleep!" she told me, laughing. Supporting her sixth system of health had given Daphne's brain the resources it needed to find her breakthrough.

If we harness our intuition effectively, it can guide our lives, helping us to make choices that best serve ourselves and others. And the better we get at knowing how to evoke our intuition, the more we can make use of this powerful ally. Sometimes we perceive our intuition outright, cued by something we see, hear, or experience; sometimes we receive its messages during stillness, contemplation, or dreams. Either way, intuition can often point the way to optimal health and a fulfilling life.

BALANCE YOUR INSIGHT

As with the LOVE and the TRUTH, it's difficult to see how you could have too much INSIGHT. Your first impulse might be "Bring it on! I'll take some more insight any day." Yet, as with all good things, you can indeed have too much INSIGHT, or rather, an INSIGHT system that is overactive, causing you to be wired, plagued by too many thoughts, and unable to stop thinking. Schizophrenia, bipolar disorder, multiple personality disorder, obsessive-compulsive disorder, and ADHD are only the most extreme examples of an overactive INSIGHT system. A person without a clinical diagnosis might also feel "I can't turn my mind off" or "Once I get started down a train of thought, I find it almost impossible to stop."

An underactive INSIGHT, by contrast, might cause you to feel slow, foggy, tired, and unable to think deeply. A balanced INSIGHT might be a better goal, although, as with all the systems, each of us will have our own version of it.

Yet sometimes an excess of the INSIGHT can be associated with genius, vision, or the kind of extraordinary insight that lights up new areas of knowledge. Perhaps a little obsessiveness, a little extra drive, can lead us to conceive new ideas that are truly valuable. And perhaps an underactive INSIGHT might be our opportunity to slow down, reset, and recharge, to take it easy for a while, to "go soft" and unfocus.

So explore the following lists, but allow your intuition and deeper sight to guide you. This is your opportunity to find out what type of INSIGHT is right for you.

A person with a healthy INSIGHT
- spends a healthy amount of time in reflection and contemplation relative to action and doing;
- enjoys healthy, positive thought patterns;
- is able to quiet their mind and redirect their thoughts as needed;
- is balanced in intellect and intuition rather than relying solely on either;

- is receptive to their intuitive voice, bodily senses, and instinct;
- can see the underlying meanings of situations;
- is able to bridge the practicality of daily living with the deeper themes of meaning and purpose, aware of both real details and symbolic images;
- has good attention to tasks;
- sleeps well, probably seven to eight hours per night on average;
- feels rested and refreshed upon waking;
- enjoys even, stable moods;
- has a sharp mind and good memory;
- doesn't overdo any food or beverage stimulants or depressants; and
- is not currently struggling with food addictions.

A person with an underactive INSIGHT
- might rely upon caffeinated beverages to help with focus, concentration, and thinking;
- looks to food and substances to *stimulate* their mind and thinking;
- oversleeps or sleeps a lot, frequently more than nine hours;
- doesn't remember dreams or claims they don't dream;
- feels fatigued early in the night;
- goes to bed early, but may wake up throughout the night;
- falls asleep throughout the day and likes short naps;
- has moods that shift slowly and can get stuck in one mood;
- lacks mental sharpness and often has a poor memory;
- might experience problems with blurry vision;
- might often feel that their mind "goes blank";
- tends to think through problems more slowly;
- might have difficulty being logical and/or learning new concepts;
- is not very good at thinking on their feet;
- is out of touch with their intuition;
- doesn't feel imaginative and doesn't consider themselves to be a visual person (has difficulty with guided imagery exercises); or
- finds it difficult to "see" into the future and tends to focus on the past.

A person with an overactive INSIGHT

- craves chocolate and is often a classic "chocoholic";
- has their moods quickly changed by foods;
- might have food addictions;
- might drink alcohol to calm down and is often particularly fond of red wine;
- can be an overly intuitive or an overly intellectual eater, either ignoring logic or ignoring their own instincts;
- might not be able to easily focus, becomes hyperactive easily, or might even have attention deficit hyperactivity disorder (ADHD) or tendencies in that direction;
- suffers from insomnia or restlessness during sleep;
- might sleep fewer than six hours per night;
- experiences volatile moods and quick mood shifts;
- seems to remember everything and might even have a photographic memory;
- might be prone to eye infections or inflammation;
- might get migraines or other types of headaches;
- thinks quickly on their feet;
- tends to overanalyze their life choices;
- is a visionary and thinks in the future more than in the past;
- dreams vividly;
- can be very moody or just shifts moods quickly;
- eats foods or takes substances to reduce their mental anxiety and overthinking; or
- is "always thinking," making it difficult to reflect, sleep, or meditate.

SPICE UP YOUR LIFE:
HOW THE INSIGHT DETOX WORKED FOR JANELLE

When I first met Janelle, she was at her wit's end.

"I'm a mess," she told me frankly. "I feel like my brain has just stopped working." And indeed, Janelle had a long list of frustrating symptoms: frequent migraines, sleep issues, memory loss, and a general sense of being foggy and unfocused.

A successful entrepreneur in her early sixties, Janelle worked long, hard hours to keep her business running in a challenging economy. She had been married for forty years to her husband, Edward—"steady Eddie," she called him with a sigh, describing him as "a wonderful man, but after forty years, you know. Not much magic left."

I had some nutritional prescriptions for her. I suggested that she eat a cup of blueberries each day, to benefit from their anthocyanins, a class of antioxidants found in blue-purple foods. As you'll see in what follows, anthocyanins can have a remarkable ability to restore brain health. Other patients had enjoyed significant improvements in memory and focus after increasing their consumption of blue-purple foods, and I expected Janelle to derive similar benefits.

I also recommended that she stop drinking her habitual glass or two of red wine before bed, since that seemed to be disrupting her sleep as well as triggering her headaches. While red wine can have some nutritional benefits, it can be challenging for many people because of the sugar content, alcohol, sulfites, and tannins.

Finally, because Janelle's life seemed so stressful, I suggested she take up meditation. I thought meditation would also help with her migraines, memory problems, and sleep issues.

But what concerned me most about her situation was the sense of boredom and "blah" that underlay the stress. "I feel like life has lost its savor," she said at one point. "When I was younger, everything was so exciting. Now it's as though nothing interesting will ever happen again."

I looked at my notes about her diet. I realized that she had loaded up her daily choices with highly spiced foods, like copious cups of black chai tea; additional infusions of caffeine from coffee, soda, and energy drinks; and lots of chocolate, which also contains caffeine. The excessive caffeine and chocolate were probably triggering headaches and creating sleep issues, and even the spices might have been too stimulating to let her relax and sleep at the end of the day. What struck me, though, was the possibility that she was responding to her sense of "blah" with spicy and stimulating foods. The problem wasn't really with her diet; she needed to spice up her life.

As we talked through these issues, Janelle realized that she had a few more choices than she had previously thought. Although her business required hard work and devotion, she could make the most of her free time by choosing new and interesting activities: a visit to a local Zen temple, a walk in a nearby botanical garden, a daylong whale-watching trip. She could also spice up her marriage by choosing some new activities with her husband.

"Eddie and I loved to visit amusement parks," she told me. "Isn't that silly? Our favorite was the roller coaster." Sharing even the small thrill of a scary ride seemed like the chance to rediscover some of the lost excitement in her marriage. Janelle also decided to take a salsa class with her husband, although initially he wasn't too keen on the idea. Eventually learning some sensual dance moves offered another chance to spice things up and recover the zest in their relationship.

Janelle's situation was a reminder of the power of Whole Detox. Neither the nutritional advice nor the life advice was enough on its own. Janelle needed to choose the right foods and avoid the wrong ones so she could support the biochemistry of her brain. But she also needed to look at the life issues that were driving her food choices, weighing down her thoughts, and draining her emotions. Nutrition, meditation, and life choices all worked together to remove the barriers to Janelle's INSIGHT and restore the savor to her life.

FOODS TO SUPPORT YOUR INSIGHT

INSIGHT-full foods can help clear your head, lift your mood, and give you access to your brain's intuitive capacity. If you're feeling foggy, depressed, unfocused, or anxious, the right foods can help to balance and support your brain:

- Whole foods and a Mediterranean diet (lots of fruits and vegetables, fresh fish, healthy fats, and whole grains) have been shown to reduce cognitive decline and to help the brain regulate energy expenditure, so both brain and body feel energized and strong throughout the day.
- Flavonoid-rich foods significantly reduce anxiety. They actually work in similar ways to the class of relaxants known as benzodiazepines (a type of tranquilizer that includes valium).

- Low-glycemic and low-sugar meals support cognition; by contrast, high-glycemic foods can impair your ability to think, reason, and focus within hours of eating. As we saw earlier, high-glycemic foods also generally lead to excess production of insulin, which can put you at greater risk of dementia over time. A growing number of studies show a close connection between type 2 diabetes and lower cognitive performance, cognitive decline, and/or dementia, suggesting a relationship between high-glycemic foods, excess insulin, and several related challenges to your brain.

- Natural sweeteners, such as raw honey and maple syrup, are the preferred choice. A number of animal studies have suggested a link between artificial sweeteners—particularly aspartame—impaired memory performance, and increased brain oxidative stress.

- Low-heat cooking and steaming help you avoid advanced glycation end products (AGEs), the crispy, crusty parts of food that result from high-heat cooking and frying.

- Low toxin loads from organically grown produce contain more phytonutrients, the vitamins and other nutrients found in plants. These phytonutrients support the health of your entire body, including your brain. And the herbicides and pesticides that cling to nonorganic produce have been shown to disrupt hormonal function and metabolic pathways (creating weight gain).

- Coconut oil has been shown to attenuate the effects of amyloid-beta, a brain-based protein associated with dementia. Coconut oil also seems to support the function of mitochondria, the cells' powerhouses, making coconut oil extremely supportive of brain cell health.

Generally, the more you can reduce inflammation—through both food choices and cooking methods—the more you promote gut and immune health, which in turn creates the biochemicals that your brain needs to generate a calm, optimistic mood and focused, sharp thought.

HIGH-FLAVONOID FOODS THAT HELP REDUCE ANXIETY

- Acai berries
- Arugula
- Bilberries
- Blackberries
- Black raspberries
- Black tea
- Blueberries
- Cacao beans
- Carob flour
- Cocoa, unsweetened
- Concord grapes
- Cranberries
- Currants
- Elderberries
- Green tea
- Kale
- Kumquats
- Mustard greens
- Parsley
- Radicchio
- White tea

Mood-Lifting Foods

Every meal you eat has the ability to put you into an uplifting mood or a downward spiral. The modern Western diet of processed and sugary foods is associated with a negative affect, which can be fearful, upset, nervous, or distressed, whereas a diet based on fresh fruit and vegetables, whole grains, fish, and healthy fats is associated with a positive mood, which can be inspired, alert, excited, enthusiastic, and determined.

Of course, no one diet is right for everyone. But once you're aware of how diet can affect your mood, you can tap into your intuition, your experience, and your knowledge to choose the foods that will best support you.

Sometimes hormonal changes, such as the menstrual cycle, lead us to crave certain foods, most likely in an effort to balance out a deficiency or an excess. Choosing foods that support the sixth system of health can help to balance both mood and hormones. The recipes for these three days of Whole Detox will give you a good start, pointing you toward the consciousness you need to create an effective, seamless dance between food and mood. Throughout Whole Detox, I counsel you away from unhealthy, processed foods, but who knows? Perhaps giving in to an occasional craving might be just what you need once in a while. Harness your intuition, honor your experience, and absorb the nutritional information in this book. Then you'll be able to choose—meal after meal, day after day—the foods that are right for you.

Foods That Contain Caffeine

As I mentioned earlier, caffeinated products (teas, coffee) are not part of Whole Detox. However, I do want to cover some basics about caffeine that you can use after you complete the program. Some people seem to be unaffected by caffeine, while others get jittery and nervous after ingesting it. Caffeine is metabolized in the liver, so if you want to know whether you can tolerate caffeine—and how much—your liver will let you know. Go with your physiological responses initially. If you feel wired for hours after a morning cup of coffee, your liver is a slow metabolizer and caffeine is probably not for you. If moderate amounts of caffeine give you a mental boost and an emotional lift—and if you are sleeping well each night—your liver is probably a fast metabolizer and you can handle and even benefit from some caffeine.

In fact, an increasing body of research suggests that caffeine could have numerous mental benefits. Studies show that it might prevent cognitive decline, reduce the incidence of dementia, and perhaps even be used to treat such neurological conditions as dementia and Parkinson's disease.

Of course, caffeine can have its downside, especially when we consume too much of it. For many people, caffeine disrupts sleep, provokes anxiety, and promotes headaches. However, as your detox continues, your liver becomes stronger and more efficient, and that might also affect your tolerance. On the other hand, too much caffeine can stress your liver, disrupting its ability to detox.

What's your takeaway? Once again, each of us is unique. Some substances—like white sugar and tobacco—are pretty much bad for everyone. Caffeine, though, has more varied effects. So when it comes to caffeine after your twenty-one-day Whole Detox, use both your mind and your intuition to know how much is good for you! And, when in doubt, just stay off it for the most part, having it only on an occasional basis.

Foods That Contain Cocoa

Certain foods lift our mood and maybe even re-create the bliss of being in love. Yes, I'm talking about chocolate, or, more specifically, foods that contain cocoa, which has a remarkable effect on our neurotransmitters and is one of the most powerful psychoactive foods.

What gives cocoa its power? A class of compounds called methylxanthines. The most common of these, theobromine, may work together with caffeine to create an enhanced effect when you consume dark chocolate. To make matters even better, the polyphenols and flavonols in the cacao plant help protect both brain matter and the cardiovascular system. Cocoa also contains flavonoids, a type of antioxidant that can help to open up the blood vessels, lowering blood pressure and inducing relaxation.

As you just read, a certain amount of caffeine can be good for us, stimulating the brain and sharpening our focus. A 1.5-ounce piece of dark chocolate contains 30 milligrams of caffeine—about a third of what you would find in a cup of coffee. Once again, use your own judgment about what relationship to chocolate works for you.

If you do tolerate chocolate, you will love the delicious, unsweetened cocoa-containing recipes in this phase of Whole Detox. After your twenty-one-day detox is over, you can also fight that late-afternoon slump with a small square of dark chocolate, which can help revive your brain and bliss out your mood. I suggest approaching your cocoa/chocolate experience with a clear intention, such as *This chocolate is infused with joy* or *When I have finished this chocolate, I will feel relaxed and joyous.* A study by researchers at the Institute of Noetic Sciences found that when people ate chocolate laden with intention, they experienced a better mood than those who ate chocolate with no intentions attached. A similar study, entitled "Metaphysics of the Tea Ceremony," had two groups of participants drink tea twice a day for seven days.

One group's tea had been "treated" with good intentions by three Buddhist monks, while the other group's tea was untreated. The groups were then asked to rate their mood and to indicate which group they thought they had been in. Those who had been given treated tea saw far greater improvements in mood. Those who believed their tea had been treated experienced even greater improvements in mood, but only if they actually had been given the treated tea.

If you are going to make hot chocolate, be sure you buy organic cocoa, because the conventional kind is laden with pesticides. Cocoa can also be high in heavy metals, such as lead, cadmium, and nickel, so contact your cocoa manufacturer about the heavy metal levels in their products.

COCOA + COCONUT = BRAIN POWER

Coconut has a number of brain benefits, especially in the form of young coconut water, a delicious drink that you can add to your juices, smoothies, and sauces as well as enjoy fresh. This beverage is full of electrolytes, like potassium, and might even help prevent Alzheimer's disease in menopausal women. Try mixing green tea or blueberry juice with coconut water and adding shredded coconut, flaxseed meal, or nut milks.

For an extra brain boost, mix cocoa and coconut. Both foods are well known for their brain benefits, and they add delicious flavor and texture to frozen treats, smoothies, puddings, and even granola. Mmmm, healthy, tasty fuel for your brain—what more could you ask for?

Foods That Help Your Brain to Remember and Learn

If you're concerned about keeping your brain sharp, these foods can help:

- Omega-3 fatty acids, which are found in wild salmon, flaxseeds, chia seeds, berries, tropical fruits, squash, and walnuts
- Turmeric in powder and raw root forms
- Flavonoids from cocoa, green tea, ginkgo biloba, citrus fruits, red wine, and dark chocolate
- Short-chain saturated fats from foods like coconut oil

- B vitamins, found in plant sources
- Vitamin B12, found in animal sources or taken as a supplement
- High-quality proteins that provide vitamins and minerals for the brain, including nuts, seeds, and whole-grain cereals

Now, at this point you're probably wondering where I stand on red wine after your twenty-one-day Whole Detox, since I suggested that Janelle cut out her late-night habit of having a glass or two. As with caffeine and cocoa, it depends. Some people have bad reactions to all of these substances; others do very well with them; still others have a varied relationship, able to enjoy some quantities of some substances at some times. So, once again, I refer you back to your own intuition. Your body will tell you whether, when, and how much you can consume these mood-altering foods. Just be aware of your body when drinking wine rather than mindlessly drinking— this is often when we get into trouble.

SPICE SAVVY

Turmeric contains a potent anti-inflammatory compound called curcumin. Black pepper contains piperine, an alkaloid with various protective properties. And when these two spices are paired together, there is synergy: more curcumin gets into the body than it does by itself. Try grinding some black pepper and mixing it with turmeric powder. To create a magical trio, add in some fat, like coconut oil or extra-virgin olive oil, because the fat helps the absorption too.

Foods That Contain Healthy Fats

I don't want to call you a "fathead," but I will tell you that about 60 percent of your brain is composed of fat! You want that brain fat to be nourished by the healthiest possible dietary fats, including lots of unsaturated omega-3s. Healthy fats keep your neurotransmitters flowing fluidly, supporting a good, positive mood. Studies have shown that people who are depressed may be influenced by the amount of omega-3 fats in their diet. You can feed your brain more healthy oils as well as magnesium by including more nuts in your meals. For example, blend walnuts with fresh herbs and sea salt to form a crumble and add it on top of salads, soups, and wraps. Don't go nuts—eat nuts!

Some other fabulous fats are the short- and medium-chain triglycerides. Coconut oil seems to have some therapeutic application for people with faulty memory, because it provides them with a suitable energy source when their brain cannot use glucose. Like other food items, however, please don't overdo it; coconut oil should never be your sole source of dietary fat! Make sure that you get the full spectrum of oils available on the market for the different cooking applications and tailored to your Seven Systems of Full-Spectrum Health. As we discussed in the TRUTH chapter, remember that variety is paramount in nutrition. Always shake things up a bit: the spices you use, the oils you cook with, and the vegetables you prepare. Variety helps keep neurons flexible and plastic!

Herbs and Spices: Jewels of the Plant Kingdom

You might recall that we discussed spices in the FIRE chapter, because several spices can help with digestion and warming a meal up for better metabolism. Similarly, we bring in spices here since they connect to brain function too. In fact, perhaps that is no surprise, considering there is a direct link between the gut and the brain (the FIRE and the INSIGHT).

Healing diets in the Mediterranean, India, North Africa, and elsewhere use an abundance of herbs and spices to restore the body and brain: oregano, dill, tarragon, ginger, black peppercorns, rosemary, and turmeric, to name only a few. Herbs and spices have been referred to as the "jewels of the plant kingdom" because they have a multitude of properties that cheer us up, pique our taste buds, and support our health, including anti-inflammatory, anti-cancer, and free-radical-quenching effects.

Even modest amounts of a spice or an herb can have a potent effect on your palate, your body, and your brain. You may not need large amounts to see substantial impact.

Curries are especially good for your brain, because they include curcumin, among other spices. Populations that eat more curry tend to have better scores on cognition tests. That shouldn't surprise us, because curcumin is well recognized for its antioxidant and anti-inflammatory action that reduces the buildup of the protein known as amyloid-beta, which is found in greater concentrations in demented brains. You will see curry and turmeric throughout the Whole Detox recipes so you can benefit from the way these two spices support your body and your mind.

Another healthy spice is cinnamon, which helps your body respond to insulin better (it is referred to as an "insulin sensitizer"). As you've already seen, excess insulin can disrupt brain function and put you at risk for dementia.

So tap into your kitchen pharmacy of herbs and spices! Sprinkle some saffron threads over your favorite dessert. Add a dash of ground cinnamon to your morning coffee. Put some zing in your salads by sprinkling them with crushed herbs and black pepper. Add fresh mint to your tea or a sprinkling of nutmeg on your steamed green beans. Spices can partner well with vegetables, legumes, whole grains, and meats—let your intuition guide you!

BLUE-PURPLE FOODS AND YOUR INSIGHT

As Janelle discovered, berries can have a remarkable power to heal the brain. Animal studies have found that berries—particularly the deep blue-purple kinds—help animals learn and improve their memory. When wild blueberry juice was given to nine older adults with memory changes, they demonstrated improved learning, word recall, and even a trend toward better mood after twelve weeks compared with those who drank a berry placebo beverage.

We used to believe that berries had their brain-healing power simply because they were concentrated antioxidants. And indeed, both berries and purple grapes are excellent sources of several antioxidants. Most notably, you have probably heard of resveratrol, a revered antioxidant in deep blue-purple foods that boosts energy and fights aging through its effects on our metabolic pathways.

Over and above the antioxidant effect, however, berries do support cognitive function. Recent research has shown that blueberries and strawberries influence various types of learning and memory, with berry compounds targeting specific regions of the brain.

Blueberries in particular have extraordinary effects on brain function.

They promote neuronal plasticity; that is, they help the brain change and grow in response to the demands made upon it. The more you make a conscious effort to learn and remember, the more your brain alters in response to this activity, and the tiny blueberry provides chemical support for that response.

Blueberries also have cell-signaling effects; that is, they play a role in how cells respond to inflammation. And they are engaged in the communication between neurotransmitters, the brain chemicals that modulate thought and emotion. Here is just a small sample of the exciting research into blue foods and the brain:

- Blueberries support neuronal and cognitive function, protecting the brain against the effects of aging and stress.
- In animal studies, blueberry extracts seemed to improve spatial memory and possibly helped to reverse age-related cognitive and behavioral decline.
- Concord grape juice seemed to support brain function in older humans, improving memory in those with mild memory decline or other types of cognitive impairment.

SUPPORT YOUR INSIGHT WHILE YOU EAT

- Use your eyes. See the colors of the food you purchase and the food you eat. Give yourself an eyeful before you begin to fill your belly.
- Eat intuitively. The hunches you have about what you need might be wiser than any nutritionist.
- Stay out of ruts. Habits are the enemy of insight and intuition; when you go on autopilot, you aren't really paying attention. Notice your body's signals and let them guide your choice of food.
- Meditate before a meal. It helps you clear the mental clutter and come into a place of peace.
- Notice your mood. See which foods change how you feel—whether they bring you calm, joy, or focus or make you more depressed, anxious, aggressive, wired, or foggy.

SUPPORT YOUR INSIGHT WHILE YOU SLEEP

One of the most important things you can do for your brain is to get lots of healthy, restorative sleep. While everybody needs different amounts of sleep, most of us need between seven and nine hours. You might also find that your need for sleep varies depending on what you're eating, how much exercise you get, and how much stress you're under. Most people underestimate their need for sleep—and most people don't get enough. I strongly urge you to make time for at least nine hours of sleep each night for a week and notice how long you actually sleep. Then commit to getting that much sleep every night.

A sadly common myth is that you can skimp on sleep during the week and then make up for it on the weekend. Unfortunately, our brains don't work that way. They are harmed every time you get insufficient sleep, and you don't restore that harm by sleeping longer one or two days a week.

If you're having trouble getting restorative sleep, completing Whole Detox is likely to help. Here are some suggestions to get you started:

- Cut out stimulants, even early in the day. No caffeinated coffee or tea, no chocolate, and no energy drinks.
- Avoid sweet foods and alcohol, especially after dinner.
- Unplug the electronics—computer, TV, and phone—at least two hours before bedtime.
- Make sure you are sleeping in a dark, cool room with no distractions. Blackout curtains and/or a sleep mask can help you shut out even the tiniest sliver of light, which will deepen your sleep and have you waking up refreshed.
- Invest in a good, comfortable mattress, one that is the right degree of hardness or softness for your taste. Many mattresses are loaded with chemicals and flame retardants, which give off toxic fumes you absorb while you sleep. Make sure you have a nontoxic mattress.

DETOXING YOUR INSIGHT: WHAT TO CHOOSE
- Blue-purple berries, which reduce inflammation in the brain
- Spices like turmeric and curry, which protect the brain from damage
- Deep, quality sleep, which fuels your dreaming and restores and heals your body
- Respect for your intuition through attending to your feelings, mood changes, and dreams
- A journaling practice to capture the wisdom of your inner world

DETOXING YOUR INSIGHT: WHAT TO AVOID
- Foods that disrupt sleep, especially excessive alcohol, caffeine, and processed sugar
- Foods that impair cognition, such as too much processed sugar or high-glycemic-index foods
- Too many stimulants, whether in your food or in your life
- A busy mind cluttered with too many thoughts

ENVISION YOUR INSIGHT

We each have our own unique INSIGHT—and our own unique way of supporting it. For some of us, stimulants are helpful sources of inspiration; others need to avoid stimulants or face anxiety, brain fog, and depression as the brain goes on a roller coaster full of exhausting peaks and crashes. For most of us, there is some kind of happy medium, the degree of stimulation that is helpful to us, although that happy medium might change depending on what kinds of stress we face and what kinds of mental, emotional, and creative demands we encounter.

Likewise, each of us has our own ways of accessing our intuition. Some of us are skilled at understanding the messages in our dreams and even at evoking dreams to tell us what we need to know. Others rely on meditation. Still others seem to know how to find quiet times—a walk, a long shower or bath, a drive in the car—to tune out the chatter of daily life and make a still space for our soft inner voice to speak.

Do you know how your intuition best speaks to you? If you do, I urge you to make enough time for yourself to benefit from this priceless resource. If you do not, I encourage you to explore your relationship with this special part of your being. Supporting your INSIGHT could be the wisdom you need to enhance both your health and your life.

CHAPTER 9

THE SPIRIT

*Never underestimate the power of dreams and the influence of the human spirit.
We are all the same in this notion: The potential for greatness lives within each
of us.*

—WILMA RUDOLPH

*The new physics provides a modern version of ancient spirituality. In a Universe
made out of energy, everything is entangled; everything is one.*

—BRUCE LIPTON

UNDERSTANDING THE SPIRIT	
Anatomy	Pineal gland, nervous system
Functions	Electromagnetic fields, life force
Living	Cleansing, circadian rhythms, purpose, meaning
Eating	Fasting, cleansing foods, natural white foods

THE SCIENCE OF THE SPIRIT

The SPIRIT as "Energy"

The SPIRIT begins with the life force that animates us into motion and
invigorates every cell in our body. That life force goes by many names: cellular intelligence, vitality, chi, qi, prana, perhaps even electricity, which radi-

ates through the network of interlacing nerves that threads through the spinal column out to every square inch of our flesh.

Sometimes the word "energy" is used to evoke the SPIRIT, such as "My energy is off today" or "I could feel the energy in the stadium mount as the home team began to win." That is a popular and unscientific use of the term "energy," yet it evokes a palpable presence that is both invisible and strongly felt. We can *feel* the energy even though we can't quite define it. And in recent decades, a growing number of scientists *have* tried to define it.

For some scientists, quantum physics seems to offer a way to grasp the notion of the SPIRIT. Quantum physics is the study of invisible particles involved in an interaction, such as generating a signal or charge. We can't see subatomic particles, but we can measure their effects. Likewise, we can't see the energy we might derive from looking up at the stars or imagining the human family, but is there something real about that energy nonetheless, something that materially affects our bodies and their biochemistry? Is there some force out there—some type of energy—that affects our minds and bodies?

I'm far from the only one asking these questions. This is one of the hottest new domains of physics, and slowly—very slowly—this research is beginning to make its way into modern medicine. Little by little, the notion of an "energetic field" is beginning to gain currency.

The SPIRIT and Light

Another way to explore the SPIRIT is via research into light. Fascinating new studies now reveal that living matter either conserves or releases light, depending on its health state. For example, foods that are decaying or under stress tend to give off more light, as measured in photons (the particles of light). It's as though the stress causes the food to release its vital energies—its light. By contrast, the practice of meditation or relaxation leads to the conservation of light—to the preservation of vital energies.

On some level, we know this intuitively. You can look at a friend—or at yourself in the mirror—and when the person is healthy, you see an almost literal glow. A person who is sick, depressed, or simply exhausted looks duller, more subdued. It is fascinating to imagine that these observations are not simply intuitive readings of facial expression or body language but actual perceptions of the amount of light being emitted.

Slowly but surely this insight into light and photon emission, too, is entering conventional medicine. Light medicine therapies are now finding their way into mainstream medical offices, with lasers of red, green, or blue light being used to achieve a wide variety of medical goals.

The SPIRIT and Electromagnetic Fields

Yet another approach to the SPIRIT is to consider electromagnetic fields (EMFs), invisible but potent clouds of charged particles that both respond to the environment and affect it. These fields can be sensed and measured, but not seen.

Some electromagnetic fields seem to help reduce pain and inflammation, with beneficial effects on such conditions as osteoarthritis, fibromyalgia, depression, and high blood pressure. Others may be harmful to human (and animal) health, particularly the ones emitted by high-voltage power lines and possibly also the cumulative effects of EMFs from appliances, electronic equipment, and the environmental effects of electrical production, telecommunications, and broadcasting.

Over the past two decades, our exposure to these fields has skyrocketed, as we surround ourselves with computers, cell phones, and other forms of electronics that are with us night and day, not to mention the environmental increase of power stations, broadcast facilities, cell phone towers, and Wi-Fi. While electromagnetism in small doses might actually have positive effects, as seen with pulsed electromagnetic field (PEMF) therapy, some scientists believe that this massive and continuous exposure increases our risk of cancer and other serious disorders. Moreover, the twenty-four-hour electronic daylight disrupts our circadian rhythms and has been shown to interfere with healthy sleep.

The flickering blue light of our computer screens disrupts the pineal gland and interferes with our production of melatonin, the hormone that makes us sleepy and keeps us in deep, restful sleep. Melatonin puts us to sleep, while cortisol, the stress hormone, wakes us up. An overexposure to electronics, especially after sundown, disrupts our melatonin–cortisol balance and plays havoc with our sleep patterns.

EMFs, meanwhile, potentially disrupt the tiny electrical currents that activate our biochemistry. Much of human anatomy, including the heart, is dependent upon electricity. Exposure to external sources of electricity—especially given how much of it we are exposed to—could disrupt our internal electrical "wiring."

POTENTIAL SOURCES OF EMFs

- Household and office wiring
- High-tension electric cables and towers
- Electric power lines
- Substations, transformers
- Radio and television transmission towers
- Cell phone masts/towers
- Cell phones
- Bluetooth and headphone devices
- Cordless phones, baby monitors
- Wi-Fi routers and wireless devices
- Wi-Fi hot spots
- Computers, laptops
- Microwave ovens
- Electric clocks, razors, blankets, hair dryers
- Fluorescent and compact fluorescent lighting
- Airport radar and telecommunication equipment
- Airport body scanners
- Military radars, radio frequencies, and extreme low frequencies
- Smart meters

EMFs affect humans in a variety of ways, depending on the type of field. Scientists have found some correlation between EMFs and a number of disorders, including childhood and adult leukemia, neurodegenerative diseases (such as amyotrophic lateral sclerosis, or ALS), miscarriage, and clinical depression although the results are inconclusive.

NEGATIVE EFFECTS OF EMFs

- A meta-analysis investigating studies published on EMFs between 1993 and 2007 showed slight increases for risk in brain cancer and leukemia compared with past studies.

- A meta-analysis conducted in 2008 by *Occupational and Environmental Medicine* analyzed a huge body of research and concluded that "EMFs may have a small impact on human attention and working memory."

- A 2006 study entitled "Mobile Phone Emissions and Human Brain Excitability" discovered that cell phones do significantly affect human brain excitability.

- Another study from the same year found a correlation between geomagnetic storm activity and the rates of suicide, suggesting that "perturbations in ambient electromagnetic field activity impact behaviour in a clinically meaningful manner. The study furthermore raises issues regarding other sources of stray electromagnetic fields and their effect on mental health."

However, as I touched on earlier, a particular type of EMF—a *pulsing electromagnetic field* (PEMF)—seems to offer exciting new benefits for people with chronic diseases. Here's a quick sampling of this research:

POSITIVE EFFECTS OF PEMF THERAPY

- A 2014 study in *Biological Psychiatry* found "rapid mood-elevating effects" resulted from low-field magnetic stimulation of subjects with depression.

- Another 2014 study discovered that PEMF therapy could be helpful when administered to patients with shoulder impingement syndrome.

- A 2013 study concluded that PEMF treatment "might be linked to improvements in peripheral resistance or circulation."

- In 2009, an article in the *Clinical Journal of Pain* found that low-frequency PEMF therapy "might improve function, pain, fatigue, and global status in [fibromyalgia] patients."

- A study reported in the *Journal of Alternative and Complementary Med-*

icine in 2009 reported that magnetic field therapy, specifically Bio-Electro-Magnetic-Energy-Regulation (BEMER), had beneficial effects on the energy levels and other functioning of patients with multiple sclerosis.

- A 2009 study conducted in India suggests that PEMF therapy might be a viable treatment for arthritis.

So, what should we conclude?

First, I think it's significant that PEMFs offer an unseen and yet powerful way of treating a number of chronic disorders that don't have good conventional treatments, including autoimmune conditions like fibromyalgia, multiple sclerosis, and arthritis. The potential benefit of PEMF therapies suggests that work with the SPIRIT offers an exciting new frontier in medical practice.

At the same time, I can't believe that constant overexposure to EMFs is good for us. I can't give you a definitive answer here, but I can give you my best recommendation, which is to reduce your exposure as much as you can. Every few months, do a "techno detox": unplug all electrical appliances, giving yourself a break both from electromagnetism and from the constant barrage of demands on your attention—even a day off periodically might make a difference. At the very least, your SPIRIT will benefit from the peace and quiet of uninterrupted living.

The SPIRIT and the Endocrine System

Grounding the SPIRIT in the body is our pineal gland, which distinguishes between light and dark, day and night, sunlight and moonlight. The pineal gland is the part of our brain that responds to light, and it may be involved in seasonal affective disorder (SAD), the depression that can result from insufficient exposure to light during the winter months.

Significantly, when the pineal is nourished with sufficient doses of bright light, SAD may ease or even dissipate altogether. Clearly this intangible—light, made only of photons—nonetheless has an important role in nourishing our physical selves. Since white is the color associated with the seventh system of health, I find it fascinating that bright white light is so healing to the pineal gland. (For more on white light and its medical uses, see "The Power of White," page 204.)

On the other hand, if your pineal gland is exposed to white light at the wrong time of day—if you see bright white light during the nighttime hours or have your sleep broken with bright light—it is prevented from producing sufficient quantities of melatonin, a hormone that helps regulate our sleep–wake cycle and is also an integral antioxidant.

People who don't get enough melatonin often develop health problems. For example, female shift workers tend to have greater rates of breast cancer, perhaps because they are working at night and sleeping during the day— exactly the opposite of what our bodies evolved to do. And indeed, cancer cells appear to proliferate in the absence of melatonin, while melatonin's protective effects seem to be extinguished by short-term exposure to bright white light at night. Ideally, you'll follow the rhythms of nature, but taking melatonin supplements, wearing a sleep mask, and darkening your room as much as possible can help reduce stress on your system during late nights and travel.

When your circadian rhythms are in sync with the planet's cycle of light, you can more readily maintain a sense of vitality and renewal. And when you feel "off," unbalanced, out of sync, out of sorts, it's often the seventh system that needs some support. Maybe you need more time in the sunlight (low vitamin D has become a widespread epidemic). Perhaps you need a darker room in which to sleep. Or perhaps you need some time to reflect on your life's purpose—the reason you get up in the morning, the relationships and commitments that get you through the day. As we have seen throughout this book, bringing together the different dimensions of a system can have transformative effects. The same is true of the seventh system, with its components of pineal gland, circadian rhythms, meaning, and purpose.

The SPIRIT and Well-Being

Fundamental to the notion of the SPIRIT is the profound connectedness that links us with all other humans and, indeed, all forms of life. It is this feeling of connection and integration that gives us our sense of purpose and meaning: because we are part of something larger than ourselves, what we do *matters*. And evidence shows that healing outcomes are dramatically improved among people who experience a deep connection with others or who believe strongly in some kind of greater purpose. This outlook seems to be particularly important for those with life-threatening diseases, including cancer.

Traditional religion is one way to access this larger sense of connectedness and purpose—but only one. Meditation, walking in nature, or any experience that takes you out of yourself can be an opportunity to feel that connection and enjoy its health benefits. You can dwell within the SPIRIT through the simple act of looking up at a nighttime sky in awe at how immense our universe is, or snorkeling in the ocean to discover the divine mystery of a whole other world that lives below us. Humans seem to have an innate attraction to being part of a greater whole, which is why Whole Detox is essential. Zooming out to see our lives from a distant vantage point—our place in the grandest possible scheme of things—will ultimately help us to zoom in and address any toxic barriers that keep us from becoming our fullest and most satisfying selves.

A growing body of research has demonstrated the links between mental health and spiritual awareness. For example, a 2014 Brazilian study found a correlation among patients undergoing dialysis. While "the stress of living with a terminal disease has a negative effect on . . . mental health," the researchers found that spiritual well-being was "the strongest predictor of mental health." Significantly, those dialysis patients who experienced that connection were also likely to sleep better and to have less psychological distress.

THE POWER OF WHITE

Throughout this book, we've explored the specific attributes of each color of the rainbow. White light, however, contains all the colors of the spectrum, much like the SPIRIT includes the entire spectrum of our lives and life itself.

Significantly, white light seems to be therapeutic in treating various types of depression. The SPIRIT is all about connection, and I view depression as the condition of being disconnected—from your emotions, from the people you love, from the web of life itself. It will be interesting to see what further research discovers about the benefits of white light, but here's a quick rundown of some of its successes so far:

- In 2011, a team of Swiss researchers found that five weeks of bright white light treatment improved depression during pregnancy.
- A 2001 study published in the *Journal of Investigative Medicine* revealed that bright light could be used to treat "circadian phase disturbances"— that is, irregular wakefulness and sleepiness—among the elderly.
- In 2011 Dutch psychiatric researchers found that both blue-enriched white light and bright white light might possibly be effective in treating SAD.
- Furthermore, a 2004 Danish study affirmed that bright light could perhaps be a helpful treatment even in *nonseasonal* depression when used in conjunction with antidepressants.
- A University of California, San Diego, study also found that bright light therapy combined with antidepressants and "wake therapy" could be effective in treating depression. Wake therapy is basically waking up depressed patients on the theory that too much sleep makes the depression worse. As you can see, there are close links between depression, light, and circadian rhythms—as you might expect from the themes of the seventh system— but we are only beginning to develop the research to fully understand them.
- Even bulimia nervosa might benefit from light therapy, according to a 1994 article published in the *American Journal of Psychiatry*. Some bulimics feel worse and binge more during the winter months, but the study found that "bright white light therapy [might possibly be] . . . an effective short-term treatment for both mood and eating disturbances associated with bulimia nervosa."

Would *you* like to benefit from the power of white? Spend at least ten minutes each day outdoors in the sunlight, or if you live in a wintry, cloudy climate, invest in a full-spectrum lamp and spend ten minutes a day basking in its glow. Immersion in full-spectrum light will help adjust your circadian rhythms, ground you on the planet, and support your nervous system.

GET TO KNOW YOUR SPIRIT

Although it can be challenging to define the SPIRIT, I'd like to suggest a few elements of this crucial system of health. Indeed, many of my nonreligious patients are surprised to discover that they do in fact have a fulfilling spiritual connection, and this connection sustains them in their efforts to cope with health and life challenges.

One aspect of the SPIRIT is the sense of *connectedness*: to all humanity, to our planet, to the universe itself. This bond extends outward to these grand dimensions, but it also extends inward, to a sense of the tiniest atomic particles and the deepest, most inward thoughts.

This connectedness can be a great comfort, especially in times of sorrow. When we feel lonely, hurt, or rejected, our sense of SPIRIT can remind us that we are never truly alone, that we are always a beloved member of the human family, kin to all living creatures, woven into the fabric of the universe. The sense of a human family inspired heroes like Nelson Mandela, who survived three decades in prison because his relationship to a larger world gave purpose and meaning to his plight.

Purpose and *meaning* fall under the SPIRIT, as they sustain us throughout life's challenges. Purpose—the sense that we are pursuing something larger than ourselves—gives us the motivation to continue when the going gets tough. Meaning—the sense that there is a reason, a value, to our efforts—gives savor to both good times and bad, so that we become larger than ourselves.

The challenge of this openness to the world, however, is that we can become overwhelmed by the pain and misery that is so prevalent on our planet. If I feel truly connected to all humanity, how can I enjoy my dinner when I am keenly aware that others are starving? How can I eat a living creature that perhaps was raised and slaughtered in pain? How can I find peace, joy, and meaning on a planet whose air and water and soil are slowly being poisoned? Feeling overwhelmed by the world's sorrows can lead some people to shut down, willing to disconnect rather than to feel the pain of connection.

These are not easy issues, and I don't pretend to have the answers. What I will say is that both scientific research and my own clinical experience show me the undeniable value of a spiritual life, whether you find that life through meditation, family, community, politics, religion, science, or any other means. If a scientist marvels at the intricacy of the atomic structure and the vastness of the ever-expanding universe, that sense of awe and wonder provides a gratifying sense of the SPIRIT, as much as the mystic who speaks to a Higher Power, the activist who plugs into history, the artist who is devoted to their creations, or the individual who simply savors a quiet walk in the woods. Although opening to the larger world can be painful, it also transforms our anatomy, flooding our body with relaxation chemicals, awakening us to our own possibilities, and giving us a reason to live.

If this notion appeals to you, I invite you to look for where the SPIRIT appears in your life and, if necessary, to unfold your daily life into more spiritual opportunities. Meditate. Spend some quiet time in a beautiful place, indoors or outdoors. Plunge into an activity you find absorbing, that takes you out of yourself. Open yourself to the possibility of connectedness and allow yourself to be refreshed, in body as well as SPIRIT.

When you balance your inner world with the outer, your reward is an increase in harmony and health. Medical researchers Dr. Nicholas Christakis at Yale University and Dr. James Fowler at the University of California, San Diego, have demonstrated the scientific validity of what they call being "connected." Their research suggests that our connections to other people can have a powerful effect on our body weight, our eating habits, and our happiness. That's the exact message of the seventh system of health: none of us is only an individual. Rather, we are the sum of all our precious connections, to our social networks and to our environment.

BALANCE YOUR SPIRIT

Of all the challenges in balancing each system, perhaps the trickiest to navigate is balancing the SPIRIT. How do we balance being grounded firmly in our body, on this planet, in the present moment, and also feel the pull of dissolving into the SPIRIT, into infinity and eternity?

And yet, as anyone who meditates will attest, it is this balance—this partaking of both body and SPIRIT, both now and forever, both here and everywhere that can refresh the SPIRIT, rekindle our purpose, and keep us facing life's challenges with serenity and strength. During good times, we can plunge fully into the pleasures of the moment—while remaining aware that they will not last forever and we should savor them to the fullest while we can. During bad times, we can honor our grief—while knowing that "this too shall pass" and we are part of a larger whole that can sustain us through our individual sorrows.

This type of balance is not easy to attain, but it can ground and stabilize us even while it helps us rise into the airy realms of the SPIRIT. Review the following descriptions of a SPIRIT that is balanced, underactive, or overactive, and consider what balance looks like for you.

A person with a healthy SPIRIT
- is both grounded in earthly matters and open to the spiritual nature of their life;
- appreciates a spiritual orientation to their life;
- is aware of their body's needs, their individual growth, and the larger world;
- knows how to put spirituality into perspective in their life, equally integrating it with other areas of living;
- makes time for meditation, prayer, or simply opening to the silence;
- feels connected with all of life but is not overwhelmed by the world's misery;
- sees everything in life as a divine lesson, but is not preoccupied or doctrinaire;
- is aware of others' states of being;
- has a strong sense of the meaning and purpose in their life;
- reflects upon the meaning of life;
- is seen as peaceful, humble, and thoughtful;
- is free from chronic, severe neurological complaints;
- is generally vital;
- is open to the use of energy medicine and other techniques for healing;
- is aware of their surroundings and moderately but not overly affected by them;
- feels connected to both their physical body and their spiritual self;
- is in generally good health;
- eats the right amount of food for their body and rarely forgets to eat;
- lives and eats based on an awareness of their interconnection with all of life;
- sees eating as a beautiful, divine miracle that nourishes body and soul; and
- will eat organically grown foods when possible.

A person with an underactive SPIRIT

- is relatively insensitive to their internal and external environments;
- feels connected to the physical body and disconnected from the soul;
- might appear overly gruff and judgmental;
- doesn't connect with people well;
- is not particularly drawn to natural settings;
- expresses doubt about the existence of something greater than themselves or a divine presence;
- is not especially interested in spiritual issues;
- sees life more as work or a chore than as a meaningful, special experience;
- lacks faith in others and themselves;
- sees life as physical and for our physical enjoyment, even to the point of excess;
- acts more than reflects;
- lacks a sense of purpose or calling;
- might feel lost or lonely;
- is unconcerned with toxins in food and regularly eats foods known to be toxic;
- tends to overeat rather than undereat and enjoys indulgent meals;
- might eat in response to toxic emotions and thoughts;
- has a dull sense of pain or is impervious to pain;
- might be numb or have dulled sensations; or
- is not fond of energy medicine modalities: has an "If I can see it, I believe it" mentality.

A person with an overactive SPIRIT

- might be acutely sensitive to pain;
- might suffer from neurological issues, such as tremors, epilepsy, neuropathy, pain, or Parkinson's disease;
- is drawn toward energy medicine modalities;
- is extremely sensitive—maybe even hypersensitive—to everything in the environment;
- feels detached from their physical body;

- might have let their health suffer due to neglect;
- might appear ungrounded, flighty, fragmented, or like someone who lives in their own world;
- is so concerned with spirituality that their bodily needs may be neglected;
- enjoys spending much of their time in meditation or prayer;
- feels so connected to all life and the planet that they are affected by everything;
- is overly sensitive to others' states of being;
- sees everything in life as divine and as a lesson to be learned;
- sees everything they encounter as full of meaning and purpose;
- is strongly purpose driven, to the point of being overly narrow and controlled by their mission rather than truly living it;
- spends time preoccupied with deep reflection on the meaning of life;
- might be overly concerned with toxins in food and will choose only organically grown foods;
- might be obsessed with cleanliness and purity;
- might have a large number of food sensitivities;
- might forget to eat; or
- sticks to simple meals, often not involving pleasure or joy.

BALANCE BODY AND SPIRIT:
HOW THE SPIRIT DETOX WORKED FOR MY PATIENTS

My patients' experiences make clear how challenging it can be to balance the SPIRIT—and how rewarding. Here are three examples of how detoxing the SPIRIT can transform a person's health—and their life.

Lucy was suffering from ulcerative colitis when she came to me. Her vitamin D was low and she had excessively high levels of her homocysteine and high-sensitivity C-reactive protein—all indicators of serious inflammation.

I knew that any conventional nutritionist would focus on Lucy's diet and intestinal health, prescribing probiotics to replenish her intestinal bacteria, glutamine to repair her gut wall, and supplements to support her immune system and bring down inflammation. And surely, I believed that the right foods and supplements would help her. But I didn't think they were enough.

Lucy struck me as someone who felt a bit lost or adrift. There was a vague, helpless quality to the way she described herself and her symptoms, but I felt that a ravaging anger was simmering underneath. When I asked her about her childhood, that anger began to seep through.

She told me that her mother had been ill with breast cancer all through Lucy's childhood and had died when Lucy was just fourteen. It fell to Lucy to be "the little mother" to her two younger brothers. Although she frequently felt inadequate to the challenge of being a parent, the one thing she could do, she told me, was cook for her family. "That was the one time I felt like I had anything to give." I was struck by the way she believed she could give material things—hot meals and nourishing food—but not spiritual or emotional nourishment.

Lucy told me, she did indeed feel adrift now, purposeless. It was as though her life had stopped when her mother's did, as though it had fallen to her to fulfill her mother's role at an age when she had been far too young to do so. I wondered if she felt disconnected from the SPIRIT, able to focus only on the physical, a choice that might have seemed the only option when she was young but was costing her dearly now.

When Lucy completed her Whole Detox Spectrum Quiz—the seven-part form that by now you have completed too—the area that came up extremely low was the SPIRIT. I knew that if I only worked with her on diet and supplements, I would be shortchanging her. She might get a little bit better, but without addressing the seventh system of health, she would never be truly well.

She and I had many long talks about finding purpose and meaning, about tapping into something larger than the body and the mundane tasks that needed doing to keep the body alive. Slowly and reluctantly, she began to take a yoga class and attend a meditation workshop. To her great surprise, she enjoyed this other way of relating to her body and she found the meditation far more satisfying than she had expected. "It's as though I've been thirsty all my life and finally someone handed me a glass of water" is how she put it to me.

Now Lucy is looking at what kind of life she truly wants—what work will satisfy her, what relationships will bring her joy. "I still don't have any of the answers," she told me in our last appointment, "but at least I've finally started to ask the questions."

Nathan was a once-vigorous man in his early thirties, prematurely gray and wrinkled. A night manager at an all-night restaurant, he was used to starting work at ten P.M. and going to bed at ten A.M. This "reverse life" wore on him, and his diet didn't help: it was full of sweet and starchy "quick energy" foods that he felt he needed to keep him going.

When he came to me, we talked about the well-established toll that shift work takes on the human body. Our bodies are meant to connect to the planet in a profound way, awake when the sun is up and asleep when the sky is dark. Violating this relationship can seriously disrupt a person's health.

Nathan began to realize that his night work was destroying his health. He got a job with normal hours and struggled to establish a more regular day–night pattern. Getting in tune with his circadian rhythms made a world of difference for him. He lost his belly fat, got his energy back, and felt ten years younger.

Magda was a tall, thin woman who was struggling with a severe case of asthma. When I met her, I thought she was almost too thin; there was a gaunt, starved look about her, and indeed, she told me she often forgot to eat or simply "didn't feel like it." She wasn't anorexic and she had never been diagnosed with an eating disorder; she just wasn't very interested in food.

The more we talked, the more I thought Magda fit the profile of someone with an overactive SPIRIT. She seemed almost obsessed with turning everything into a lesson or an occasion to "practice being my higher self." She worried continually about suffering children, abused animals, the destruction of natural habitats, feeling each story as though it were happening to her.

I admired her intense spiritual commitment. But I was concerned that her focus on the SPIRIT appeared to come at the expense of her body. I thought that small, regular meals would help her to feel grounded—rooted. (Yes, we've come full circle, from the SPIRIT to the ROOT!) I also thought that a steady, reliable source of high-fiber, healthy food, with lots of fresh fruits and vegetables ("the fruits of the earth"), would help to soothe the anxiety that so often triggered her asthma and would give her a solid, strong home for her overactive SPIRIT.

Magda saw her spiritual connection as the foundation for her life, but she agreed that maybe it was time for a bit of balance. She decided to take a class in West African dance—a physical, grounded form of movement that was also a way of celebrating the SPIRIT with every fiber of her body. Losing herself in dance was a spiritual experience for her, but it was also a way to relate more fully to her body and to feel love for her muscles, bones, and sinews as well as the less physical parts of herself. Dancing brought her a profound joy that balanced the sorrow she felt for the suffering planet.

Of course, I also suggested dietary changes and several supplements for Magda, and I know they helped alleviate her asthma and restore her immune system (asthma reflects a severely challenged immune system). But, as with Lucy and Nathan, just looking at food and supplements would have been only a partial solution. We are whole beings, and we need a whole detox—an approach that speaks to every single one of our Seven Systems of Full-Spectrum Health. When my patients removed their seventh-system barriers, their detox took a great leap forward, and their health took off.

FOOD TO FEED THE SPIRIT

Whatever your notion of the SPIRIT, I invite you to think about the ways in which something in you seems to reach beyond your immediate circumstances to more meaningful relationships—with your family, your community, your planet. I invite you as well to consider the ways that "SPIRIT-filled" foods can boost your health and inspire your life.

Cleansing Foods

The SPIRIT is about purification and clarification—getting clear of the physical fray so we can focus on what is really important. In detox, this means getting clear of any "noise" that interferes with our system—any preservatives, toxins, or problem foods that disrupt our body's harmony and keep us from feeling clear.

As a result, I place an even greater emphasis on cleansing foods as we venture into the SPIRIT. Of course, our bodies are meant to cleanse themselves—not unlike a self-cleaning oven! But we live in a world with such an enormous toxic burden that sometimes we need to give them a little help. Even before we are born, we take on some toxicity from our mother's toxic burden, and our own toxic burden only grows from there, thanks to pollution, unhealthy foods, and lack of activity.

Let's turn that process around! Lay down your toxic burden and shed the toxic barriers that are holding you back. To achieve this noble mission, however, you need the help of your primary detox organ: the liver.

Feed your liver with such herbs as milk thistle as well as with the spectrum of compounds in whole plant foods. In particular, alkalizing greens (such as parsley, fennel, kale, and cilantro), lemon, and sesame products (such as tahini) help the liver do its job. For the gut, insoluble fiber is ideal for sweeping toxins out of the body, via nonstarchy vegetables, berries, and legumes. You won't believe how good these cleansing foods can make you feel!

THE BODY AS A WHOLE: THE MANY PATHS OF TOXIN EXCRETION

- *Breathing:* Deep breathing or vigorous aerobic activity helps to expel toxins from your lower lungs.
- *Defecating:* Voiding the bowels at least once a day rids your body of waste and eliminates all the toxins that go with it. Ideally, you should be clearing your bowels two or three times a day.

- *Urinating:* Passing toxins through the urine we expel is another way to detox. But if the kidneys are stressed by environmental toxins and an unhealthy diet, they won't do an optimal job of getting rid of the daily burden of poison our food and environment thrust upon us.
- *Sweating:* Perspiration allows you to release toxins through your pores. But if your skin is layered with too many personal care products, and if you aren't exerting yourself enough to break a sweat, you miss out on this opportunity for detox.

Intermittent Fasting

Our bodies need food to restore and replenish themselves. But paradoxically, intermittent fasting can actually help your cells revitalize and rejuvenate. Occasionally depriving your cells of food—say, for twelve to sixteen hours at a time one day a week—can support better function of the mitochondria, the powerhouse that generates energy for the cells. Food restriction also helps your body lower the rate of cellular death.

Fasting of this type can significantly improve metabolic efficiency. You don't need as much sleep and your body begins to need less food. It's as though you're practicing, one day a week, for a time when you need no food at all and can live entirely on the SPIRIT.

As long as we live and breathe, occasionally going without food can actually be good for the body as well as the SPIRIT. Here's a small sampling of research on the benefits of fasting and calorie restriction:

Prolonged fasting seems to reduce levels of a hormone called IGF-1 (insulin-like growth factor–1), a substance that contributes to aging and perhaps to some cancers. Researchers believed that by reducing IGF-1, fasting contributed to cell renewal and regeneration.

Similar research found that fasting supported stem cell regeneration. We used to believe that stem cells were irreversibly destroyed by the aging process. Apparently, calorie restriction helps to reverse the effects of aging.

Fasting seemed to improve the mood of depressed and aging men. Researchers observed "significant decreases in tension, anger, confusion, and total mood disturbance and improvements in vigor."

DETOX SUPERSTARS

Detox superstars help the liver in multiple ways, through all the phases of detox. These foods include pomegranate, green tea, curcumin, cruciferous vegetables, and artichoke hearts. And medicinal mushrooms like reishi should be incorporated into some regular meals for their immune-modulating ability.

Make sure to give your mushrooms and vegetables their daily dose of light. Exposing cut, sliced mushrooms to sunlight increases their vitamin D content. Vegetables actually have their own circadian rhythms, so placing them in contact with sunlight rather than leaving them in a dark refrigerator promotes the formation of phytonutrients, according to a recent study.

Pure Foods

As you rid your physical body of toxins and debris, you strengthen it to allow for more openness to your SPIRIT. One way to lessen your toxic burden is to avoid taking it on in the first place! To support your SPIRIT, stay away from foods that have been contaminated with artificial ingredients or additives, including artificial sweeteners, dyes, preservatives, and coloring. When we load ourselves up with these synthetic ingredients, we challenge the nervous system, which is really quite sensitive and one of the first body systems to be impacted by toxin burden. If your nervous system is challenged in this way, you might develop neurological symptoms: headaches, hyperactivity, and the inability to focus on a task.

Instead, aim for clean, pure food: organically grown fruits and vegetables, meat from free-range animals, and wild-caught fish. Both your body and your SPIRIT will be relieved.

Clarifying Broths

The detox process gives your organs a chance to heal and restore, so look for foods that won't tax them unduly. Broths are easy to digest, nourishing, and soothing—an ideal support for a weary SPIRIT. Additionally, broths tend to be alkalizing due to the presence of electrolytes from vegetables, so they will help your body to naturally detox through a gentle shift in pH.

WASH YOUR ORGANIC VEGETABLES!

Even organically grown produce needs to be washed—and thoroughly. And thick-skinned fruits—avocados, oranges, lemons, limes—need to be washed so any residue from growing or transport is kept out of your kitchen. Get a U-shaped vegetable brush—they don't cost much—and scrub away the waxes, pesticides, insecticides, and herbicides that so frequently coat food. Make sure you rinse the brush well, and replace it or disinfect it with a white vinegar rinse every two to three months. Buy a brush with natural bristles and a wooden handle so you can recycle it when you're ready to replace it.

WHITE FOODS AND YOUR SPIRIT

By this time, you know when I say "white," I don't mean white rice, white flour, and certainly not white sugar. I'm talking about foods that are naturally white, not pale as the result of their natural fiber being processed away. The white color in refined foods indicates that the food has been drained of its life force—so how could it ever nourish you?

It never ceases to amaze me how our food culture strips bountiful nutrients away from foods that were already perfect in nature and then adds human inventions like preservatives. Why not leave the foods in their delicious, healthy, natural state? Are we trying to outwit Mother Nature? Do we actually think we can improve upon the original food?

Healthy, whole, white foods help cleanse and clarify the seventh system. Think ripe pears (especially good for moistening the lungs), cauliflower (cleanses the liver), coconut products (good, accessible energy sources for your intestines), onions and garlic (cleanse the blood and liver), cabbage (cleanses the liver and, when fermented, is excellent for the gut), and white beans (high in fiber).

SUPPORT YOUR SPIRIT WHILE YOU EAT

- Invite your SPIRIT to the table. Take a few moments to meditate, to feel gratitude, or to think about the purpose of this meal (to replenish your body, prepare you for a challenging task, share time with loved ones).

- See the cosmos in your plate. Your food began as a seed, planted in a field, tended by a caring farmer and workers, bathed in sunlight and moonlight, and visited by a multitude of insects. The seed transformed into a vegetable, which was eventually picked by someone's loving hand and then transported to a store or farmers' market. Someone chose the vegetable and then prepared it—perhaps you or someone at the restaurant where you ate. Savor the interrelationships that come along with the food.
- Get some exposure to the sun (indirectly or directly). The healing power of the sun is immense; it radiates and provides nourishment to all life. Before eating, allow your plateful of food to bask in the sun for a couple of minutes so it becomes invigorated with the high photonic energy of solar radiance. If you, too, bathe in the sun, even for a short time, you'll boost your body's production of vitamin D.
- Breathe deeply. Oxygen is the major component your body uses to access the energy in the glucose molecule, and every cell in your body depends upon glucose. Moreover, breathing into the low belly rather than shallowly helps to clear the body of toxins while delivering the raw material to burn food for energy. As you breathe, imagine yourself harnessing all the energy within the food.
- Experience love. The more we consume it, the more it grows, enabling others to be fed. The more love we are able to receive, the more we feed both the SPIRIT and the body. Enjoy love in all its many facets: love of the self, of others, of nature, of the planet, of whatever you perceive as larger than yourself.
- Cleanse your environment. Allow yourself to notice the people, situations, places, tasks, and events that are toxic for you—that create barriers to your total health and fulfillment. Then do whatever you can to remove or avoid these environmental toxins.

RESTORE YOUR SPIRIT WITH ENERGY MEDICINE

Energy medicine is recognized by the National Center for Complementary and Alternative Medicine, which is part of the National Institutes of Health. Although for years this approach to healing was scorned by conventional practitioners, energy medicine is now rapidly gaining acceptance within hospitals, clinics, and institutes. For example, many premier cancer centers now offer acupuncture and other alternatives to supplement conventional treatments. As a matter of fact, I would say that "alternative" medicine is not alternative anymore!

ENERGY MEDICINE THAT ADDRESSES THE SPIRIT

- Acupuncture
- Distant healing
- Flower essences
- Healing Touch
- Homeopathy
- Qigong
- Reiki
- Tai chi

As interest in energy medicine has grown, so has research into various alternative techniques. So far, much of the research is inconclusive, but some intriguing studies and some promising results suggest that addressing the SPIRIT in the form of energy may have significant effects.

In a 2009 study conducted at Kaiser Permanente, the giant Californian health-care organization, a group of people were offered treatment by Healing Touch, which, as the name suggests, involves the transfer of healing energy from a certified practitioner's hands. Many participants found that the frequency, intensity, or duration of the pain lessened after only a few treatments, and, perhaps even more important, they also "experienced profound shifts in their view of themselves, their lives, and their potential for healing and transformation." The researchers concluded that "energy healing can be an important addition to pain management services." Other research has found that Healing Touch can reduce pain in older adults, improve pain and mobility in people with arthritis, and soothe pain for those suffering from spinal cord injuries. Healing Touch might even have some effect upon the symptoms of cancer.

Another form of energy medicine is Reiki, a Japanese healing practice that involves being touched on the skull, shoulders, chest, and back. Numerous studies have suggested that Reiki creates health benefits, including relaxation, improvement in symptoms, prevention of symptoms, better mood, greater well-being, and a decrease in salivary cortisol levels, indicating a reduction in stress. Some research indicates that Reiki changes the functioning of an autonomic nervous system—the part of the nervous system that produces stress and relaxation responses—shifting the balance from unhealthy stress to a healthier state of relaxation.

Perhaps the most well-studied form of energy medicine is acupuncture, a centuries-old Chinese practice that involves stimulating energy pathways (meridians) with tiny needles. Dozens of published studies indicate acupuncture's effectiveness in treating chronic pain as well as many other conditions.

I find the emerging field of energy medicine to be quite exciting, especially for those domains in which conventional medicine has not been entirely effective, such as relieving chronic pain. The success of these therapies is yet another indication of the power of the SPIRIT, and the necessity of incorporating the SPIRIT into our quest for health.

DETOXING YOUR SPIRIT: WHAT TO CHOOSE
- Rest and rejuvenation for a wired nervous system
- A sense of awe regarding something larger than yourself: nature, the human family, the cosmos, or whatever moves you
- Regular cleansing practices
- Bright white light in your living space
- Peaceful contemplation and reflection on your life's calling or your path
- Quality time in nature: in a forest, on a beach, in the mountains, in the desert

DETOXING YOUR SPIRIT: WHAT TO AVOID
- Disruptive electromagnetic fields
- Activities that change subtle nerve function, such as too much use of your computer or cell phone
- Overeating or forgetting to eat
- Disruptions in your sleep–wake cycle
- Anything that causes physical pain
- Situations that make you chronically nervous

CONNECT TO YOUR SPIRIT

One of the most helpful books I've ever read was Dan Buettner's *The Blue Zones: 9 Lessons for Living Longer from the People Who've Lived the Longest*. Buettner decided to search the planet for the healthiest, longest-lived people and figure out what their secret was. Not surprisingly, the nine healthiest communities he identified ate clean, natural food; lots of fresh fruits and vegetables; significant amounts of healthy fats; and low amounts of animal proteins. They tended to be vigorous and physically active as well.

Perhaps more surprisingly to people used to thinking of health in strictly physical terms, the Blue Zones people enjoyed strong communities and a deep sense of purpose and engagement. They were part of something larger than themselves—a community as well as a spiritual world, which included ancestors and a whole system of belief—and this larger world both called forth their best efforts and ensured support when they faltered. Clearly, this spiritual dimension was an integral part of their long lives and optimal health. I invite you to detoxify the SPIRIT in your life—to remove the barriers to your SPIRIT—and complete this final phase of your Whole Detox.

CHAPTER 10

HOW TO GET THE MOST FROM YOUR WHOLE DETOX

Now that you've read all about the Seven Systems of Full-Spectrum Health, you're ready to start putting your knowledge into action. In seven three-day segments, you'll dive deeply into each one of the seven systems. Each day has its own unique theme:

DAILY DETOX THEMES

The ROOT	
Day 1	Body Awareness and Instinct
Day 2	Community
Day 3	Protein
The FLOW	
Day 4	Emotions
Day 5	Creativity
Day 6	Fats and Oils
The FIRE	
Day 7	Stress
Day 8	Thoughts
Day 9	Carbohydrates and Sugar
The LOVE	
Day 10	Self-Care
Day 11	Movement
Day 12	Vegetables

The TRUTH	
Day 13	Truths
Day 14	Affirmations
Day 15	Liquid Foods
The INSIGHT	
Day 16	Moods and Cognition
Day 17	Visualizations
Day 18	Spices
The SPIRIT	
Day 19	Connection
Day 20	Meditation
Day 21	Fasting

Each day, you'll address the day's theme using seven different approaches:

- Following the Whole Detox meal plans
- Keeping the Whole Detox Emotion Log
- Recording your limiting thoughts in a journal
- Engaging in physical movement
- Speaking specific affirmations
- Visualizing certain imagery
- Meditating

In fact, each approach corresponds to one of the Seven Systems of Full-Spectrum Health:

1. The ROOT: meal plans
2. The FLOW: Whole Detox Emotion Log
3. The FIRE: limiting thoughts
4. The LOVE: movement
5. The TRUTH: affirmations
6. The INSIGHT: visualizations
7. The SPIRIT: meditations

Let's take a closer look.

1. MEAL PLANS

Every day you will eat delicious, nourishing, colorful meals that support one of the seven systems. For the first three days of your detox, you'll focus on red foods and foods that support the ROOT: protein and minerals. For the next three days, you'll focus on orange foods and foods that support the FLOW: healthy oils and fats, tropical foods, and hydrating foods. For the three days after that, you'll focus on yellow foods and foods that support the FIRE: whole grains, legumes, and yellow spices. And so on.

The exciting thing about the Whole Detox meals is that they give you the chance to really explore each of the seven colors. You'll have the opportunity to experience for yourself how eating red foods, proteins, and minerals strengthens your ROOT, how consuming orange foods and healthy fats helps your emotions to FLOW, how eating the right kinds of yellow foods helps rebalance your FIRE.

When your Whole Detox is over, I'll want you to consume the rainbow: to include some of each of the seven colors every single day. But during your detox, you'll take it one color at a time, so you can have a good long visit with each. Think of these twenty-one days as a journey into the rainbow, where you can explore each color's effect on your mind, body, and spirit.

2. THE WHOLE DETOX EMOTION LOG

Every night before you go to bed, you'll complete the Whole Detox Emotion Log, noting the emotions you experienced that day. This is a simple exercise—you can take a look at the log on pages 381–83 to see just how simple—but its effects can be profound.

First, checking in with your emotions can be a transformative experience. Many of us focus so much on just getting through the day that we forget to pause, breathe, and ask ourselves how we feel. Our emotions get pushed aside, buried, or dumped into stagnant swamps, an underlying current of anger, sadness, anxiety, or frustration that we barely notice anymore but that saps our vitality and creativity nonetheless. We rush by the moments of excitement, satisfaction, and joy too, ignoring how we feel in favor of what we must do. The Whole Detox Emotion Log will help you to slow down a bit each day to reflect on your personal FLOW.

Second, by tracking your emotions on a daily basis, you'll have the opportunity to notice the patterns that shape your emotional life. Do you spend most of your days angry, frustrated, or sad? What makes you happy? What brings you peace? Are there activities or people who uplift you? Do certain situations routinely annoy you or bring you down? Becoming aware of how you feel over time can be a profound awakening.

Once you are aware, you can start asking questions. What can you do to spend more time feeling excited, inspired, or content? Do you have opportunities to alter patterns that aren't serving you? Is there an emotional message you've been unwilling to hear, such as I thought Margo was my friend, but I really don't enjoy my time with her or Every time I take a walk, I feel happy and uplifted? Learning how you feel gives you the opportunity to take the actions that serve you best.

The Whole Detox Emotion Log also gives you the chance to connect feelings to food. Do you find yourself craving sugar after a stressful day? Do you seek comfort food after a rough time with a friend? Do you finish your workday drained and dehydrated? These are the insights that begin to emerge from the simple act of noting your emotions.

3. LIMITING THOUGHTS

One of the things that sap our energy is limiting thoughts: If someone else needs help, I can't say no. Nobody cares what I think. I'm not good at learning new things. These—as much as heavy metals, pesticides, and xenoestrogens—are toxic barriers that weigh us down, sapping energy that might be used for better things.

Every day of your Whole Detox you have the chance to identify one of these toxic barriers and break through it. Each day I suggest three possible limiting thoughts relating to that day's theme. You can choose the thought that rings the most true for you or identify one of your own. Then you have the chance to spend five minutes journaling about that thought: how it has limited you, when you first began to think that way, what your life might be like without that toxic barrier.

I remember hearing years ago that we have from sixty thousand to eighty thousand thoughts each day—and a majority of them are negative! Imagine how those limiting thoughts are choking your internal flame and how much more brightly you would burn with better fuel. After all, we don't have infinite energy. Limiting thoughts weigh heavily upon us, putting out energy that could otherwise be used for better things.

As always, the first step is awareness: identify a thought that has been holding you back and give yourself a little time to reflect upon it. As you let go of limiting thoughts, you'll be able to replace them with expansive, positive, empowering thoughts—thoughts that better fit your current reality and serve you for a more fulfilling future. For many of my workshop participants, this has been one of the most exciting approaches within Whole Detox. I am eager to see what it brings for you.

4. MOVEMENT

Each day, you'll engage in some gentle movement. This might be a yoga pose, a walk in the woods, or some other type of movement that connects you to the day's specific theme. On your first ROOT day, for example, you'll take a walk, feeling the earth beneath your feet. On your first FLOW day, you'll go for a swim and flow with the water. On your first FIRE day, you'll do a tai chi "push hands" movement, designed to connect you with your solar plexus and your fiery drive to define your space. Through using your body, you will connect more intimately to each system.

Moving allows you to expand your lungs, keep your circulation flowing, breathe deeply, and engage your heart. Movement keeps nutrients circulating throughout your body, nourishing your organs, bones, muscles, and nerves. It expands your sense of possibilities, freeing you to go where you will and to carry your burdens lightly. It is a profound form of self-love—it's no accident those endorphins released by exercise leave you feeling happy and well cared for!

Many of us have difficulty making time for the self-care involved in daily movement. Although we spend hours rushing around to serve others—boss, clients, coworkers, family, friends—we find it hard to move just for ourselves. So for twenty-one days you'll have the chance to practice moving in ways that are primarily designed to benefit you and no one else.

Accordingly, for every movement I prescribe, I want you to do only as much as you feel comfortable with—no pain, no strain, no suffering, just small movements that allow your body to expand and breathe at its own pace. Do make time for the movement, but don't push it. Just allow your body to enjoy the movement that is your birthright.

If you've already got your own exercise program—whether yoga, running, weights, or anything else—that's terrific. You're welcome to continue whatever activities you choose. Just don't neglect the movement assignments in your Whole Detox, because each one has a very specific purpose, and I'd hate for you to miss any of them. The goal with these movements is not fitness or weight loss; it's a bodily recognition of each day's theme and each of the seven systems. Believe me, I've chosen each day's movement very carefully, and you'll get the full benefit of Whole Detox by completing each type of movement on the day it's prescribed. Allow yourself to be surprised by what you discover throughout the twenty-one days.

5. AFFIRMATIONS

An affirmation is a simple statement affirming a positive attribute of your life: "I am rooted fully in my physical body," "My moods are balanced and my thinking is clear and precise," "I am fulfilled with the abundance of life." When you fully engage with an affirmation, you find that it begins to become true for you, subtly transforming negative self-talk into positive and empowering truths.

Each day, I provide you with an affirmation you can use to identify with that day's theme, or you can feel free to write one of your own. Just be sure that you use only positive language: "I am free" rather than "I am not restricted." Be sure, too, that you phrase your affirmation as a fact, not as a wish, a hope, or a future possibility: "I am free" rather than "Someday I will be free" or "I want to be free."

I've used affirmations for years with patients and workshop participants, and I've always been surprised at how effective and transformative they can be. Science has begun to validate those perceptions with a growing body of research on the positive effects of affirmations. They are an integral part of many therapeutic techniques, and I am excited to include them as part of Whole Detox.

Many of my patients have asked me how they can repeat a statement that does not seem true to them. "What if I don't feel fully rooted in my body?" one of my patients asked me, regarding the Day 1 affirmation for the ROOT. "It's not true, so how can I say it is?"

My answer is that we are mining another possibility, another version of the truth. If you lived in the least toxic, most positive version of your life, the affirmation would be true. By asserting that it is true ("fake it until you make it"), you create the opportunity for it to become true.

If you find yourself feeling unsure or skeptical, why not experiment for twenty-one days and find out just how well affirmations might work for you? Say the words out loud, see how they affect your body and your emotions, and live in the vision they inspire. Use your voice to speak this truth, and see how healing it can be to connect to this alternate vision of yourself. Give yourself a chance to reprogram toxic beliefs into healing truths, and discover what possibilities begin to open up.

6. VISUALIZATIONS

The process of visualization is simple. Each day, I provide you with a brief description of an empowering image related to the day's theme. Using that image as a starting point, let your mind's eye conjure up the details, allowing your insight and imagination to take you on a visionary journey. You might be invited to visualize colors, places in your body, or even images of nature. Spending some time engaged with healing imagery can be a rich opportunity to explore a facet of yourself, your life, or your future.

Most of us spend at least some time daydreaming, fantasizing, or projecting our hopes, fears, and wishes into the future. Visualizing is no different, except that each day I give you a specific image with which to begin. Take the image and run with it—let your mind flesh out the vision and see where your insight and imagination take you. Before you can manifest what you want in your life, you have to envision it, so your twenty-one days of visualization will give you some good practice in using this effective tool.

As with affirmations, there is a huge body of research confirming the benefit of visualization as a transformative technique. My patients and work-shop participants have confirmed that this approach unlocks new insights, sometimes inspiring major life changes, other times allowing for a richer and more satisfying experience of the lives they already have. In fact, next to all the recipes they love, this is their favorite part of Whole Detox. Leverage this technique just a few minutes a day to show you a new vision, and you might be amazed at the possibilities that open up.

7. MEDITATIONS

You will meditate, taking a few minutes each day to be in solitude and silence to allow meaning and purpose to surface. Many of us think of med-itation in a somewhat limited way: sitting, eyes closed, motionless. That is one way of meditating, but not the only one, and within Whole Detox I give you a much more varied buffet of meditation choices. Once again, each day's meditation embodies the system and theme of that day, allowing you to explore them more deeply.

A great deal of research supports the many benefits of meditation and also indicates that meditation has the greatest benefits for those who prac-tice regularly. My hope is that your twenty-one-day habit of daily medita-tion will enable you to become a consistent meditator so you, too, can enjoy these benefits.

If you are already engaged in a meditation practice, you can continue or not throughout this time, but either way, please follow my daily prescription. I want you to have the full spectrum of Whole Detox, and every meditation has been designed to give you the most complete, tailored experience.

One of the most intriguing findings in recent years has been the discov-ery that these mind–body practices actually transform genetic expression. While we can't change the composition of our DNA, we can absolutely change the way our genes manifest in our bodies and our lives—and med-itation is one of the most effective tools for doing so. (Diet, exercise, and other lifestyle choices also have this effect.) And so we come full circle, as the spirit meets the body. We leave the body and the self to come back forti-fied, energized, and inspired, ready to pursue our life's purpose and to savor the meaning of life.

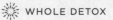

THE POWER OF SYNERGY, PART II

As you saw in chapter 2, Whole Detox draws profoundly on the power of synergy, making the most of how our seven systems constantly affect one another. I've designed your twenty-one days of Whole Detox to maximize the benefits of synergy, so every one of your seven systems is engaged on every day.

Many of my workshop participants start Whole Detox believing that the most important component is the food. Yes, of course the food is important—but the other six modalities are equally important. For the investment of about thirty minutes each day in addition to your meal preparation activities, you can benefit from the full spectrum of the seven systems, detoxing not just one part of your self but your *whole* self. I urge you to take full advantage of your twenty-one days by following the entire prescription—and allowing yourself to be surprised. Welcome to Whole Detox! You're in for a wonderful, colorful rainbow ride.

A DAY OF WHOLE DETOX

Feel free to organize your day as best suits your schedule. You can get into a routine for twenty-one days or make each day different—whatever works best for you. Here's one possible version of a Whole Detox day just to get you started:

Morning
- Begin the day with your *affirmation*. That way you can repeat it to yourself throughout the day.
- If you can, take a few minutes before breakfast to complete the *visualization* exercise. This imagery, together with your affirmation, will set the tone for your day.
- *Breakfast*

Midday
- *Lunch*
- On your lunch break, take a few minutes to identify and journal

about a limiting thought. For the rest of the day, notice how that thought appears and imagine how you might break through it.

Afternoon
- Snack

Evening
- Before you eat dinner, complete the movement portion of your day.
- Dinner
- As the day winds down, take time to meditate.
- As you prepare for bed, note the day's emotions in your Whole Detox Emotion Log.

FOODS FOR WHOLE DETOX: AN OVERVIEW		
Foods	**Yes to these**	**No to these**
Fruits	Organic whole fruits, unsweetened, fresh and frozen	Fruit products with added sugars
Vegetables	All raw, frozen, sautéed, fermented, steamed, roasted vegetables	Corn; breaded, fried, or creamed vegetables
Legumes	All fresh, frozen, or dried beans/peas; hummus	Soybean products: soy milk, soy sauce, soybean oil in processed foods, soy yogurt, tempeh, tofu, textured vegetable protein
Animal proteins	Organic, free-range game and poultry; organic, grass-fed, pasture-raised lean beef; wild-caught fish	Breaded fish sticks, canned meals, pork in all forms (e.g., hot dogs), shellfish
Nuts and seeds	Nuts, unsweetened nut milks, and unsweetened nut butters; seeds and unsweetened seed butters	Peanuts and peanut butter

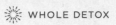

Foods	Yes to these	No to these
Protein powders	Hemp, pea, rice, and whey (whey protein powder for omnivores only)	Soy
Grains	Gluten-free grains: amaranth, arrowroot, buckwheat, millet, gluten-free oats, quinoa, rice (brown, purple/black, wild), tapioca, teff	Barley, cornmeal and corn starch, Kamut, oats, rye, spelt, triticale, wheat
Dairy and milk alternatives	Unsweetened milk alternatives: almond, cashew, coconut, hazelnut, hemp, rice	All dairy products, including yogurt
Eggs	Egg replacer	Eggs
Oils	Almond, avocado, flaxseed, grapeseed, hempseed, extra-virgin olive, pumpkin, rice bran, safflower and sunflower (high-oleic preferred), sesame, walnut	Butter, margarine, mayonnaise, processed oils, salad dressings, shortening, spreads
Sweeteners	Blackstrap molasses, dates and date syrup, honey (raw preferred), pure maple syrup, ripe fruits and fruit concentrates, stevia	Agave nectar; artificial sweeteners; evaporated cane juice; high-fructose corn syrup; refined, white, and brown sugars
Herbs and spices	All herbs and spices	Gluten-containing herbs and spices, herbs and spices with fillers
Other	Apple cider vinegar, balsamic vinegar, raw cacao and cacao nibs, unsweetened cocoa powder, coconut aminos	Barbecue sauce, chocolate, chutney, ketchup, relish, salad dressings, soy sauce, teriyaki
Beverages	Unsweetened fruit and vegetable juices; uncaffeinated herbal teas; filtered, distilled, mineral, and seltzer water	Alcohol, coffee and other caffeinated beverages (try to avoid decaf too), soft drinks

THE WHOLE DETOX MEALS: ADDITIONAL SUPPORT

Some Detox Challenges

By the time you finish Whole Detox, you're going to feel terrific. But some people experience a few challenges during the first few days of the program as their bodies adjust to the switch in food.

If you do experience transition issues, you'll probably have the most difficult time during the first two to three days, with another week or so of minor challenges. You can make the transition easier, however, by letting go of caffeine and processed sugar gradually over four to five days before beginning the program. Each day, cut back a little on your caffeine and sugar intake until you are down to zero. If you drink caffeinated coffee or tea, you might cut it with decaf, going from one-quarter decaf to half decaf to three-quarters decaf to all decaf.

Letting go of caffeine and sugar can produce headaches and irritability. Other withdrawal symptoms you might experience on Whole Detox include sleep problems, changes in temperature (feeling hotter or colder), lightheadedness, mood swings, joint or muscle aches, changes in your bowel habits, and changes in your body odor or breath. They won't last long, though, and as the program continues, you'll feel better and better.

Get Ready for Whole Detox

- Read through the program. Get a quick overview so you know what to expect.
- Check out the list of food staples on pages 239–40 and make sure you're well stocked. The list of where to get foods and some basic kitchen equipment, located in Resources, will also help you prepare. Ideally, you'll have plenty of glass containers and stainless-steel cookware.
- You might want to avoid any strenuous physical activity, since your body might need some time to adjust to the dietary changes. Judge for yourself and adjust accordingly.
- Relax and enjoy the process. Listen to your body, get some rest, and don't let the detox be "toxic" for you!

Omnivore or Vegan?

I've created Whole Detox meals with two options:

- The omnivore approach focuses primarily on clean, lean meats and seafood, vegetables, and fruits, with very few legumes, whole grains, nuts, and seeds.
- The vegan option includes vegetables, fruits, legumes, whole grains, nuts, and seeds.

I personally embrace all eating paths since everyone's needs are so different. You should feel free to choose; for any given meal, pick from either column. (However, the shopping lists have been organized for each plan separately, so if you want to mix and match, make sure you buy the right foods.)

TIPS FOR THE OMNIVORE APPROACH

- Choose organic, 100-percent grass-fed meats; organic, free-range poultry; and wild-caught fish. Avoid fish that contain high levels of mercury (see Resources).
- Don't overcook your meat; you'll lose too many nutrients.
- Trim any visible fat, which is a ready-made repository for toxins.

TIPS FOR THE VEGAN APPROACH

- If you are eating beans/legumes from cans, make sure to rinse them well, and choose brands stored in bisphenol-free cans.
- Rather than buy food in cans, it would be best if you could buy dry legumes and whole grains in bulk and soak them to reduce their cooking time.
- Check out the section below for a simple way of making beans.

WHOLE DETOX, BEANS, AND LEGUMES

Sure, it's quicker to open a can, rinse the beans, and eat them. However, when you cook them from scratch, you avoid the potential toxins that reside in most canned foods, along with the extra salt, sugar, and other preservatives (e.g., sulfites) that are often added. If you plan ahead, you can have beans in your freezer in serving sizes, ready to defrost and add to one of your recipes. Or you can just cook what you need for the next three to six days and store them in the fridge. All it takes is a little upfront work to make your life easier through Whole Detox.

Here are some simple instructions for cooking beans (makes about 5 cups cooked beans):

> 1 pound dried beans, any kind (the least expensive option is to buy them in bulk and rinse them well); this amount of beans will provide you with about 5 cups of cooked beans.
>
> Optional: 1 bay leaf, 1 to 2 whole garlic cloves, ½ onion, and/or chopped carrots and celery
>
> 2 to 3 teaspoons sea salt, plus more to taste

The night before you plan to cook the beans (or during the day if you will cook them in the evening), pick through them and discard any shriveled ones. Then place the beans in a large bowl and cover them with a few inches of water. Leave them on the counter to soak overnight (or for 6 to 8 hours). Soaking will reduce their cooking time and help them cook more evenly. (Note that lentils and split peas need no soaking. Just rinse them and they are ready to cook.)

By the next day, the beans will have absorbed much of the water and nearly doubled in size. Strain them and rinse them gently. Discard the soaking water.

Transfer the beans to a heavy cooking pot, such as a Dutch oven. Add any of the optional ingredients you like and cover the beans with about 1 inch of water. Bring the pot to a boil over medium-high heat, reduce the heat to a gentle simmer, and cook the beans partially covered for about 1 hour. You may need to add more water, so check them frequently. Soaked beans can take 1 to 2 hours to cook, but they average about an hour. Cooking time depends on their size and variety.

Add the sea salt when the beans are just barely tender yet still too firm to eat. Try not to add the salt too early as it will lengthen the cooking time and toughen the beans. Continue simmering the beans until they are as tender and creamy as you like them. Add more salt to taste.

Cool the beans and transfer them in their cooking liquid to storage containers in portion sizes for your recipes. In general, beans will keep for one week refrigerated, or they can be frozen for up to three months.

Please note: If you intend to use your beans in a soup, it's best to slightly undercook them initially and finish cooking them in the soup itself. Once you've scooped up all your beans, this liquid makes a great base for soups and quick sauces.

Allow Time to Prepare

Each recipe involves only thirty minutes of cooking time, and many of the recipes require less. I have made it as efficient as possible by having you make enough for leftovers and then incorporate the leftovers into your next day's meals. For some people following Whole Detox, the recipes provide too much extra food. Feel free to scale back if you find that you need less. Conversely, feel free to proportionally increase the recipe if you need more. You may have extra food left over before the end of the twenty-one days; in those cases, you may use the extra food in place of recommended snacks or meals.

Don't Go Hungry

This isn't a diet program, and I don't want you counting calories or going hungry. I also don't want you eating more than your body needs. I've provided serving sizes for each recipe, but you don't have to follow them. Make more if you find yourself hungry; make less if you feel like you're eating too much.

Rotate Your Protein

You'll notice that protein powder is included in every smoothie. I've provided you with a list of suggested protein powders, and feel free to use any of them, but don't use one type for all twenty-one days. The more you rotate your food choices, the healthier you'll be. Repeating food choices can create food reactions. And practicing diversity ensures that you get a broader spectrum of nutrients.

Keep It Fresh

Select fresh foods rather than canned or frozen whenever you can. Also whenever possible, choose organically grown fruits and vegetables to reduce your toxin load. And even with organic produce, wash your fruits and vegetables thoroughly with a scrub brush and biodegradable soap.

If you must buy some conventionally grown produce, focus on organic choices for the following items:

- Apples
- Celery
- Cherry tomatoes
- Collard greens
- Cucumbers
- Grapes
- Hot peppers
- Kale
- Nectarines
- Peaches
- Potatoes
- Snap peas
- Spinach
- Strawberries
- Sweet bell peppers

Why these items? Because the Environmental Working Group says they are currently the most contaminated. So if you must buy conventionally grown produce, at least avoid these items on EWG's "Dirty Dozen Plus" list. This list is updated every year, so make sure you check in periodically—they even have an app for your phone (www.ewg.org/foodnews/).

Know Your Oils
Read oil labels carefully, and choose only those that are obtained by a cold-pressed method.

Drink Purified Water
Drink about half your body weight in ounces, up to 100 ounces each day. Make sure your water is filtered and please avoid plastic containers.

Be Comfortably Active
Physical activity is part of your Whole Detox program. If you already have an exercise plan, you can stick to it if you have the energy to do both, or you can just follow the recommended activities for twenty-one days. Whatever you do, don't stress or strain. This is a time for rest, recov-

ery, and healing. You'll be rewarded with boatloads of energy when your detox ends.

Choose the Right Blender

Make sure you have a high-speed blender for your morning smoothie. See Resources for suggestions regarding equipment.

What About Supplements?

I don't prescribe supplements during Whole Detox. However, if your health-care provider has asked you to take supplements, make sure you work with that person to determine whether you need to continue taking them during the program. Usually, people continue with their typical supplement routines, and if they want to add in dietary supplements tailored to detox, they check in with their health-care provider.

ALMOST THERE!

There are just a few more things to do as you prepare for Whole Detox:

- *Get your house ready.* Clear your kitchen so you have room to cook. Make sure the places you plan to eat and serve food are clear and uncluttered as well. Ideally, you would clean up your entire house to keep your mind clear and your body ready to detox, but if that feels like an overwhelming chore, just focus on the cooking and eating areas.
- *Get your network ready.* Let your friends and family know you'll be trying a new way of eating for twenty-one days. Ask for their support and encouragement. You might even invite them to do Whole Detox with you!
- *Get your mind ready.* Think your way through the next three weeks. Will you be taking food to work? When will you go shopping? Are your Emotion Log and journal by your bed? What do you need to do to make Whole Detox go as smoothly as possible? Envisioning your twenty-one days will help you anticipate and solve any challenges that might arise.

Shopping for Whole Detox

I strongly recommend shopping every three days for Whole Detox, buying just the foods that you need for your next phase. Your foods will be extra fresh and delicious, and you'll have the added benefit of focusing specifically on each phase.

If every three days just isn't practical for you, you can combine two phases into one trip and shop every six days instead. The following are your Whole Detox meal plans and shopping lists, organized phase by phase, with an initial Whole Detox Staples list for pantry items that will serve you all the way through.

SHOPPING LIST: WHOLE DETOX STAPLES

Many grocery stores stock organic foods. If you have trouble finding any ingredient in a recipe, there are several websites that carry organic foods and some unusual items as well. Fresh produce should be organic when possible, and if you need to, as I mentioned before, refer to EWG's "Dirty Dozen Plus" list of the most pesticide-laden produce that it's most important to purchase as organically rather than conventionally grown.

The following staple nonperishable foods will be used frequently during your Whole Detox. Regardless of which type of meal plans you follow, have these products on hand before you start your detox:

- Garlic bulbs, approximately 2 to 3 bulbs
- Ginger, fresh, about a 6-inch root
- Lemons (about 8–10 medium) and limes (about 2–3)
- Apple cider vinegar, organic
- Balsamic vinegar, no sugar added (contains natural sugars)
- Coconut oil, virgin, organic
- Flaxseed oil, cold-pressed, organic (store in the refrigerator)
- Olive oil, unfiltered (if possible), extra-virgin, organic
- Sesame oil, cold-pressed, organic
- Almond milk, unsweetened (boxed variety, or about 32 fluid ounces)
- Coconut milk, full-fat, 2 bisphenol-free cans, 13.5 ounces each

- Coconut milk, unsweetened, 2 boxes, 32 fluid ounces each
- Coconut water, unsweetened, 1 carton, 32 fluid ounces
- Coconut aminos
- Honey
- Chia seeds, about ½ cup
- Hemp seeds, about ¼ cup
- Flaxseed meal, about ¾ cup
- Protein powders (Ideally, as I touched on earlier, you will rotate protein powders, using as many different types as possible. Buy enough for a total of twenty-one servings. Serving sizes vary with each brand of powder, but aim for about 12 to 15 grams of protein per serving. Be sure there are no added sugars.) Choices include the following:

Hemp	Rice
Pea	Whey (for omnivores only)

- Spices and herbs, dried (These should be purchased in small amounts either in bulk or in small containers. Choose organic when possible.)

Bay leaves	Nutmeg, ground
Black pepper	Onion powder
Cardamom, ground	Oregano, ground
Cayenne pepper, ground	Paprika
Chili powder	Parsley flakes
Cinnamon, ground	Pumpkin pie spice
Cloves, ground	Red pepper flakes, crushed
Cumin, ground	Rosemary
Cumin seeds	Sage
Curry powder	Sea salt
Dill	Tandoori seasoning (typically includes
Fennel seeds	a combination of garam masala,
Garlic powder	garlic, ginger, onion, and cayenne
Ginger powder	pepper)
Lavender buds	Thyme
Mustard seeds	Turmeric powder

- Vanilla extract

YOUR DAILY PLAN

Breakfast: a high-protein smoothie with fruits and vegetables
Lunch: a salad with protein
Afternoon snack: fruit or vegetable paired with nuts or a protein spread
Dinner: a warm meal with vegetables, protein, and a small amount of grain
  (if applicable)

Your morning smoothie is quick and easy to make, so you should have plenty of time to prepare it, even on a day when you're heading off to work while helping your family get ready for their days too! If you want to have your smoothie later in the day instead and prepare one of the meals for breakfast, you may consider that too. However, I like smoothies first thing in the morning due to their ease and the ability to get a lot of nutrients in one sitting first thing in the morning. I suggest preparing your lunch salad and protein at the same time. That way you'll have it with you at the office; or if you work at home, you'll be able to relax during lunchtime, enjoying the fruits of your morning labors!

※

CHAPTER 11

WHOLE DETOX 21-DAY PROGRAM

DAY 1: THE ROOT—BODY AWARENESS AND INSTINCT

I think that what we're seeking is an experience of being alive, so that our life experiences on the purely physical plane will have resonances within our own innermost being and reality, so that we actually feel the rapture of being alive.

—JOSEPH CAMPBELL

Meal Plan

	Omnivore	Vegan
Breakfast	Rooty Toot-Toot Shake	Rooty Toot-Toot Shake
Lunch	Terra Salad and Beef Burger	Terra Salad and Kidney Beans
Snack	Apple with Almond Butter	Apple with Almond Butter
Dinner	Tandoori Chicken with Kale and Red Bell Pepper	Tandoori Chickpeas with Kale and Red Bell Pepper

Whole Detox Emotion Log

At the end of the day, track any emotions that you had on the Whole Detox Emotion Log.

Thought Pattern Activity

The following are some limiting thoughts that relate to the ROOT:

I am unprotected.

My body is a burden, and I wish I didn't have to take care of it.

I am out of touch with my bodily instincts.

Pick the limiting thought that seems to ring most true for you. If none of the examples feel true, write down your own limiting thought as it relates to the ROOT.

Next, set your timer for five minutes. Spend that time journaling on that thought, how it has affected your life, and how you feel when you have that thought.

Movement

Take a fifteen-minute walk outdoors. If you have a dog, take her or him with you. Breathe in the fresh air. Survey the landscape. Feel the earth beneath your feet.

Affirmation

Spend three minutes saying aloud the following affirmation:

I am rooted fully in my physical body.

Feel how your body responds to these words. You can also create your own statement. Feel free to write it on a beautiful notecard or a plain Post-it note and put it in your immediate environment for the day.

Visualization

Set a timer for three minutes. During that time, close your eyes and visualize yourself being completely rooted in your physical body. Imagine your body is like a tree, spanning its roots down through your feet and having your arms wide and open to the possibilities of your physical world. Feel yourself being stable and grounded.

Meditation

For three minutes, meditate with your eyes closed while standing with your feet firmly planted on the earth and your hands at your sides.

DAY 1 RECIPES

Breakfast

ROOTY TOOT-TOOT SHAKE

Dedicated to my father
Serves 1

¾ cup purified water

Juice of 1 small lemon, about 1 tablespoon

½ medium raw beet, diced, unpeeled (save the other ½ for tomorrow's lunch)

2 to 3 beet green leaves

½ medium red apple, sliced (keep the peel on; save the other ½ for today's snack)

½ tablespoon chia seeds

1 scoop protein powder of your choice (hemp, pea, rice, or whey for omnivores)

⅛ teaspoon turmeric powder

Dash of ground black pepper

1 to 2 ice cubes (optional)

Put all the liquid and whole food ingredients into a high-speed blender first, followed by the dry ingredients, then blend everything until a fluid consistency is reached. Add more water if needed. Drink immediately.

NUTRITION INFORMATION PER SERVING

Calories	Protein (g)	Carbs (g)	Fat (g)	Sat Fat (g)	Unsat Fat (g)	Fiber (g)
226	27	23	7	4	0.2	2

Lunch

TERRA SALAD AND BEEF BURGER *(OMNIVORE)* OR KIDNEY BEANS *(VEGAN)*

Serves 1

FOR OMNIVORES:

1 Beef Burger (recipe follows)

FOR VEGANS:

¾ cup cooked kidney beans

FOR BOTH:

2 handfuls roughly chopped red- and green-leaf lettuce, about 2 cups

1 tablespoon diced red onion

4 radishes, sliced

1 tablespoon unhulled sesame seeds

FOR THE RASPBERRY VINAIGRETTE:

3 tablespoons balsamic vinegar

3 tablespoons extra-virgin olive oil

8 red raspberries

½ teaspoon crushed red pepper flakes

Place all the salad ingredients in a serving bowl.

With an electric hand mixer or food processor, mix together all the vinaigrette ingredients. Spoon half the vinaigrette over the salad. (Save the other half for tomorrow's lunch.)

Vegans, serve the salad with the kidney beans on the side or tossed in with the greens.

Omnivores, serve it with the following Beef Burger.

BEEF BURGER

⅓ pound organic, grass-fed ground beef

2 tablespoons diced red onion

¼ teaspoon turmeric powder

½ teaspoon dried rosemary

Dash of ground black pepper

Dash of sea salt

1 teaspoon extra-virgin olive oil

In a bowl, mix together the ground beef, onion, turmeric, rosemary, pepper, and salt until everything is well combined. Form the mixture into a hamburger patty.

Heat the olive oil in a pan, and pan-fry the burger from 7 to 10 minutes on each side.

NUTRITION INFORMATION PER SERVING

	Calories	Protein (g)	Carbs (g)	Fat (g)	Sat Fat (g)	Unsat Fat (g)	Fiber (g)
Omnivore	441	33	12	29	5	19	3
Vegan	436	15	42	24	3	17	12

Snack

APPLE WITH ALMOND BUTTER
Serves 1

½ medium red apple (leftover from breakfast), sliced

2 tablespoons almond butter

Spread the apple slices with almond butter and enjoy!

NUTRITION INFORMATION PER SERVING

Calories	Protein (g)	Carbs (g)	Fat (g)	Sat Fat (g)	Unsat Fat (g)	Fiber (g)
243	5	18	19	2	16	4

Dinner

TANDOORI CHICKEN *(OMNIVORE)* OR CHICKPEAS *(VEGAN)* WITH KALE AND RED BELL PEPPER
Serves 2

FOR OMNIVORES:

2 4-ounce organic, free-range, boneless, skinless chicken breasts, cubed

FOR VEGANS:

1½ cups cooked chickpeas

FOR BOTH:

1 tablespoon coconut oil

1 tablespoon tandoori seasoning

Dash of ground black pepper

½ teaspoon sea salt

1 garlic clove, minced

2 tablespoons diced red onion

¾ cup unsweetened, full-fat coconut milk

4 handfuls roughly chopped kale, about 4 medium to large leaves

½ large red bell pepper, thinly sliced into strips

Juice of ½ lemon

1 teaspoon extra-virgin olive oil

Melt the coconut oil in a frying pan set over medium-high heat. Add the tandoori seasoning, pepper, and salt, and stir the spices for a few seconds before adding the garlic and onion. Continue to stir the mixture until the onion becomes soft and translucent. Add the coconut milk, and mix it in well before stirring in either the chicken (*omnivore*) or chickpeas (*vegan*). Cover the pan and let the mixture simmer on medium heat for 7 to 10 minutes.

Meanwhile, in a saucepan, steam the kale and the red bell pepper until the kale becomes wilted and bright green (don't let it lose its color!). Remove the vegetables from the heat, and transfer them to a serving plate. Drizzle them with lemon juice and olive oil.

When the chicken or chickpeas are ready, spoon half of them onto the serving plate with the vegetables. (Save the other half for tomorrow's lunch.) Serve immediately.

NUTRITION INFORMATION PER SERVING

	Calories	Protein (g)	Carbs (g)	Fat (g)	Sat Fat (g)	Unsat Fat (g)	Fiber (g)
Omnivore	461	33	20	30	23	5	4
Vegan	507	14	46	33	23	7	10

DAY 2: THE ROOT—COMMUNITY

The power of community to create health is far greater than any physician, clinic, or hospital.

—MARK HYMAN, M.D.

Meal Plan

	Omnivore	Vegan
Breakfast	Red Berry Smoothie	Red Berry Smoothie
Lunch	Beet and Swiss Chard Salad with Tandoori Chicken	Beet and Swiss Chard Salad with Tandoori Chickpeas
Snack	Red Bell Pepper with Paprika Hummus	Red Bell Pepper with Paprika Hummus
Dinner	Grounding Chili	Grounding Chili

Whole Detox Emotion Log

At the end of the day, track any emotions that you had on the Whole Detox Emotion Log.

Thought Pattern Activity

The following are some limiting thoughts that relate to the ROOT:

I don't feel connected to people around me.
My family doesn't understand me.
I don't belong anywhere.

Pick the limiting thought that seems to ring most true for you. If none of the examples feel true, write down your own limiting thought as it relates to the ROOT.

Next, set your timer for five minutes. Spend that time journaling on that thought, how it has affected your life, and how you feel when you have that thought.

Movement

Do some physical activity that involves you being in a community setting; for example, go to a class at the gym or walk with friends.

Affirmation

Spend three minutes saying aloud the following affirmation:

I belong to communities that are nourishing.

Feel how your body responds to these words. You can also create your own statement. Feel free to write it on a beautiful notecard or a plain Post-it note and put it in your immediate environment for the day.

Visualization

Set a timer for three minutes. During that time, close your eyes and visualize yourself being completely surrounded by people who nourish, protect, and love you. See roots connecting you to each of them.

Meditation

Engage in a full-length mirror meditation by focusing on your image in a mirror without judgment. For three minutes, meditate on your physical self and see how your features, expressions, posture, and clothing reflect your community, family, tribe, and social network.

DAY 2 RECIPES

Breakfast

RED BERRY SMOOTHIE
Serves 1

½ cup strawberries
¼ cup red raspberries
¾ cup unsweetened coconut milk
(boxed variety)

1 scoop protein powder of your choice
(hemp, pea, rice, whey for omnivores)
1 tablespoon bee pollen granules
(optional)
Water and ice as needed

Put all the liquid and whole food ingredients into a high-speed blender first, followed by the dry ingredients, then blend everything until a fluid consistency is reached. Add more water if needed. Drink immediately.

NUTRITION INFORMATION PER SERVING

Calories	Protein (g)	Carbs (g)	Fat (g)	Sat Fat (g)	Unsat Fat (g)	Fiber (g)
247	28	18	6	4	0.1	4

Lunch

BEET AND SWISS CHARD SALAD WITH TANDOORI CHICKEN *(OMNIVORE)* OR CHICKPEAS *(VEGAN)*
Serves 1

2 handfuls finely chopped Swiss chard,
about 2 medium to large leaves
½ medium raw beet, grated, unpeeled

4 strawberries, sliced
1 tablespoon raw sunflower seeds

Toss together in a serving bowl all the salad ingredients with either the chicken (*omnivore*) or chickpeas (*vegan*). Pour yesterday's remaining raspberry vinaigrette over the bowl's contents and serve.

NUTRITION INFORMATION PER SERVING

	Calories	Protein (g)	Carbs (g)	Fat (g)	Sat Fat (g)	Unsat Fat (g)	Fiber (g)
Omnivore	576	38	38	34	23	6	10
Vegan	622	19	64	37	23	7	16

Snack

RED BELL PEPPER WITH PAPRIKA HUMMUS
Serves 1

½ cup hummus
½ teaspoon freshly squeezed lemon
  juice

½ teaspoon paprika
¾ large red bell pepper, cut into thin
  slices

Stir into the hummus the lemon juice and paprika, then use hummus as a dip for the red pepper slices.

NUTRITION INFORMATION PER SERVING

Calories	Protein (g)	Carbs (g)	Fat (g)	Sat Fat (g)	Unsat Fat (g)	Fiber (g)
229	10	23	12	2	9	9

Dinner

GROUNDING CHILI
Serves 2

FOR OMNIVORES:

½ pound organic, free-range, lean
  ground turkey

FOR VEGANS:

1½ cups cooked adzuki beans
¼ cup purified water

FOR BOTH:

1 tablespoon extra-virgin olive oil
½ medium red onion, diced
2 garlic cloves, minced
1 teaspoon ground cumin

1 teaspoon chili powder
1 teaspoon paprika
Dash of sea salt
Dash of ground black pepper

6 shiitake mushrooms

1 cup chopped cauliflower

1 carrot, scrubbed and chopped

2 medium tomatoes, diced

2 tablespoons uncooked quinoa (red variety preferred)

2 cups low-sodium tomato juice

1 cup purified water

In a large soup pot set over low to medium heat, heat the olive oil and sauté the onion and garlic until the onions become soft, about 2 to 3 minutes. Add the cumin, chili powder, paprika, salt, and pepper.

Omnivores, add the turkey and brown it for about 5 to 7 minutes.

Vegans, add the adzuki beans plus about ¼ cup water, so the beans don't burn, and cook the mixture for about 2 to 3 minutes.

Both omnivores and vegans, then add the mushrooms, cauliflower, carrot, tomatoes, quinoa, tomato juice, and additional cup of water. Cook the mixture for about 8 to 10 more minutes, stirring consistently. Season to taste.

Spoon up half the chili and serve warm. (Save the other half for tomorrow's lunch.)

NUTRITION INFORMATION PER SERVING

	Calories	Protein (g)	Carbs (g)	Fat (g)	Sat Fat (g)	Unsat Fat (g)	Fiber (g)
Omnivore	417	28	36	18	4	12	9
Vegan	469	21	79	9	1	6	21

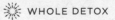

DAY 3: THE ROOT—PROTEIN

Our cells engage in protein production, and many of those proteins are enzymes responsible for the chemistry of life.

—RANDY SCHEKMAN

Meal Plan

	Omnivore	Vegan
Breakfast	Sunrise Smoothie	Sunrise Smoothie
Lunch	Beet Root and Greens Grounding Chili	Beet Root and Greens Grounding Chili
Snack	Avocado and Walnuts	Avocado and Walnuts
Dinner	Ginger-Garlic Beef on Quinoa	Ginger-Garlic Black Beans on Quinoa

Whole Detox Emotion Log

At the end of the day, track any emotions that you had on the Whole Detox Emotion Log.

Thought Pattern Activity

The following are some limiting thoughts that relate to the ROOT:

I am ungrounded.
I feel unstable in my body.
My surroundings don't support me.

Pick the limiting thought that seems to ring most true for you. If none of the examples feel true, write down your own limiting thought as it relates to the ROOT.

Next, set your timer for five minutes. Spend that time journaling on that thought, how it has affected your life, and how you feel when you have that thought.

Movement
MOUNTAIN POSE (TADASANA)

1. Stand with your body relaxed. Your feet should be shoulder-width apart.
2. Bend your knees slightly.
3. Tilt your pelvis slightly forward.
4. Keeping your body balanced, evenly distribute your weight over the soles of your feet. Feel the ground solid beneath your feet.
5. Maintain this position for three minutes. As with all yoga poses, go to your comfortable limit. Nothing should be painful.

Practicing this barefoot and outdoors adds a connection to nature and the earth (but is not required, especially if you live in a cold climate).

Affirmation
Spend three minutes saying aloud the following affirmation:

I am anchored in my beautiful, strong, physical structure.

Feel how your body responds to these words. You can also create your own statement. Feel free to write it on a beautiful notecard or a plain Post-it note and put it in your immediate environment for the day.

Visualization
Set a timer for three minutes. During that time, close your eyes and visualize yourself feeling strong and stable in your skeletal structure. See your bones as being packed with the necessary minerals they need. Imagine your muscles as being fibrous, fit, and flexible, working well with your skeleton.

Meditation
For three minutes, invigorate and stimulate your bones with a weight-bearing, meditative activity. Take a leisurely walk outside, and as you do, contemplate each step. See each step as significant, strong, and strengthening. Make the movement your sole focus and meditation.

DAY 3 RECIPES

Breakfast

SUNRISE SMOOTHIE
Serves 1

- 1 small red apple, sliced (leave peel on)
- 1 small carrot, scrubbed and diced (leave peel on)
- 4 pink grapefruit sections (save the rest of the grapefruit for today's lunch)
- 1 teaspoon freshly squeezed lemon juice

- ½-inch piece fresh ginger, chopped
- 6 red raspberries
- ½ cup unsweetened coconut milk (boxed variety)
- 1 tablespoon flaxseed meal
- 1 scoop protein powder of your choice (hemp, pea, rice, whey for omnivores)
- Water and ice as needed

Put all the liquid and whole food ingredients into a high-speed blender first, followed by the dry ingredients, then blend everything until a fluid consistency is reached. Add more water if needed. Drink immediately.

NUTRITION INFORMATION PER SERVING

Calories	Protein (g)	Carbs (g)	Fat (g)	Sat Fat (g)	Unsat Fat (g)	Fiber (g)
402	28	41	17	11	1	9

Lunch

BEET ROOT AND GREENS WITH GROUNDING CHILI
Serves 1

- 1 small to medium raw beet, grated, unpeeled (totals about 1 cup)

- 2 beet green leaves, finely chopped
- 7 red grapes

FOR THE DRESSING:

- 3 tablespoons grapefruit juice (from the leftover grapefruit from breakfast)
- 2 tablespoons extra-virgin olive oil

- 1 teaspoon ground oregano
- Dash of sea salt
- Dash of ground black pepper

Combine the beet, beet greens, and grapes in a bowl. Stir or whisk together all the ingredients for the dressing, then pour the dressing over the salad.

Warm up yesterday's leftover Grounding Chili to serve with the salad.

NUTRITION INFORMATION PER SERVING

	Calories	Protein (g)	Carbs (g)	Fat (g)	Sat Fat (g)	Unsat Fat (g)	Fiber (g)
Omnivore	634	31	57	32	6	24	14
Vegan	469	24	100	23	3	18	26

Snack

AVOCADO AND WALNUTS
Serves 1

½ avocado (leave the pit in the other ½ and save it for tomorrow's lunch)
½ teaspoon freshly squeezed lemon juice

Dash of sea salt
1 scant handful (about 8) walnut halves (red variety preferred)

Drizzle the avocado with lemon juice and sprinkle it with salt, then eat it with the walnuts.

NUTRITION INFORMATION PER SERVING

Calories	Protein (g)	Carbs (g)	Fat (g)	Sat Fat (g)	Unsat Fat (g)	Fiber (g)
266	4	11	25	3	21	8

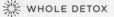

Dinner

GINGER-GARLIC BEEF *(OMNIVORE)* OR BLACK BEANS *(VEGAN)* ON QUINOA
Serves 1

FOR OMNIVORES:

    4- to 6-ounce organic, grass-fed flank steak, cut into strips

FOR VEGANS:

    ¾ cup cooked black beans

FOR BOTH:

- 1 teaspoon sesame oil
- ½ teaspoon minced fresh ginger
- ½ garlic clove, minced
- 2 tablespoons diced red onion
- 1 tablespoon extra-virgin olive oil
- 1 teaspoon chili powder
- 1 teaspoon ground cumin
- 1 teaspoon paprika
- 1 teaspoon ground oregano
- ½ teaspoon garlic powder

- ½ teaspoon onion powder
- 1 teaspoon sea salt
- 1 teaspoon ground black pepper
- 1 medium turnip, diced
- 1 medium carrot, cut into bite-size strips
- 1 cup chopped broccoli
- 1 large portobello mushroom, sliced
- ½ cup cooked quinoa (red variety preferred)

In a wok or heavy skillet set over medium heat, warm the sesame oil. Add the ginger, garlic, and onion, and stir-fry the mixture for 30 seconds.

Omnivores, add the beef strips, olive oil, chili powder, cumin, paprika, oregano, garlic powder, onion powder, salt, and pepper to the skillet, and continue stir-frying until the beef strips are cooked through, about 7 to 10 minutes.

Vegans, add the black beans, olive oil, chili powder, cumin, paprika, oregano, garlic powder, onion powder, salt, and pepper to the skillet, and continue stir-frying for 4 to 5 minutes.

Both omnivores and vegans, then add the turnip, carrot, broccoli, and mushroom, and stir-fry for another 2 to 3 minutes. Season to taste. Serve over the cooked quinoa.

NUTRITION INFORMATION PER SERVING

	Calories	Protein (g)	Carbs (g)	Fat (g)	Sat Fat (g)	Unsat Fat (g)	Fiber (g)
Omnivore	657	50	44	32	7	21	10
Vegan	543	19	72	21	3	17	18

The Seven Systems of Full-Spectrum Health

SYSTEM	ENDOCRINE GLAND	ANATOMY	PHYSIOLOGICAL ACTIVITIES	CORE ISSUES	FOODS
THE ROOT	Adrenals	• Blood cells • Bones • DNA • Immune system • Joints	• Legs and feet • Muscles • Rectum • Skin • Tailbone (coccyx)	• Enzyme activity • Flight-or-fight response • Gene expression • Protein production	• Safety • Survival • Tribe	• Dietary proteins • Immune-enhancing foods • Insoluble fiber	• Mineral-rich foods • Root vegetables • Red-colored foods
THE FLOW	Ovaries/Testes	• Bladder • Hips • Kidneys	• Large intestine • Reproductive system • Sacrum	• Cellular replication • Fat storage • Reproduction • Water balance	• Creativity • Emotions • Relationships	• Dietary fats and oils • Fermented foods • Fish and seafood • Nuts and seeds	• Tropical foods • Water • Orange-colored foods
THE FIRE	Pancreas	• Gallbladder • Liver	• Small intestine • Stomach	• Assimilation • Biotransformation • Blood sugar balance • Digestion	• Balance • Energy • Power	• Dietary carbohydrates • Healthy sweeteners • Legumes • Soluble fiber	• Whole grains • Yellow-colored foods
THE LOVE	Thymus and Heart	• Armpits • Arms • Blood vessels • Breasts • Hands	• Lungs • Lymphatic system • Shoulders • Wrists	• Breathing • Circulation • Oxygenation	• Compassion • Expansion • Service	• Leafy vegetables • Microgreens • Phytonutrients • Sprouts • Vegetables (especially green)	
THE TRUTH	Thyroid	• Cheeks • Chin • Ears • Mouth	• Neck • Nose • Throat	• Chewing • Metabolism • Hearing • Smelling • Speaking	• Authenticity • Choice • Voice	• Fruits • Juices • Sauces	• Sea plants • Soups • Teas
THE INSIGHT	Pituitary	• Brain • Eyebrows • Eyes	• Forehead • Neurons • Neurotransmitters	• Mood balance • Sleep • Thought processing	• Intuition • Reflection • Visualization	• Caffeine • Chocolate/cocoa • Mood-modulating foods	• Spices • Blue-purple foods
THE SPIRIT	Pineal	• Electromagnetic field • Energy meridians • Nervous system		• Circadian rhythms • Cleansing • Light sensitivity	• Connection • Purpose • Soul	• Fasting and detoxification practices • Photons • Toxin-free foods	

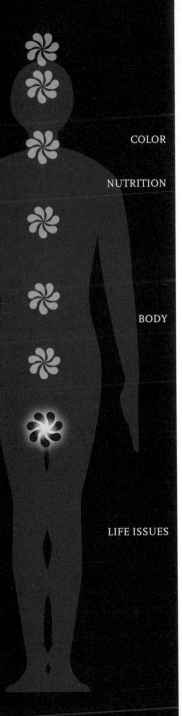

THE ROOT

COLOR Red

NUTRITION
- Protein (animal and vegetable)
- Minerals (e.g., calcium, iron, zinc)
- Red foods (e.g., cherries, pomegranates, apples)

BODY
- Protein-containing structures (e.g., muscles, skin)
- Mineral-containing structures (e.g., bones
- Immune system
- Adrenal glands and stress hormones (e.g., cortisol, adrenaline)
- Lower body from legs to feet
- DNA: individual identity, genetic identity, inheritance, and blood

LIFE ISSUES
- Safety and the ability to survive in a physical world
- Connections to people and social networks: family, communities, "tribes"
- Rootedness, groundedness: relationship to the physical earth

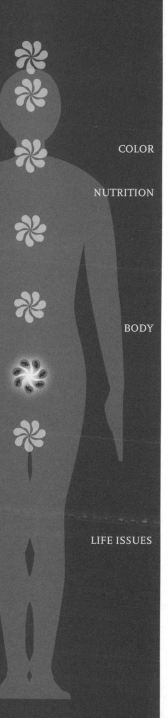

THE FLOW

COLOR   Orange

NUTRITION
- Fats and oils (unsaturated and saturated fats)
- Orange foods (e.g., carrots, sweet potatoes, citrus fruits, salmon)
- Water

BODY
- Reproductive system: ovaries, testes
- Urinary system: kidneys, bladder, urethra
- Large intestine, which pulls water from waste products

LIFE ISSUES
- Creativity: art, scientific discovery, problem-solving, new ideas, making a home beautiful, new recipes, foods from different cultures
- Fertility: producing new life, new ideas, new energy
- Partnerships or relationships with one other person

SYSTEM 3
THE FIRE

COLOR | Yellow

NUTRITION
- Carbohydrates: quick-burning sugars and starches, high-fiber foods
- Yellow foods (e.g., ginger root, yellow summer squash, banana)
- Whole grains and legumes high in fiber and B vitamins

BODY
- Digestive system: stomach, pancreas, liver, gallbladder, small intestine

LIFE ISSUES
- Drive and ambition
- Energy, power, and confidence
- Work-life balance vs. issues of burnout

SYSTEM 4
THE LOVE

COLOR — Green

NUTRITION
- Vegetables
- Green foods (e.g., spirulina, chlorella, leafy greens, broccoli, Brussels sprouts, kale)

BODY
- Heart and cardiovascular system: circulation of nutrients to care for the entire body
- Lungs and respiratory tract: associated with expansiveness and also with grief
- Thymus: adaptive immune system (responding to threats appropriately)
- Lymphatic system

LIFE ISSUES
- Compassion and service
- Self-care
- Expansion: feeling larger, more generous
- Grief
- Movement (e.g., aerobic activities like walking, dancing, jogging)

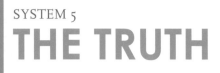

SYSTEM 5
THE TRUTH

COLOR	Aquamarine
NUTRITION	• Sea plants (e.g., nori, wakame, hijiki, dulse) • Fruits • Liquid foods (e.g., smoothies, soups, sauces, broths, stews, teas)
BODY	• Voice box (larynx) and throat • Thyroid gland • Sensory organs: ears, nose, throat, and mouth
LIFE ISSUES	• Authenticity • Voice: speaking your truth • Choices

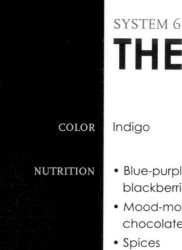

SYSTEM 6
THE INSIGHT

COLOR	Indigo

NUTRITION
- Blue-purple foods (e.g., blueberries, blackberries, kale, grapes)
- Mood-modulating foods (e.g., caffeine, chocolate, alcohol)
- Spices

BODY
- Pituitary gland, which organizes biochemicals necessary for thought and emotion
- Eyes
- Sleep
- Neurons, neurotransmitters, and brain
- Cognition and thought processing
- Mood

LIFE ISSUES
- Insight and intuition, the "inner eyes"
- Visualization
- Reflection and discernment

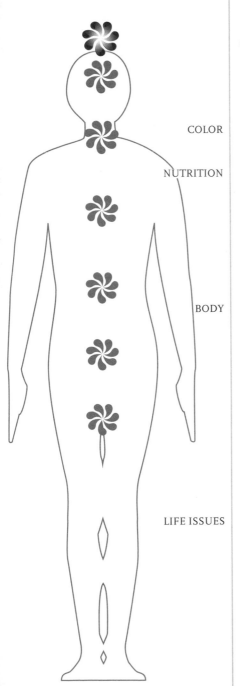

THE SPIRIT

COLOR | White

NUTRITION |
- White foods (natural, not bleached) (e.g., cauliflower, coconut products, onions, garlic, cabbage, white beans)
- Cleansing, purifying foods (e.g., lemon, organically grown foods)
- Fasting

BODY |
- Pineal gland, which modulates circadian rhythms
- Response to light
- Electromagnetic field

LIFE ISSUES |
- Spirituality
- Sense of purpose and meaning
- Feeling connected to something larger
- Awe, wonder, and gratitude

DAY 4: THE FLOW—EMOTIONS

*We all know that being able to express deep emotion can literally save a person's
life, and suppressing emotion can kill you both spiritually and physically.*

—LISA KLEYPAS

Meal Plan

	Omnivore	Vegan
Breakfast	Tropical Smoothie	Tropical Smoothie
Lunch	Shredded Carrot and Cabbage Salad with Mediterranean Cod	Shredded Carrot and Cabbage Salad with Nut-Seed Pâté
Snack	Nectarine and Macadamia Nuts	Nectarine and Macadamia Nuts
Dinner	Wild Salmon with Tangy Apricot Sauce and Greens	Creamy Carrot Coconut Curry Soup

Whole Detox Emotion Log

At the end of the day, track any emotions that you had on the Whole Detox
Emotion Log.

Thought Pattern Activity

The following are some limiting thoughts that relate to the FLOW:

How I feel isn't important.
My emotions need to be controlled.
I fear becoming lost in my emotions.

Pick the limiting thought that seems to ring most true for you. If none
of the examples feel true, write down your own limiting thought as it
relates to the FLOW.

Next, set your timer for five minutes. Spend that time journaling on
that thought, how it has affected your life, and how you feel when you have
that thought.

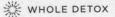

Movement

Enjoy a swim or some water aerobics! Depending upon your geographical location, you may opt to take a dip in an indoor pool. However, if you have the option, natural bodies of water are best. Swimming puts minimal stress on the joints and strengthens the cardiovascular system. Even if you don't consider yourself a great swimmer, the backstroke is one of the easier, more relaxing swimming strokes. If you don't have access to a pool of any type, making large swimming motions with your arms to engage your cardiovascular system.

Affirmation

Spend three minutes saying aloud the following affirmation:

I am open to my fullest, healthiest emotional expression.

Feel how your body responds to these words. You can also create your own statement. Feel free to write it on a beautiful notecard or a plain Post-it note and put it in your immediate environment for the day.

Visualization

Set a timer for three minutes. During that time, close your eyes and visualize yourself being in the flow of your emotional expression. Imagine any happy feelings dancing inside you and creating healthy movement. Let these happy feelings visit the places within you that feel stuck and stagnant, allowing for greater movement and ease.

Meditation

For three minutes, sit still with your hands cupped in your low belly region. Close your eyes and do a scan of your body from top to bottom, looking for stored, stuck emotions. If you find any, meditate on that place. Create a dialogue with the emotion using a journal.

DAY 4 RECIPES

Breakfast

TROPICAL SMOOTHIE
Serves 1

1 cup peach slices

1 small banana

1 cup unsweetened coconut milk
  (boxed variety)

1 tablespoon flaxseed meal

1 tablespoon unsweetened coconut
  flakes

½ teaspoon ground cardamom

½ teaspoon ground cinnamon

1 scoop protein powder of your choice
  (hemp, pea, rice, whey for omnivores)

Water and ice as needed

Put all the liquid and whole food ingredients into a high-speed blender first, followed by the dry ingredients, then blend everything until a fluid consistency is reached. Add more water if needed. Drink immediately.

NUTRITION INFORMATION PER SERVING

Calories	Protein (g)	Carbs (g)	Fat (g)	Sat Fat (g)	Unsat Fat (g)	Fiber (g)
390	28	42	13	8	0.1	7

Lunch

SHREDDED CARROT AND CABBAGE SALAD WITH MEDITERRANEAN COD (OMNIVORE) OR NUT-SEED PÂTÉ (VEGAN)
Serves 1

FOR OMNIVORES:

1 tablespoon extra-virgin olive oil

½ teaspoon ground oregano

3 ounces wild-caught cod

Juice of ½ medium lemon

FOR VEGANS:

¼ cup raw sunflower seeds, soaked for
  several hours and rinsed

¼ cup raw pine nuts, soaked for several
  hours and rinsed

2 tablespoons tahini

⅛ teaspoon ground cumin

Juice of ½ medium lemon

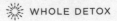

FOR BOTH:

½ cup shredded carrots

½ cup shredded red cabbage

1 handful mixed greens, about 1 cup, cut into bite-size pieces

½ avocado (saved from yesterday), cubed

Sea salt and ground black pepper to taste

FOR THE DRESSING

2 tablespoons orange juice

1 tablespoon high-oleic sunflower oil or extra-virgin olive oil

¼ teaspoon parsley flakes

In a small bowl, combine the carrots and cabbage. In another small bowl, whisk together all the dressing ingredients, then pour the dressing over the carrots and cabbage. Set the salad aside.

Omnivores, heat the olive oil in a skillet set over medium-high heat, then stir in the oregano. Gently add the cod to the skillet and squeeze the lemon juice on top. Let the cod cook until it's firm, about 5 minutes on each side. While it's cooking, arrange the mixed greens and avocado on a serving plate. Place the cooked cod on the greens, and top the cod with the salad (or put it to the side if you prefer). Season to taste.

Vegans, in a high-speed blender or food processor, blend the sunflower seeds, pine nuts, tahini, cumin, and lemon juice, adding water as needed for consistency. Arrange the mixed greens and avocado on a serving plate. Spoon the salad on top of the greens, followed by the nut and seed blend. Season to taste.

NUTRITION INFORMATION PER SERVING

	Calories	Protein (g)	Carbs (g)	Fat (g)	Sat Fat (g)	Unsat Fat (g)	Fiber (g)
Omnivore	535	19	22	44	6	46	10
Vegan	720	18	32	64	7	40	11

Snack

NECTARINE AND MACADAMIA NUTS
Serves 1

> 1 medium nectarine (or orange if you prefer)
> 1 scant handful (about 10) macadamia nuts

NUTRITION INFORMATION PER SERVING

Calories	Protein (g)	Carbs (g)	Fat (g)	Sat Fat (g)	Unsat Fat (g)	Fiber (g)
245	3	19	20	3	16	4

Dinner

WILD SALMON WITH TANGY APRICOT SAUCE AND GREENS *(OMNIVORE)*
Serves 2

> 1 tablespoon plus 2 teaspoons extra-virgin olive oil
>
> 1 8- to 10-ounce wild-caught salmon fillet
>
> 2 handfuls arugula or other leafy greens, about 2 cups
>
> 1 teaspoon freshly squeezed lemon juice
>
> 1 teaspoon dried dill

FOR THE SAUCE:

> 3 apricots, pitted and diced
>
> 3 tablespoons balsamic vinegar
>
> 1 teaspoon minced fresh ginger
>
> 1 tablespoon sesame oil
>
> 4 tablespoons orange juice (fresh-squeezed preferred)
>
> 1 teaspoon orange zest

In a skillet set over low heat, warm 1 tablespoon of the olive oil. Place the salmon in the oil with its skin side down. Cover the skillet and let the salmon cook.

Meanwhile, make the sauce. In a small saucepan set over medium heat, combine the apricots, vinegar, and ginger, and stir the mixture for about 2 to 3 minutes. Reduce the heat to low, and add the sesame oil, orange juice, and orange zest, combining everything well. Then pour this heated mixture on top of the salmon, continuing to cook until the salmon is done, turning it on each side for a total cooking time of about 7 to 10 minutes.

In a bowl, lightly toss the greens with the remaining olive oil, lemon juice, and dill. Transfer them to a serving plate, then dish half the salmon alongside them. (Save the other half of the salmon for tomorrow's lunch.)

NUTRITION INFORMATION PER SERVING

Calories	Protein (g)	Carbs (g)	Fat (g)	Sat Fat (g)	Unsat Fat (g)	Fiber (g)
470	36	14	29	5	23	1

CREAMY CARROT COCONUT CURRY SOUP *(VEGAN)*

Serves 2

2 teaspoons coconut oil

½ medium yellow onion, chopped

8 medium to large carrots, scrubbed, cut into ½-inch-thick rounds

2 teaspoons curry powder

¼ teaspoon ginger powder

1 cup purified water

2 cups organic vegetable broth

3 tablespoons almond butter

½ cup unsweetened, full-fat coconut milk (canned)

Sea salt and freshly ground pepper to taste

In a large saucepan or soup pot set over medium heat, melt the coconut oil. Add the onion, sautéing it 3 to 4 minutes, or until it becomes soft and translucent. Add the carrots, curry powder, ginger powder, and water, and let the mixture cook, stirring it constantly, for another 30 seconds. Pour in the broth, raise the heat to high, and bring the soup to a boil. As soon as it reaches a boil, reduce the heat to low and partially cover the pot. Simmer the soup about 15 minutes, preferably until the carrots are somewhat tender. Add the almond butter and the coconut milk, stirring for an additional 30 seconds, allowing the nut butter to melt slightly.

Carefully transfer the soup in batches to a high-speed blender or food processor, or use a wand mixer in the pot, and blend the soup until it's smooth. Season it with salt and pepper.

Ladle half the soup into a serving bowl and eat it while it's hot. (Save the remaining half of the soup for tomorrow's lunch.)

NUTRITION INFORMATION PER SERVING

Calories	Protein (g)	Carbs (g)	Fat (g)	Sat Fat (g)	Unsat Fat (g)	Fiber (g)
445	8	38	32	16	14	9

DAY 5: THE FLOW—CREATIVITY

Creativity involves breaking out of established patterns in order to look at things in a different way.

—EDWARD DE BONO

Meal Plan

	Omnivore	Vegan
Breakfast	Mango-Peach-Ginger Smoothie	Mango-Peach-Ginger Smoothie
Lunch	Kale and Carrot Salad with Orange Cardamom Dressing Wild Salmon with Tangy Apricot Sauce	Kale and Carrot Salad with Orange Cardamom Dressing Creamy Carrot Coconut Curry Soup
Snack	Orange Bell Pepper with Walnut Pesto	Orange Bell Pepper with Walnut Pesto
Dinner	Rosemary Lamb and Herbed Quinoa	Rosemary Lentils and Herbed Quinoa

Whole Detox Emotion Log

At the end of the day, track any emotions that you had on the Whole Detox Emotion Log.

Thought Pattern Activity

The following are some limiting thoughts that relate to the FLOW:

I'm not very creative.
I rarely have good ideas.
Creativity is for artists only.

Pick the limiting thought that seems to ring most true for you. If none of the examples feel true, write down your own limiting thought as it relates to the FLOW.

Next, set your timer for five minutes. Spend that time journaling on that thought, how it has affected your life, and how you feel when you have that thought.

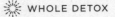

Movement

The FLOW is centered in the area just below your waist and stomach—the area where your reproductive organs, kidneys, and bladder are located. Get your energy flowing by working your hips: Spin a hula hoop around your waist for three minutes. If you don't have a hula hoop, sit on the floor, open your legs as wide as you comfortably can, and stretch with a flat back (as best you can) over to each foot. Make sure your back is as straight as you can make it—don't let it curve—as you keep your neck aligned with your back. Reach from side to side, pulling out of your hip area and giving yourself a maximal stretch forward, to the level of comfort only.

Affirmation

Spend three minutes saying aloud the following affirmation:

I am highly creative in my actions and thoughts.

Feel how your body responds to these words. You can also create your own statement. Feel free to write it on a beautiful notecard or a plain Post-it note and put it in your immediate environment for the day.

Visualization

Set a timer for three minutes. During that time, close your eyes and visualize yourself feeling the flow of the creative force. Imagine that it, similar to a waterfall, cascades over you and enters every cell of your being, making you feel more vibrant and playful in all you do and think.

Meditation

For three minutes let yourself do a flowing meditation by sitting quietly in a chair while you move your upper body in a slow, circular motion.

DAY 5 RECIPES

Breakfast

MANGO-PEACH-GINGER SMOOTHIE
Serves 1

½ mango, cored and diced (save the
  other half for tomorrow's smoothie)
1 small peach, sliced
2 Medjool dates, pitted
1 teaspoon grated fresh ginger
½ teaspoon ground cinnamon

½ cup unsweetened almond milk
1 tablespoon flaxseed meal
1 scoop protein powder of your choice
  (hemp, pea, rice, whey for omnivores)
Water and ice to blend

Put all the liquid and whole food ingredients into a high-speed blender first, followed by the dry ingredients, then blend everything until a fluid consistency is reached. Add more water if needed. Drink immediately.

NUTRITION INFORMATION PER SERVING

Calories	Protein (g)	Carbs (g)	Fat (g)	Sat Fat (g)	Unsat Fat (g)	Fiber (g)
328	28	45	6	0.1	0.4	7

Lunch

KALE AND CARROT SALAD WITH ORANGE CARDAMOM DRESSING
Serves 1

2 handfuls chopped kale, about 2 large
  leaves

½ cup grated carrots
1 tablespoon chia seeds

FOR THE DRESSING:

2 tablespoons orange juice
1 tablespoon extra-virgin olive oil
½ garlic clove, minced

¼ teaspoon ground cardamom
Dash of sea salt
Dash of ground black pepper

Arrange the kale, carrots, and chia seeds on a serving plate. In a small bowl, whisk together all the ingredients for the dressing, then pour it over the salad.

Warm up yesterday's leftover Wild Salmon with Tangy Apricot Sauce (*omnivore*; or eat the salmon at room temperature if you prefer) or Creamy Carrot Coconut Curry Soup (*vegan*) to serve with the salad.

NUTRITION INFORMATION PER SERVING

	Calories	Protein (g)	Carbs (g)	Fat (g)	Sat Fat (g)	Unsat Fat (g)	Fiber (g)
Omnivore	775	42	44	48	8	40	10
Vegan	750	16	68	51	19	31	18

Snack

ORANGE BELL PEPPER WITH WALNUT PESTO

Makes about 3 cups pesto

7 large garlic cloves

1 cup fresh basil leaves

2 cups walnut halves

½ cup raw pine nuts

2 tablespoons freshly squeezed lemon juice

1 cup extra-virgin olive oil

½ teaspoon sea salt

Dash of ground black pepper

1 orange bell pepper, sliced

Combine the garlic, basil, walnuts, pine nuts, lemon juice, olive oil, salt, and pepper in a high-speed blender or food processor, blending the mixture until it is smooth. Add additional lemon juice, olive oil, salt, or pepper to taste.

Dip the slices of orange bell pepper in some of the pesto for your snack. (Store the remaining pesto in a glass jar in the refrigerator for use in other meals over the next several days.)

NUTRITION INFORMATION PER SERVING

Calories	Protein (g)	Carbs (g)	Fat (g)	Sat Fat (g)	Unsat Fat (g)	Fiber (g)
529	7	16	51	6	43	5

Dinner

ROSEMARY LAMB *(OMNIVORE)* OR LENTILS *(VEGAN)* AND HERBED QUINOA
Serves 2

FOR OMNIVORES:

10 ounces organic, grass-fed ground lamb (makes about 6 meatballs)

FOR VEGANS:

1½ cups barely, or not fully, cooked orange/red lentils

FOR BOTH:

2 teaspoons extra-virgin olive oil

2 tablespoons chopped cashews or other nuts of choice (optional)

1½ teaspoons dried rosemary

1 teaspoon dried thyme

1 teaspoon parsley flakes

1 teaspoon dried sage

½ garlic clove, minced

Pinch of ground black pepper

1½ teaspoons freshly squeezed orange juice

½ cup cooked quinoa, cooked according to package directions (this is enough for just one serving)

Omnivores, in a mixing bowl, combine well the lamb, chopped nuts, rosemary, thyme, parsley, sage, garlic, pepper, and orange juice. Divide the mixture into six equal portions and roll each one in your hand to form 6 medium meatballs. In a skillet, heat the olive oil and brown the meatballs for 15 to 20 minutes, turning as needed.

Vegans, in a skillet set over medium heat, warm the olive oil with the partially cooked lentils. Stir in the chopped nuts, rosemary, thyme, parsley, sage, garlic, pepper, and orange juice, and cook the mixture for about 5 to 7 minutes.

Both omnivores and vegans, spoon the cooked quinoa onto a serving plate.

Omnivores, add to the plate 3 meatballs. (Save the remaining 3 meatballs for tomorrow's lunch.)

Vegans, place half the lentil mixture onto the plate with the quinoa. (Save the remaining lentils for tomorrow's lunch.)

Season to taste and serve warm.

NUTRITION INFORMATION PER SERVING

	Calories	Protein (g)	Carbs (g)	Fat (g)	Sat Fat (g)	Unsat Fat (g)	Fiber (g)
Omnivore	525	33	23	33	11	18	3
Vegan	395	18	51	14	2	9	10

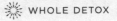

DAY 6: THE FLOW—FATS AND OILS

Thirty years of nutritional advice have left us fatter, sicker, and more poorly nourished. Which is why we find ourselves in the predicament we do: in need of a whole new way to think about eating.

—MICHAEL POLLAN

Meal Plan

	Omnivore	Vegan
Breakfast	Orange Bliss Smoothie	Orange Bliss Smoothie
Lunch	Citrus Fennel Salad Rosemary Lamb	Citrus Fennel Salad Rosemary Lentils
Snack	Avocado and Pumpkin Seeds	Avocado and Pumpkin Seeds
Dinner	Macadamia Nut-Encrusted Halibut with Mango Curry Chutney Seasoned Leeks	Wild Rice and Nut-Stuffed Orange Bell Pepper with Mango Curry Chutney Seasoned Leeks

Whole Detox Emotion Log
At the end of the day, track any emotions that you had on the Whole Detox Emotion Log.

Thought Pattern Activity
The following are some limiting thoughts that relate to the FLOW:

It's difficult to go with the flow of life.
If I eat fat, I'll get fat.
I fear fat.

Pick the limiting thought that seems to ring most true for you. If none of the examples feel true, write down your own limiting thought as it relates to the FLOW.

Next, set your timer for five minutes. Spend that time journaling on that thought, how it has affected your life, and how you feel when you have that thought.

Movement

CHILD'S POSE (BALASANA)

This is one of the most powerful poses to connect you to your breath. It is a relaxing and restorative pose that releases tension in the lower back, massages the internal organs, and gently opens the hips. Go only to the degree that you feel comfortable.

1. Kneel on a mat or blanket.
2. Separate your knees about hip-width apart and sit on your heels, if you can, or put a folded blanket or block under you to come closer down to the floor.
3. Exhale and slowly fold over. Let your forehead rest on the mat or blanket.
4. You can let your arms go back so they are resting by your feet or you can stretch your arms out in front of you, palms down.
5. Maintain this position for three minutes. Take several deep inhalations and exhalations. Feel the flow of air in your abdomen. Observe how you feel.

Affirmation

Spend three minutes saying aloud the following affirmation:

I flow freely and fluidly in every moment.

Feel how your body responds to these words. You can also create your own statement. Feel free to write it on a beautiful notecard or a plain Post-it note and put it in your immediate environment for the day.

Visualization

Set a timer for three minutes. During that time, close your eyes and visualize yourself as moving particles. See where in your body the particles are moving rapidly or too slowly. Allow all of them to come into a synchronous, rhythmic dance. Feel the freedom of this dynamic movement coursing through you.

Meditation

For three minutes, meditate in the presence of running water, such as a stream, river, or even a fountain (small or large). You can also listen to a CD playing sounds of running water. While you are in the moment, listening,

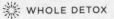
imagine that a generous flow of healthy energy moves through you at a pace that is just right.

DAY 6 RECIPES

Breakfast

ORANGE BLISS SMOOTHIE
Serves 1

½ mango, diced (saved from
yesterday's smoothie)

½ medium carrot, finely diced or grated
to make it easy to blend

½ cup freshly squeezed orange juice

½ cup unsweetened almond milk

½ teaspoon pumpkin spice powder

1 scoop protein powder of your choice
(hemp, pea, rice, whey for omnivores)

Water and ice to blend

Put all the liquid and whole food ingredients into a high-speed blender first, followed by the dry ingredients, then blend everything until a fluid consistency is reached. Add more water if needed. Drink immediately.

NUTRITION INFORMATION PER SERVING

Calories	Protein (g)	Carbs (g)	Fat (g)	Sat Fat (g)	Unsat Fat (g)	Fiber (g)
275	26	35	4	0.1	0.1	3

Lunch

CITRUS FENNEL SALAD WITH ROSEMARY LAMB *(OMNIVORE)* OR LENTILS *(VEGAN)*
Serves 1

1 orange, peeled and sectioned

½ fennel bulb, very thinly sliced (save
the other half for tomorrow's lunch;
use the fronds in the dressing)

½ avocado, sliced (leave the pit in the
other ½ and save it for today's snack)

¼ medium shallot, very thinly sliced

2 tablespoons chopped walnut halves

2 tablespoons chopped fresh mint
leaves

FOR THE DRESSING:

1 tablespoon extra-virgin olive oil
1 tablespoon apple cider vinegar
1½ teaspoons honey

1 tablespoon fennel fronds, finely
 chopped
Dash of sea salt
Dash of ground black pepper

In a bowl, gently toss together the orange sections and fennel bulb slices. Add the avocado, shallot, walnuts, and mint, and toss well. Transfer the salad to a serving plate or bowl, and set it aside.

In a small bowl, whisk together the olive oil and apple cider vinegar. Add the honey and fennel fronds, and season the mix with salt and pepper. Pour the dressing over the salad.

Warm up yesterday's leftover Rosemary Lamb (*omnivore*) or Lentils (*vegan*) to serve with the salad.

NUTRITION INFORMATION PER SERVING

	Calories	Protein (g)	Carbs (g)	Fat (g)	Sat Fat (g)	Unsat Fat (g)	Fiber (g)
Omnivore	903	36	53	63	15	45	14
Vegan	773	21	81	44	6	36	21

Snack

AVOCADO AND PUMPKIN SEEDS
Serves 1

½ avocado (saved from lunch)
Sea salt to taste

2 tablespoons roasted pumpkin seeds

Sprinkle the avocado with the salt, then eat it with the pumpkin seeds.

NUTRITION INFORMATION PER SERVING

Calories	Protein (g)	Carbs (g)	Fat (g)	Sat Fat (g)	Unsat Fat (g)	Fiber (g)
287	7	11	25	4	12	7

Dinner

MACADAMIA NUT–ENCRUSTED HALIBUT *(OMNIVORE)*
Serves 2

¼ cup brown rice flour

2 tablespoons flaxseed meal

2 tablespoons melted coconut oil, divided

¼ to ⅓ cup orange juice

¼ cup finely chopped, lightly salted macadamia nuts

2 5-ounce wild-caught halibut fillets

2 tablespoons finely chopped green onion, for garnish

In a small bowl, combine the flour and flaxseed meal, and transfer it to a shallow dish or plate. In a separate shallow dish, combine 1 tablespoon of the melted coconut oil with the orange juice. Put the macadamia nuts in a third shallow dish or on a plate.

Dip a fillet in the flour mixture, coating both sides, then in the coconut oil and orange juice mixture, and finally in the nuts, completely coating the fillet. Repeat the same with the second piece of fish.

In a skillet set over medium heat, warm the remaining tablespoon of coconut oil. Place the fillets in the skillet and cook both sides of each well, about 5 to 7 minutes total, or until done. Remove the fish from the heat.

Transfer 1 fillet to a serving plate, and sprinkle it with the green onion. Optionally, you may top it with the Mango Curry Chutney (recipe follows). (Save the second fillet for tomorrow's lunch.) Serve the halibut alongside the Seasoned Leeks (recipe follows).

NUTRITION INFORMATION PER SERVING

Calories	Protein (g)	Carbs (g)	Fat (g)	Sat Fat (g)	Unsat Fat (g)	Fiber (g)
511	34	23	33	14	26	4

WILD RICE AND NUT–STUFFED ORANGE BELL PEPPER *(VEGAN)*
Serves 2

1 tablespoon extra-virgin olive oil
½ cup chopped yellow onion
2 garlic cloves, minced
1 cup organic vegetable broth
½ cup uncooked wild rice
½ cup dried sprouted lentils
¼ cup diced celery
¼ cup carrot, sliced in ½-inch-thick rounds

¼ cup raw cashews
2 tablespoons slivered almonds
⅛ teaspoon dried rosemary
⅛ teaspoon ground oregano
Pinch of sea salt
2 large orange bell peppers, stemmed and seeded but left whole

In a large saucepan, heat the olive oil and sauté the onion and garlic until the onion is soft. Add the broth, rice, sprouted lentils, celery, and carrot. Bring the mixture to a boil, then cover the pan, reduce the heat, and let it simmer for 20 to 25 minutes, or until the rice is almost done.

Meanwhile, in a small bowl, combine the cashews, almonds, rosemary, oregano, and salt. When the rice and vegetables are ready, remove them from the heat and stir in the nut and spice mixture, then set it aside.

Fill another saucepan with a few inches of water and set the bell peppers, top side up, in the water. Bring the pot to a boil and cook the peppers for 2 to 3 minutes, or until they are slightly tender. Remove them from the water and place one on a serving plate.

Stuff the pepper with half the rice-nut mixture and spoon any excess of that half-portion around the pepper. Do the same with the second pepper, using the remaining half of the rice-nut mixture. (Save the second stuffed pepper for tomorrow's lunch.)

Serve the stuffed pepper with a dollop of Mango Curry Chutney (recipe follows) and alongside the Seasoned Leeks (recipe follows).

NUTRITION INFORMATION PER SERVING

Calories	Protein (g)	Carbs (g)	Fat (g)	Sat Fat (g)	Unsat Fat (g)	Fiber (g)
587	23	85	20	3	15	14

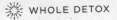

MANGO CURRY CHUTNEY

Makes about ¾ to 1 cup

- ½ tablespoon sesame oil
- ¼ teaspoon ground cayenne pepper
- 1 tablespoon curry powder
- 2 tablespoons diced yellow onion
- ½ tablespoon minced fresh ginger
- 2 tablespoons golden raisins
- 1 fresh, ripe mango, cut into strips, or ¾ cup frozen mango
- ¼ cup orange juice
- 2 tablespoons apple cider vinegar

In a small skillet, heat the oil and add the cayenne pepper, curry powder, and onion. When the onion becomes soft, add the ginger, raisins, and mango, and continue sautéing the mixture for 1 minute.

In a small mixing bowl, combine the orange juice and vinegar. Add this to the skillet, and continue simmering on low heat, stirring frequently, for 15 to 20 minutes, or until the chutney is slightly thickened. Then remove it from the heat.

After the chutney has cooled, store any leftovers in a glass jar in the refrigerator.

NUTRITION INFORMATION PER SERVING

Calories	Protein (g)	Carbs (g)	Fat (g)	Sat Fat (g)	Unsat Fat (g)	Fiber (g)
51	0.4	10	1	0.2	1	1

SEASONED LEEKS

Serves 1

- 1 tablespoon extra-virgin olive oil
- 1 cup sliced leeks
- Seasoning of your choice (oregano, dill, thyme, etc.)

In a skillet set over medium-high heat, warm the olive oil, then stir-fry the leeks for 3 to 4 minutes, adding whatever herbs or spices you desire. Serve warm.

NUTRITION INFORMATION PER SERVING

Calories	Protein (g)	Carbs (g)	Fat (g)	Sat Fat (g)	Unsat Fat (g)	Fiber (g)
125	1	9	10	1	8	1

DAY 7: THE FIRE—STRESS

Every day we have plenty of opportunities to get angry, stressed, or offended. But what you're doing when you indulge these negative emotions is giving something outside yourself power over your happiness. You can choose to not let little things upset you.

—JOEL OSTEEN

Meal Plan

	Omnivore	Vegan
Breakfast	Spice Shake	Spice Shake
Lunch	Arugula and Fennel Salad Macadamia Nut-Encrusted Halibut with Mango Curry Chutney	Arugula and Fennel Salad Wild Rice and Nut-Stuffed Orange Bell Pepper with Mango Curry Chutney
Snack	Yellow Squash with Walnut Pesto	Yellow Squash with Walnut Pesto
Dinner	Chicken and Cauliflower Curry	Fiery Curry Lentil Soup

Whole Detox Emotion Log

At the end of the day, track any emotions that you had on the Whole Detox Emotion Log.

Thought Pattern Activity

The following are some limiting thoughts that relate to the FIRE:

I can't escape being burnt out.
Life is exhausting.
I can't help eating when I'm stressed.

Pick the limiting thought that seems to ring most true for you. If none of the examples feel true, write down your own limiting thought as it relates to the FIRE.

Next, set your timer for five minutes. Spend that time journaling on that thought, how it has affected your life, and how you feel when you have that thought.

Movement

TAI CHI "PUSH HANDS"

1. Begin by standing comfortably, with your left foot about eight inches in front of your right foot. Let your body weight settle onto your back right foot.
2. Position your hands about six inches in front of your chest, with your palms facing outward. Your hands should be shoulder-width apart. Don't let them move closer together or farther apart when making the movements.
3. Slowly shift your body weight forward onto your left foot. As you move forward, stretch your arms out, making a slow, horizontal circle with your hands.
4. Bring your hands back into your chest, shifting your weight back onto your right foot. Repeat the movement, keeping the same steady motions.

Get your entire body involved, feeling the expansion and contraction. Most important, have fun!

Affirmation

Spend three minutes saying aloud the following affirmation:

I am resilient and powerful from within.

Feel how your body responds to these words. You can also create your own statement. Feel free to write it on a beautiful notecard or a plain Post-it note and put it in your immediate environment for the day.

Visualization

Set a timer for three minutes. During that time, close your eyes and visualize yourself having your inner power center fill with the color yellow. Let the light beam brightly from that inner place, giving you the sensation of warmth, cheerfulness, and empowerment.

Meditation

For three minutes, meditate on your energy and how you can bring it into balance by assessing what needs to be burnt away and what needs additional sparking.

DAY 7 RECIPES

Breakfast

SPICE SHAKE
Serves 1

¼ cup raw almonds, preferably soaked
  overnight and rinsed well
2 cups purified water
1 Medjool date, pitted
½ teaspoon turmeric powder
½ teaspoon ground cinnamon

½ teaspoon ginger powder
½ teaspoon vanilla extract
Pinch of ground nutmeg
Pinch of ground clove
1 tablespoon coconut oil
Water and ice to blend

Put all the liquid and whole food ingredients into a high-speed blender first, followed by the dry ingredients, then blend everything until a fluid consistency is reached. Add more water if needed. Drink immediately.

NUTRITION INFORMATION PER SERVING

Calories	Protein (g)	Carbs (g)	Fat (g)	Sat Fat (g)	Unsat Fat (g)	Fiber (g)
346	8	13	32	13	17	5

Lunch

ARUGULA AND FENNEL SALAD WITH MACADAMIA NUT–ENCRUSTED HALIBUT (OMNIVORE) OR NUT-STUFFED ORANGE BELL PEPPER (VEGAN)
Serves 1

1 large handful arugula, about 2 cups
½ fennel bulb, thinly sliced (saved from yesterday)
2 tablespoons raw pine nuts

FOR THE DRESSING:

1 tablespoon freshly squeezed lemon
  juice
1 tablespoon extra-virgin olive oil

¼ teaspoon dried dill
Dash of ground black pepper
Dash of sea salt

Arrange the arugula, fennel, and pine nuts on a serving plate.

In a small bowl, whisk together all the ingredients for the dressing, then drizzle it over the salad.

Warm up yesterday's leftover Macadamia Nut–Encrusted Halibut (omnivore) or Wild Rice and Nut–Stuffed Orange Bell Pepper (*vegan*) to serve with the salad. Topping your leftovers with Mango Curry Chutney is optional.

NUTRITION INFORMATION PER SERVING

	Calories	Protein (g)	Carbs (g)	Fat (g)	Sat Fat (g)	Unsat Fat (g)	Fiber (g)
Omnivore	801	39	37	59	17	47	9
Vegan	877	28	99	46	6	36	19

Snack

YELLOW SQUASH WITH WALNUT PESTO
Serves 1

- 1 small yellow summer squash, sliced
- 2 tablespoons Walnut Pesto (saved from Day 5)

Dip the squash slices in the walnut pesto and enjoy!

NUTRITION INFORMATION PER SERVING

Calories	Protein (g)	Carbs (g)	Fat (g)	Sat Fat (g)	Unsat Fat (g)	Fiber (g)
481	5	6	50	6	43	2

Dinner

CHICKEN AND CAULIFLOWER CURRY *(OMNIVORE)*
Serves 2

- 1 tablespoon extra-virgin olive oil
- ½ large yellow onion, diced
- 2 large garlic cloves, minced
- ½-inch piece fresh ginger, minced
- ½ medium yellow bell pepper, cut into 2-inch strips
- 2 tablespoons unsweetened, full-fat coconut milk

1 teaspoon honey

2 teaspoons curry powder

1 teaspoon turmeric powder

1 teaspoon tapioca flour

¼ teaspoon sea salt

Pinch of ground black pepper

2 cups chopped cauliflower

2 4-ounce organic, free-range, boneless, skinless chicken breasts, cut into 1-inch pieces

1 cup cooked white quinoa

1 tablespoon chopped fresh cilantro

1 tablespoon chopped green onions

In a large skillet set over medium heat, warm the olive oil, then add the onion, garlic, ginger, and bell pepper, and cook the vegetables, stirring occasionally, until they are soft, about 5 to 7 minutes. Stir in the coconut milk, honey, curry powder, turmeric powder, tapioca flour, salt, and pepper. Bring the mixture to a boil, then add the cauliflower and chicken pieces. Reduce the heat to low, cover the skillet, and simmer the mixture for 15 to 20 minutes, or until the chicken is cooked and the cauliflower is soft.

Spoon the prepared quinoa onto a serving plate, and top it with half the hot curry, then garnish the dish with the cilantro and green onions. (Save the remaining half of the curry for tomorrow's lunch.)

NUTRITION INFORMATION PER SERVING

Calories	Protein (g)	Carbs (g)	Fat (g)	Sat Fat (g)	Unsat Fat (g)	Fiber (g)
408	34	39	13	4	7	7

FIERY CURRY LENTIL SOUP (VEGAN)
Serves 2

1 teaspoon extra-virgin olive oil

2 large garlic cloves, minced

½ medium yellow onion, finely diced

½ cup uncooked yellow lentils, rinsed

2 carrots, sliced

1 large yellow potato, cut into 1-inch cubes

4 cups organic vegetable broth

1 teaspoon curry powder

1 teaspoon ground cumin

Dash of sea salt

Dash of ground black pepper

In a large stock pot set over medium heat, warm the olive oil, then add the garlic and onions, sautéing them until they are soft. Add the lentils, carrots, potato, broth, curry powder, cumin, salt, and pepper, and bring the mixture to a boil. Lower the heat and simmer the soup for 20 to 30 minutes, stirring occasionally, until the lentils are tender.

Serve half the soup warm. (Save the remaining half for tomorrow's lunch.)

NUTRITION INFORMATION PER SERVING

Calories	Protein (g)	Carbs (g)	Fat (g)	Sat Fat (g)	Unsat Fat (g)	Fiber (g)
414	17	79	5	0.4	2	15

DAY 8: THE FIRE—THOUGHTS

It takes but one positive thought when given a chance to survive and thrive to over-power an entire army of negative thoughts.

—ROBERT H. SCHULLER

Meal Plan

	Omnivore	Vegan
Breakfast	Sunshine Smoothie	Sunshine Smoothie
Lunch	Power-Packed Spinach Salad Chicken and Cauliflower Curry	Power-Packed Spinach Salad Fiery Curry Lentil Soup
Snack	Apple with Sunflower Seed Butter	Apple with Sunflower Seed Butter
Dinner	Turkey-Lentil Meatballs Roasted Spaghetti Squash	Seasoned Chickpeas Roasted Spaghetti Squash

Whole Detox Emotion Log

At the end of the day, track any emotions that you had on the Whole Detox Emotion Log.

Thought Pattern Activity

The following are some limiting thoughts that relate to the FIRE:

My thoughts are out of control.

I expect the worst to happen.

It's difficult to escape my negative thoughts.

Pick the limiting thought that seems to ring most true for you. If none of the examples feel true, write down your own limiting thought as it relates to the FIRE.

Next, set your timer for five minutes. Spend that time journaling on that thought, how it has affected your life, and how you feel when you have that thought.

Movement

WARRIOR POSE (VIRABHANDRASANA)

This exercise opens up your solar plexus area and hips. As with all yoga poses, go to your comfortable limit. Nothing should be painful.

1. Stand facing straight ahead with your arms at your sides.
2. Take a deep inhale, and on the exhalation, step your left foot back about three to four feet.
3. Pivot your left foot to a forty-five-degree angle, making sure it is firmly grounded on the mat.
4. Bend your right knee until the knee lines up with your right ankle and your shin is perpendicular to the floor.
5. Raise your arms above your head.
6. Take several deep inhalations and exhalations.
7. Maintain this position for one to two minutes.
8. Repeat the pose on the other side for one to two minutes.

Affirmation

Spend three minutes saying aloud the following affirmation:

Every thought I have frees me into possibilities.

Feel how your body responds to these words. You can also create your own statement. Feel free to write it on a beautiful notecard or a plain Post-it note and put it in your immediate environment for the day.

Visualization

Set a timer for three minutes. During that time, close your eyes and visualize yourself being filled with thoughts. See them as little lights. Find the ones that are burning bright and give you a sense of power and strength. Allow them to become brighter and stronger. As these bright thoughts fill you from within, you feel transformed. Possibilities seem endless; your potential is radiant.

Meditation

Sit with your thoughts for at least three minutes. Be a passive observer of the thoughts that rise and fall. When you are finished, jot down as many of the thoughts as you can remember. See which ones are coming up multiple times. Are they affirming and empowering or defeating and dismal? If the latter, create a new thought to cancel out anything that is draining to your FIRE.

Wait for a couple of hours and try again. See whether your thoughts have shifted.

DAY 8 RECIPES

Breakfast

SUNSHINE SMOOTHIE
Serves 1

1 small banana

1 cup pineapple juice

1 teaspoon freshly squeezed lemon
 juice

1-inch piece fresh ginger, grated

1 scoop protein powder of your choice
 (hemp, pea, rice, whey for omnivores)

Water and ice to blend

Put all the liquid and whole food ingredients into a high-speed blender first, followed by the dry ingredients, then blend everything until a fluid consistency is reached. Add more water if needed. Drink immediately.

NUTRITION INFORMATION PER SERVING

Calories	Protein (g)	Carbs (g)	Fat (g)	Sat Fat (g)	Unsat Fat (g)	Fiber (g)
341	25	57	2	0.1	0.1	3

Lunch

**POWER-PACKED SPINACH SALAD WITH CHICKEN AND CAULIFLOWER CURRY
(OMNIVORE) OR FIERY CURRY LENTIL SOUP (VEGAN)**
Serves 1

1 large handful spinach, about 2 cups
1½ tablespoons hemp seeds

1 tablespoon chia seeds
1 tablespoon minced shallot

FOR THE DRESSING:

1 tablespoon freshly squeezed lemon
juice
½ teaspoon honey

1½ tablespoons extra-virgin olive oil
½ teaspoon mustard seeds
Dash of sea salt

In a serving bowl, combine the spinach leaves with the hemp seeds, chia seeds, and shallot. Set the bowl aside.

In a small bowl, whisk together all the dressing ingredients, then drizzle the dressing over the salad.

Warm up yesterday's leftover Chicken and Cauliflower Curry (omnivore) or Fiery Curry Lentil Soup (vegan) to serve with the salad.

NUTRITION INFORMATION PER SERVING

	Calories	Protein (g)	Carbs (g)	Fat (g)	Sat Fat (g)	Unsat Fat (g)	Fiber (g)
Omnivore	667	38	37	41	8	28	10
Vegan	784	25	97	35	4	23	21

Snack

APPLE WITH SUNFLOWER SEED BUTTER
Serves 1

1 Golden Delicious apple, sliced

2 tablespoons sunflower seed butter

Spread the apple slices with the sunflower seed butter and enjoy!

NUTRITION INFORMATION PER SERVING

Calories	Protein (g)	Carbs (g)	Fat (g)	Sat Fat (g)	Unsat Fat (g)	Fiber (g)
265	6	31	15	2	13	9

Dinner

TURKEY-LENTIL MEATBALLS *(OMNIVORE)*

Serves 2 (makes 6 large meatballs)

1 tablespoon high-oleic sunflower oil or extra-virgin olive oil

½ medium yellow onion, finely chopped

1 garlic clove, minced

¼ cup finely chopped celery

¾ cup finely chopped kale

8 ounces organic, free-range ground turkey

½ cup cooked French green lentils

¼ cup almond meal (other nut meal or nut flour can be substituted, such as hazelnut)

¼ cup finely chopped fresh parsley

1 tablespoon Dijon mustard

1 teaspoon ground ginger

1 tablespoon flaxseed meal

1½ teaspoons sea salt

Freshly ground black pepper to taste

Preheat the oven to 400°F.

In a large skillet, heat the oil, then add the yellow onion and garlic, sautéing them for about a minute. Add the celery and kale, and continue sautéing until the vegetables soften.

In a large bowl, combine by hand the turkey, lentils, almond meal, parsley, mustard, ginger, flaxseed meal, salt, and pepper. Form the mixture into 6 1½-inch round balls, and place the meatballs on a parchment-lined baking sheet.

Bake the meatballs for 25 minutes, until they are lightly browned.

Enjoy 3 meatballs with a serving of the Roasted Spaghetti Squash (recipe follows). (Save the remaining 3 meatballs for tomorrow's lunch.)

NUTRITION INFORMATION PER SERVING

Calories	Protein (g)	Carbs (g)	Fat (g)	Sat Fat (g)	Unsat Fat (g)	Fiber (g)
223	15	12	13	2	6	5

SEASONED CHICKPEAS *(VEGAN)*

Serves 2

1 tablespoon extra-virgin olive oil

1 tablespoon cumin seeds

1 shallot, finely chopped

1 garlic clove, minced

1½ cups cooked chickpeas

Zest and juice of ½ lemon

2 tablespoons finely chopped fresh parsley

2 tablespoons finely chopped fresh thyme

Pinch of sea salt

Freshly ground black pepper to taste

In a large sauté pan, gently heat the olive oil, then stir in the cumin seeds, heating them for 1 to 2 minutes. Add the shallot and garlic, and sauté them for 3 to 4 minutes, stirring frequently. Add the chickpeas, stirring until all the ingredients are warmed and blended together.

Remove the pan from the heat, and stir in the lemon zest and juice, parsley, and thyme. Season the mixture with salt and pepper.

Spoon half the chickpeas onto a serving plate, alongside a serving of Roasted Spaghetti Squash (recipe follows). (Save the other half of the chickpeas for tomorrow's lunch.)

NUTRITION INFORMATION PER SERVING

Calories	Protein (g)	Carbs (g)	Fat (g)	Sat Fat (g)	Unsat Fat (g)	Fiber (g)
226	8	29	9	1	6	7

ROASTED SPAGHETTI SQUASH

Serves about 4

1 small spaghetti squash

1 tablespoon extra-virgin olive oil, plus more for drizzling

Sea salt and freshly ground black pepper to taste

Preheat the oven to 400°F.

Cut both ends off the squash, then cut the squash in half lengthwise. Scoop out the seeds and discard them. Drizzle the flesh of each half with the olive oil and sprinkle each with salt and pepper to taste.

Place the squash halves flesh side down in a glass baking dish filled with about ½ inch of water. Roast the squash in the oven for about 20 to 25 minutes, or until it is tender. Insert a knife in the center to check for doneness. Be careful not to overcook them.

When they are ready, remove them from the oven, discard the water, and use a fork to gently scrape out the flesh of both halves of the squash.

Place about a quarter of the "spaghetti" flesh into a large serving bowl. Drizzle it with a little more olive oil, and serve it with 3 Turkey-Lentil Meatballs (omnivore) or half the Seasoned Chickpeas (vegan). (Save the remaining squash flesh for any future snack or meal or for others in your family to enjoy; no more is required in your twenty-one-day program.)

NUTRITION INFORMATION PER SERVING

Calories	Protein (g)	Carbs (g)	Fat (g)	Sat Fat (g)	Unsat Fat (g)	Fiber (g)
93	2	15	4	0.6	3	3

DAY 9: THE FIRE —CARBOHYDRATES AND SUGAR

Everybody's got their poison, and mine is sugar.

—DERRICK ROSE

Meal Plan

	Omnivore	Vegan
Breakfast	Pineapple-Banana Spiced Smoothie	Pineapple-Banana Spiced Smoothie
Lunch	Quinoa, Amaranth, and Pine Nut Salad Turkey-Lentil Meatballs	Quinoa, Amaranth, and Pine Nut Salad Seasoned Chickpeas
Snack	Yellow Bell Pepper with Walnut Pesto	Yellow Bell Pepper with Walnut Pesto
Dinner	Sesame-Tahini Chicken	Black Beans with Tahini

Whole Detox Emotion Log

At the end of the day, track any emotions that you had on the Whole Detox Emotion Log.

Thought Pattern Activity

The following are some limiting thoughts that relate to the FIRE:

The only thing that picks me up is sugar.
I have difficulty finding sweetness in life.
I need quick energy to fuel my quickly moving life.

Pick the limiting thought that seems to ring most true for you. If none of the examples feel true, write down your own limiting thought as it relates to the FIRE.

Next, set your timer for five minutes. Spend that time journaling on that thought, how it has affected your life, and how you feel when you have that thought.

Movement

Stomach crunches: Lie on your back on a mat or blanket and place your hands behind your head. Bend your knees and lift your feet off the floor, pointing your toes toward the ceiling. Contract your stomach muscles and curl your tailbone, lifting your lower back slightly off the floor toward the ceiling. Return to the starting position and repeat for one to three minutes or until you feel a comfortable "burn." Know your limits! Exert yourself, but not to the point where it becomes painful.

Affirmation

Spend three minutes saying aloud the following affirmation:
My life is saturated with sweetness.

Feel how your body responds to these words. You can also create your own statement. Feel free to write it on a beautiful notecard or a plain Post-it note and put it in your immediate environment for the day.

Visualization

Set a timer for three minutes. During that time, close your eyes and visualize yourself inviting a thick, shining liquid of joy to coat your outer being. Then let every cell of your being on the inside feel relaxed and soothed, saturated with the syrupy sweetness of joy.

Meditation

For three minutes, meditate on the word "sweetness." What comes forth? End your meditation by making a list of all the ways you can make your life sweeter without indulging in dietary sweeteners.

DAY 9 RECIPES

Breakfast

PINEAPPLE-BANANA SPICED SMOOTHIE

Serves 1

1 cup unsweetened coconut milk
   (boxed variety)
½ cup pineapple chunks, frozen or fresh
1 small banana
½ tablespoon coconut oil
1 teaspoon turmeric powder

½ teaspoon ground cinnamon
½ teaspoon ground ginger
1 teaspoon chia seeds
1 scoop protein powder of your choice
   (hemp, pea, rice, whey for omnivores)
Water and ice to blend

Put all the liquid and whole food ingredients into a high-speed blender first, followed by the dry ingredients, then blend everything until a fluid consistency is reached. Add more water if needed. Drink immediately.

NUTRITION INFORMATION PER SERVING

Calories	Protein (g)	Carbs (g)	Fat (g)	Sat Fat (g)	Unsat Fat (g)	Fiber (g)
391	26	38	16	11	2	5

Lunch

QUINOA, AMARANTH, AND PINE NUT SALAD WITH TURKEY-LENTIL MEATBALLS (*OMNIVORE*) OR SEASONED CHICKPEAS (*VEGAN*)

Serves 1

½ cup cooked quinoa
½ cup cooked amaranth

Pinch of sea salt
¼ medium cucumber, diced

½ medium shallot, diced

¼ cup chopped fresh cilantro

¼ cup chopped fresh basil

1½ tablespoons extra-virgin olive oil

1 tablespoon freshly squeezed lemon juice

2 tablespoons raw pine nuts

Dash of ground black pepper

In a medium bowl, combine the quinoa and amaranth with a pinch of salt. In a separate bowl, toss together the cucumber, shallot, cilantro, basil, olive oil, and lemon juice, then add this to the quinoa-amaranth mixture, combining the salad well. Sprinkle in the pine nuts, and season with pepper to taste.

Serve the salad, warm or cold, with yesterday's leftover Turkey-Lentil Meatballs (*omnivore*) or Seasoned Chickpeas (*vegan*).

NUTRITION INFORMATION PER SERVING

	Calories	Protein (g)	Carbs (g)	Fat (g)	Sat Fat (g)	Unsat Fat (g)	Fiber (g)
Omnivore	794	28	64	49	6	37	12
Vegan	797	21	81	45	5	37	14

Snack

YELLOW BELL PEPPER WITH WALNUT PESTO
Serves 1

1 yellow bell pepper, sliced

2 tablespoons Walnut Pesto (saved from Day 5)

Dip the yellow bell pepper slices in the walnut pesto and savor!

NUTRITION INFORMATION PER SERVING

Calories	Protein (g)	Carbs (g)	Fat (g)	Sat Fat (g)	Unsat Fat (g)	Fiber (g)
529	7	16	51	6	43	5

Dinner

SESAME-TAHINI CHICKEN *(OMNIVORE)*

Serves 1

¼ cup uncooked organic long-grain brown rice

½ cup water or organic broth (vegetable or chicken)

¼ cup cubed yellow squash

1 tablespoon freshly squeezed lemon juice

2 4-ounce organic, free-range, boneless, skinless chicken breasts, cubed

Dash of sea salt

Dash of ground black pepper

1 tablespoon sesame oil, divided

½ tablespoon rice vinegar

1 teaspoon minced fresh ginger

1 garlic clove, minced or pressed

2 tablespoons chopped green onions

½ tablespoon unhulled sesame seeds

1 tablespoon tahini

Use a rice cooker to cook the rice with the squash, if one is available. If not, combine the rice with the ½ cup water or broth in a medium saucepan. Toss in the cubed squash, and bring the pot to a boil over medium-high heat. Reduce the heat to low and simmer the mixture, covered, until the rice is tender and the water has been absorbed, 30 to 40 minutes.

While the rice is cooking, in a medium bowl, pour the lemon juice over the chicken breasts and sprinkle them each with salt and pepper.

In a heated skillet, warm ½ tablespoon of the sesame oil, then add the chicken breasts and pan-fry them on medium heat until they are cooked through. Remove them from heat, and set aside half of the chicken. (Save the other half for tomorrow's lunch.)

In a small bowl, whisk the remaining ½ tablespoon sesame oil with the rice vinegar, ginger, and garlic. When the rice and squash have finished cooking and fully cooled, pour the oil and vinegar mixture into the rice and squash, tossing to coat everything. Add the green onion, then the cooked chicken, or keep the chicken on the side if you prefer.

Sprinkle the dish with the sesame seeds and drizzle the chicken with the tahini before serving.

NUTRITION INFORMATION PER SERVING

Calories	Protein (g)	Carbs (g)	Fat (g)	Sat Fat (g)	Unsat Fat (g)	Fiber (g)
526	35	47	22	3	16	4

BLACK BEANS WITH TAHINI *(VEGAN)*

Serves 2

2 teaspoons extra-virgin olive oil

½ medium red onion, diced

2 garlic cloves, minced

½ teaspoon ground cumin

1½ cups cooked black beans

1 large romaine lettuce heart

2 teaspoons minced, fresh cilantro

½ avocado, diced or sliced

2 tablespoons tahini

In a medium saucepan set over medium heat, warm the olive oil, then add the onion, garlic, and cumin, stirring the mixture for 2 to 3 minutes, or until the onion is soft and translucent. Add the black beans and simmer them until they are warmed through.

On a serving plate, arrange the romaine heart, then spoon half the beans alongside. (Save the remaining half of the beans for tomorrow's lunch.) Garnish the dish with the cilantro and avocado, and drizzle the romaine with tahini.

NUTRITION INFORMATION PER SERVING

Calories	Protein (g)	Carbs (g)	Fat (g)	Sat Fat (g)	Unsat Fat (g)	Fiber (g)
410	16	44	21	3	17	17

DAY 10: THE LOVE—SELF-CARE

Taking good care of you means the people in your life will receive the best of you rather than what's left of you.

—CARL BRYAN

Meal Plan

	Omnivore	Vegan
Breakfast	Emerald Smoothie	Emerald Smoothie
Lunch	Greenie Genie Salad Sesame-Tahini Chicken	Greenie Genie Salad Black Beans with Tahini
Snack	Kiwi and Pistachios	Kiwi and Pistachios
Dinner	Anchovies, White Beans, and Asparagus	White Beans and Asparagus

Whole Detox Emotion Log

At the end of the day, track any emotions that you had on the Whole Detox Emotion Log.

Thought Pattern Activity

The following are some limiting thoughts that relate to the LOVE:

If someone else needs help, I can't say no.
It's selfish to take care of myself or to put myself first.
I think it's wrong to spend time on me.

Pick the limiting thought that seems to ring most true for you. If none of the examples feel true, write down your own limiting thought as it relates to the LOVE.

Next, set your timer for five minutes. Spend that time journaling on that thought, how it has affected your life, and how you feel when you have that thought.

Movement

Focus on your heart and chest area by doing "doorway" stretches: Stand in a doorway within your living or work space and use one arm at a time to push against the doorframe while allowing the chest to expand forward. Alternate arms and repeat the movement for three minutes.

Affirmation

Spend three minutes saying aloud the following affirmation:

Love extends through me and is received by me in equal measure.

Feel how your body responds to these words. You can also create your own statement. Feel free to write it on a beautiful notecard or a plain Post-it note and put it in your immediate environment for the day.

Visualization

Set a timer for three minutes. During that time, close your eyes and visualize your heart as a flower. Reflect on a moment you felt loved and see the flower expanding open. Then connect to a memory in which you gave love to someone and see the flower continue to expand. Visualize your heart "flower" being nourished and opened by this wonderful exchange of giving and receiving love.

Meditation

You will need about ten minutes for this activity. Draw your heart on a piece of paper. Inside the heart, write the names of activities, foods, and people you find to be supportive. Outside the heart, write the names of activities, foods, and people that must remain on the outside of your heart. Meditate for four minutes on your final drawing. Do you find too much on the outside and not enough on the inside? Meditate on four ways you can be more nourishing toward yourself.

DAY 10 RECIPES

Breakfast

EMERALD SMOOTHIE
Serves 1

½ cup unsweetened decaffeinated green tea

½ cup unsweetened coconut milk (boxed variety)

¼ cup apple juice

¼ avocado (leave the pit in the rest and save it for today's and tomorrow's lunches)

¼ cup lightly steamed kale (about 4 large leaves)

½ green apple, sliced (save the rest for today's lunch)

1 scoop protein powder of your choice (hemp, pea, rice, whey for omnivores)

Water and ice to blend

Put all the liquid and whole food ingredients into a high-speed blender first, followed by the dry ingredients, then blend everything until a fluid consistency is reached. Add more water if needed. Drink immediately.

NUTRITION INFORMATION PER SERVING

Calories	Protein (g)	Carbs (g)	Fat (g)	Sat Fat (g)	Unsat Fat (g)	Fiber (g)
310	26	26	12	4	6	7

Lunch

GREENIE GENIE SALAD WITH SESAME-TAHINI CHICKEN *(OMNIVORE)* OR BLACK BEANS WITH TAHINI *(VEGAN)*

Serves 1

1 cup chopped broccoli

1 large handful microgreens, about 1 cup

½ green apple (saved from breakfast), sliced

½ avocado (saved from breakfast; save the remaining ¼ for tomorrow's lunch)

4 to 5 walnut halves

FOR THE DRESSING:

1 tablespoon avocado oil

1 tablespoon decaffeinated green tea

1 teaspoon freshly squeezed lime juice

Salt to taste

In a serving bowl, toss together the broccoli, greens, apple, avocado, and walnuts. In a separate small bowl, whisk together all the dressing ingredients and pour the dressing mixture over the salad.

Warm up yesterday's leftover Sesame-Tahini Chicken (omnivore) or Black Beans with Tahini (vegan) to serve with the salad.

NUTRITION INFORMATION PER SERVING

	Calories	Protein (g)	Carbs (g)	Fat (g)	Sat Fat (g)	Unsat Fat (g)	Fiber (g)
Omnivore	535	33	26	36	5	29	12
Vegan	820	23	70	56	7	45	29

Snack

KIWI AND PISTACHIOS

Serves 1

1 kiwi fruit

1 handful unsalted, raw, shelled pistachios, about 3 tablespoons

NUTRITION INFORMATION PER SERVING

Calories	Protein (g)	Carbs (g)	Fat (g)	Sat Fat (g)	Unsat Fat (g)	Fiber (g)
173	5	16	11	1	8	4

Dinner

ANCHOVIES *(OMNIVORE)*, WHITE BEANS, AND ASPARAGUS *(VEGAN)*
Serves 1

FOR OMNIVORES:

    4 anchovies (Vital Choice brand
       preferred)

    ½ cup cooked Great Northern beans

FOR VEGANS:

    ¾ cup cooked Great Northern beans

FOR BOTH:

    5 asparagus stalks, tough ends
       removed, cut into bite-size pieces

    1 tablespoon avocado oil

    1 garlic clove

    1 tablespoon minced green onion

    2 tablespoons minced fresh parsley

    5 green olives, sliced

    2 tablespoons raw pine nuts

Omnivores, drain any oil from the anchovies (if applicable), and cut them into bite-size pieces. Set them aside.

Both omnivores and vegans, steam the asparagus for 3 to 4 minutes or until it is bright green.

In a skillet set over medium heat, warm the avocado oil, then add the garlic and green onion, sautéing them for 1 to 2 minutes. Add the asparagus, parsley, beans, and anchovies (omnivore). Sauté for an additional 1 to 2 minutes.

Remove from the heat and transfer the mixture to a serving plate. Sprinkle the dish with the olives and pine nuts.

NUTRITION INFORMATION PER SERVING

	Calories	Protein (g)	Carbs (g)	Fat (g)	Sat Fat (g)	Unsat Fat (g)	Fiber (g)
Omnivore	470	18	32	33	3	27	8
Vegan	498	18	43	31	3	26	11

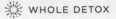

DAY 11: THE LOVE—MOVEMENT

Every breath we take, every step we make, can be filled with peace, joy, and serenity.

—THICH NHAT HANH

Meal Plan

	Omnivore	Vegan
Breakfast	Green Love Smoothie	Green Love Smoothie
Lunch	The Heart Salad	The Heart Salad
Snack	Seasoned Kale Chips	Seasoned Kale Chips
Dinner	Hearty Turkey Breast Super Spinach	Steamed Nutty Greens with Brown Rice

Whole Detox Emotion Log

At the end of the day, track any emotions that you had on the Whole Detox Emotion Log.

Thought Pattern Activity

The following are some limiting thoughts that relate to the LOVE:

It takes too much energy for me to move.
I have no time to exercise.
I can't do exercises as I'd like, so I don't want to do them at all.

Pick the limiting thought that seems to ring most true for you. If none of the examples feel true, write down your own limiting thought as it relates to the LOVE.

Next, set your timer for five minutes. Spend that time journaling on that thought, how it has affected your life, and how you feel when you have that thought.

Movement

Create a movement that represents you. Find a quiet place and play your favorite music. Sing along if you like! Immerse yourself in the rhythms and melodies. Let your body move organically and breathe deeply. Don't think about it. Don't hesitate for fear you'll look foolish. Express your inner love and merge with the music.

Affirmation

Spend three minutes saying aloud the following affirmation:

Love moves through my heart and blood vessels.

Feel how your body responds to these words. You can also create your own statement. Feel free to write it on a beautiful notecard or a plain Post-it note and put it in your immediate environment for the day.

Visualization

Set a timer for three minutes. During that time, close your eyes and visualize your heart. Place your attention there and see your heart as a green, healthy plant. Imagine that you "feed" your heart love, and each time you do so, it grows leaves, stems, and tendrils that extend throughout your arms and legs. You feel refreshed and healed by the soothing green energy moving through you.

Meditation

For three minutes, engage in a breath-focused meditation: Place both your hands over your heart and, as you inhale, feel your breath expanding your heart chambers and branching blood vessels, relaxing them and making them feel soft and supple. As you exhale, release all the tension held in your circulatory system into your hands while you open your hands up in front of you, palms facing outward. Continue with this pattern of breath until you feel relaxed and heart centered.

DAY 11 RECIPES

Breakfast

GREEN LOVE SMOOTHIE
Serves 1

1 kiwi fruit, peeled and sliced
½ small cucumber, peeled and sliced
1 large handful spinach leaves, about
   1½ cups
1 cup unsweetened coconut water

1 tablespoon raw cacao nibs
1 tablespoon chia seeds
1 scoop protein powder of your choice
   (hemp, pea, rice, whey for omnivores)
Water and ice to blend

Put all the liquid and whole food ingredients into a high-speed blender first, followed by the dry ingredients, then blend everything until a fluid consistency is reached. Add more water if needed. Drink immediately.

NUTRITION INFORMATION PER SERVING

Calories	Protein (g)	Carbs (g)	Fat (g)	Sat Fat (g)	Unsat Fat (g)	Fiber (g)
313	30	31	9	3	2	11

Lunch

THE HEART SALAD
Serves 1

FOR OMNIVORES:
   4 ounces lox

FOR VEGANS:
   ¼ cup cooked cannellini beans
   ¼ cup cooked lima beans

FOR BOTH:
   2 large handfuls spinach leaves, about
    3 cups
   ¼ avocado, diced (saved from
    yesterday)
   ¼ cup broccoli sprouts
   ¼ teaspoon fresh dill

   ¼ cup sliced strawberries, sliced in half
    to resemble heart shapes
   2 tablespoons toasted slivered almonds
   Dash each of sea salt and ground
    black pepper

FOR THE DRESSING:

    1 tablespoon flaxseed oil   ½ tablespoon balsamic vinegar

    1 tablespoon extra-virgin olive oil

Wash the spinach leaves and put them into a large serving bowl. Add the avocado, broccoli sprouts, and dill, and lightly toss everything. Top the salad with the strawberries and almonds.

Add all the dressing ingredients to a jar with a lid or a shaker cup, and shake to combine them well. Drizzle the salad with the dressing.

Omnivores, eat the salad with the lox; vegans, with the beans.

NUTRITION INFORMATION PER SERVING

	Calories	Protein (g)	Carbs (g)	Fat (g)	Sat Fat (g)	Unsat Fat (g)	Fiber (g)
Omnivore	587	27	19	47	6	39	9
Vegan	562	13	39	42	5	36	15

Snack

SEASONED KALE CHIPS

Serves 2 or more

    2 bunches green curly-leaf kale,   Sea salt

        washed and dried   1 teaspoon turmeric powder

    2 tablespoons avocado oil

Preheat the oven to 375°F.

Stem the kale by tearing the leafy greens from their tough stems, then tear the greens into smaller pieces, discarding the stems. In a large bowl, toss the leaves with the avocado oil, then add the salt and turmeric, and coat everything well.

Lightly oil two large baking sheets. Spread the leaves evenly on the sheets, and bake them in the oven for 5 minutes. Stir and turn the leaves, and continue baking for another 3 to 5 minutes, or until the leaves are crispy. Watch to be sure the chips do not burn.

(Save half the chips for tomorrow's snack.)

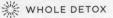
NUTRITION INFORMATION PER SERVING

Calories	Protein (g)	Carbs (g)	Fat (g)	Sat Fat (g)	Unsat Fat (g)	Fiber (g)
174	3	13	14	2	12	6

Dinner

HEARTY TURKEY BREAST *(OMNIVORE)*
Serves 2

1 tablespoon extra-virgin olive oil

¼ cup chopped green onions

1 garlic clove, minced

½ cup chopped spinach

¼ cup chopped shiitake mushrooms

1 teaspoon dried rosemary

1 teaspoon dried sage

Sea salt and ground black pepper to taste

2 4- to 5-ounce organic, free-range, boneless turkey breasts

Parchment paper

Kitchen twine

Preheat the oven to 375°F.

In a medium skillet, heat the olive oil, then sauté the onions, garlic, spinach, mushrooms, rosemary, and sage until the onions and mushrooms have softened slightly. Season with salt and pepper to taste. Remove the vegetables from the heat and set them aside.

Carefully slice each turkey breast lengthwise and spread open the breasts fully. Cover the meat with parchment paper, then pound it with a wooden or metal mallet (or rolling pin) until each piece is about ¼-inch thick. Trim the breasts until they are roughly a rectangle shape.

Spread a thin layer of the sautéed vegetables on each turkey breast. Tightly roll the breasts lengthwise and secure them using kitchen twine.

In a roasting pan or baking dish, add a thin layer of water, then lay the stuffed breasts in the water. Roast them for about 20 to 25 minutes, or until the turkey is slightly browned. Serve warm with Super Spinach (recipe follows).

(Save one roasted breast for tomorrow's lunch.)

NUTRITION INFORMATION PER SERVING

Calories	Protein (g)	Carbs (g)	Fat (g)	Sat Fat (g)	Unsat Fat (g)	Fiber (g)
192	29	2	8	1	6	0.4

SUPER SPINACH *(OMNIVORE)*
Serves 1

2 large handfuls spinach, about 3 cups   1 teaspoon hemp seeds, or to taste
1 teaspoon sesame oil

In a large skillet, bring about ¼ cup water to a boil. Add the spinach and
let it cook until it is wilted, about 2 minutes. Reduce the heat, and add the
sesame oil. Sprinkle hemp seeds on top as desired. Serve warm.

NUTRITION INFORMATION PER SERVING

Calories	Protein (g)	Carbs (g)	Fat (g)	Sat Fat (g)	Unsat Fat (g)	Fiber (g)
89	3	8	6	1	4	3

STEAMED NUTTY GREENS WITH BROWN RICE *(VEGAN)*
Serves 2

1 small bunch asparagus, about 12   2 tablespoons chopped fresh cilantro
stalks, tough ends removed   ½ teaspoon ground oregano
½ cup sliced Brussels sprouts, about   1 tablespoon Walnut Pesto (saved from
6 or 7   Day 5)
¾ cup cooked brown rice   Sea salt and ground black pepper to
½ avocado, cubed   taste
2 teaspoons apple cider vinegar   1 tablespoon avocado oil

Steam the asparagus and Brussels sprouts until they are tender.

In a bowl, combine the rice, avocado, vinegar, cilantro, oregano, and
pesto. Salt and pepper the mixture to taste.

Arrange half the cooked asparagus and Brussels sprouts around the edge
of a serving plate, and drizzle them with the avocado oil. Spoon half the
rice mixture into the center of the plate. (Save the other half of the rice and
vegetables for tomorrow's lunch.)

NUTRITION INFORMATION PER SERVING

Calories	Protein (g)	Carbs (g)	Fat (g)	Sat Fat (g)	Unsat Fat (g)	Fiber (g)
322	8	32	20	3	17	9

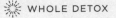

DAY 12: THE LOVE—VEGETABLES

Don't eat vegetables because they are good for you. Eat them for one reason alone. Because they are gorgeous.

—JILL DUPLEIX

Meal Plan

	Omnivore	Vegan
Breakfast	Mint-Green Smoothie	Mint-Green Smoothie
Lunch	Cucumber Salad Hearty Turkey Breast	Cucumber Salad Steamed Nutty Greens with Brown Rice
Snack	Seasoned Kale Chips	Seasoned Kale Chips
Dinner	Almond Salmon with Swiss Chard	Rosemary-Roasted Cauliflower with Spinach and Tahini

Whole Detox Emotion Log

At the end of the day, track any emotions that you had on the Whole Detox Emotion Log.

Thought Pattern Activity

The following are some limiting thoughts that relate to the LOVE:

I feel closed off.
It is difficult for me to recover from hurt.
I can't get beyond my grief.

Pick the limiting thought that seems to ring most true for you. If none of the examples feel true, write down your own limiting thought as it relates to the LOVE.

Next, set your timer for five minutes. Spend that time journaling on that thought, how it has affected your life, and how you feel when you have that thought.

Movement

COBRA POSE (BHUJANGASANA)

This exercise opens up the heart. It is also a good shoulder strengthener. As with all yoga poses, go to your comfortable limit. Nothing should be painful.

1. Lie on your stomach on a mat or blanket with your feet extended out and the tops of your feet and forehead touching the mat.
2. Set your hands under your shoulders and your forearms on the floor, parallel to each other. Inhale and lift your upper torso and head away from the floor into a mild backbend.
3. You may stay in this pose for a minute or so, and then, if you are able, take a deep breath, lift your head and upper body further, almost straightening your arms.
4. Keep pressing the tops of your feet into the mat and let your pubic bone drop down into the mat to stabilize your lower back. Keep your hands pressed firmly against the mat.
5. Breathe out.
6. Continue engaging your legs and pushing your pelvis into the mat. Make sure your arms are not fully straightened, because this may hyperextend your elbows.
7. Take several deep inhalations and exhalations. Feel your chest opening.
8. Maintain this position for a minute or so. Bend your arms, lower your torso, and rest.
9. Repeat the pose for one to two minutes.

Affirmation

Spend three minutes saying aloud the following affirmation:

I am open to accepting love in my life.

Feel how your body responds to these words. You can also create your own statement. Feel free to write it on a beautiful notecard or a plain Post-it note and put it in your immediate environment for the day.

Visualization

Set a timer for three minutes. During that time, close your eyes and visualize your heart expanding out to meet people in your life who are healing and nourishing, and who love you. Feel your heart field magnify and reach out several feet around you. Bask in the green glow of this magnificent love and healing.

Meditation

For three minutes, shift your consciousness from your head to your heart. Imagine your heart filling with love. To come into this place, you may need to "feel" love from a previous memory or experience, or simply conjure it up.

DAY 12 RECIPES

Breakfast

MINT-GREEN SMOOTHIE
Serves 1

½ cup unsweetened almond milk
1 cup cubed honeydew melon
¼ cup raw almonds
4 to 5 fresh mint leaves

1 scoop protein powder of your choice
(hemp, pea, rice, whey for omnivores)
Water and ice to blend

Put all the liquid and whole food ingredients into a high-speed blender first, followed by the dry ingredients, then blend everything until a fluid consistency is reached. Add more water if needed. Drink immediately.

NUTRITION INFORMATION PER SERVING

Calories	Protein (g)	Carbs (g)	Fat (g)	Sat Fat (g)	Unsat Fat (g)	Fiber (g)
407	33	25	21	1	15	6

Lunch

CUCUMBER SALAD WITH HEARTY TURKEY BREAST *(OMNIVORE)* OR STEAMED NUTTY GREENS WITH BROWN RICE *(VEGAN)*
Serves 1

1 small cucumber, peeled
½ cup shredded green cabbage
½ cup chopped broccoli
2 tablespoons unsalted, raw, shelled pistachios
½ avocado, sliced

1 tablespoon freshly squeezed lime juice
1 tablespoon extra-virgin olive oil
Sea salt and ground black pepper to taste

With a vegetable peeler or spiralizer, slice the cucumber into "noodles."

In a bowl, toss the noodles with the cabbage, broccoli, pistachios, avocado, lime juice, and olive oil. Season with salt and pepper to taste. Serve immediately.

Warm up yesterday's leftover Hearty Turkey Breast (omnivore) or Steamed Nutty Greens with Brown Rice (vegan) to serve with the salad.

NUTRITION INFORMATION PER SERVING

	Calories	Protein (g)	Carbs (g)	Fat (g)	Sat Fat (g)	Unsat Fat (g)	Fiber (g)
Omnivore	747	38	27	57	8	48	13
Vegan	751	17	57	56	8	46	22

Snack

SEASONED KALE CHIPS (LEFTOVER FROM YESTERDAY'S SNACK)
Serves 1

NUTRITION INFORMATION PER SERVING

Calories	Protein (g)	Carbs (g)	Fat (g)	Sat Fat (g)	Unsat Fat (g)	Fiber (g)
174	3	13	14	2	12	6

Dinner

ALMOND SALMON WITH SWISS CHARD *(OMNIVORE)*
Serves 2

2 tablespoons almond meal (make
your own by grinding up almonds in
a blender)

2 tablespoons extra-virgin olive oil,
divided

2 3- to 4-ounce wild-caught salmon
fillets

1 garlic clove, minced

1 small bunch (about 5 large leaves)
Swiss chard, stemmed and roughly
chopped

1 tablespoon balsamic vinegar

Sea salt and ground black pepper to
taste

Preheat the oven to 375°F.

In a small bowl, combine well the almond meal and 1 tablespoon of the olive oil. Spread the almond paste over both the salmon fillets, then set the fillets in a glass baking dish and bake them for 15 to 20 minutes, or until they are just cooked through.

Meanwhile, in a sauté pan set over medium heat, warm the remaining tablespoon of olive oil, then add the garlic, and cook it for about 1 minute. Add the chard and cook it until it wilts, about 3 to 4 minutes. Toss the chard with the vinegar, and add salt and pepper to the mixture to taste.

Arrange the Swiss chard on a serving plate, top it with one of the salmon fillets, and eat the dish warm. (Save the second fillet for tomorrow's lunch.)

NUTRITION INFORMATION PER SERVING

Calories	Protein (g)	Carbs (g)	Fat (g)	Sat Fat (g)	Unsat Fat (g)	Fiber (g)
454	36	11	30	4	18	3

ROSEMARY-ROASTED CAULIFLOWER WITH SPINACH AND TAHINI *(VEGAN)*
Serves 2

3 cups chopped cauliflower

2 garlic cloves, minced

1 tablespoon extra-virgin olive oil

2 teaspoons dry rosemary powder

2 tablespoons raw pine nuts

Sea salt and freshly ground black
pepper to taste

2 large handfuls spinach, about 3 cups

1 tablespoon tahini

Preheat the oven to 425°F.

In a large mixing bowl, combine the cauliflower with the garlic and olive oil, ensuring all the cauliflower is coated with oil. Sprinkle the mixture with the rosemary and pine nuts, and season it with salt and pepper to taste.

On a baking sheet, spread the cauliflower evenly, then roast the pieces, uncovered, for 20 to 25 minutes, or until the tops and edges are lightly browned.

Serve half the cauliflower immediately on top of either fresh or wilted spinach, and drizzle everything with tahini. (Save the other half of the cauliflower for tomorrow's lunch.)

NUTRITION INFORMATION PER SERVING

Calories	Protein (g)	Carbs (g)	Fat (g)	Sat Fat (g)	Unsat Fat (g)	Fiber (g)
221	6	16	17	2	14	6

DAY 13: THE TRUTH—TRUTHS

If you tell the truth, you don't have to remember anything.

—MARK TWAIN

Meal Plan

	Omnivore	Vegan
Breakfast	Soothing Melon Smoothie	Soothing Melon Smoothie
Lunch	Kale and Mango Salad Almond Salmon	Kale and Mango Salad Rosemary-Roasted Cauliflower
Snack	Toasted Nori	Toasted Nori
Dinner	Thai Coconut Chicken	Thai Coconut Chickpeas

Whole Detox Emotion Log

At the end of the day, track any emotions that you had on the Whole Detox Emotion Log.

Thought Pattern Activity

The following are some limiting thoughts that relate to the TRUTH:

I don't know what is true for me.
It's difficult to tell the truth.
I fear what my life might be like if I spoke my truth.

Pick the limiting thought that seems to ring most true for you. If none of the examples feel true, write down your own limiting thought as it relates to the TRUTH.

Next, set your timer for five minutes. Spend that time journaling on that thought, how it has affected your life, and how you feel when you have that thought.

Movement
Tune in to your authentic voice through chanting, humming, or singing during your activities today.

Affirmation
Spend three minutes saying aloud the following affirmation:

I speak my truth freely.

Feel how your body responds to these words. You can also create your own statement. Feel free to write it on a beautiful notecard or a plain Post-it note and put it in your immediate environment for the day.

Visualization
Set a timer for three minutes. During that time, close your eyes and visualize all the words locked within your throat that you may not have said. See your throat as a cluttered canal. Let the words that most connect to your truth come forward. Imagine that they arrive on the tip of your tongue. Keeping your eyes closed, say them out loud. Repeat this process as many times as you need to, allowing your truth to come forward and be expressed.

Meditation
For at least three minutes, meditate using sound by chanting each vowel sound: "*ah*," "*ee*," "*eye*," "*ooh*," "*eww.*" To do this, breathe in deeply, and on the exhale, release "*ah*," then repeat the rhythm of breaths with the other vowel sounds.

DAY 13 RECIPES

Breakfast

SOOTHING MELON SMOOTHIE
Serves 1

1 small banana

½ cup cubed cantaloupe

½ cup cubed honeydew melon

1 tablespoon flaxseed meal

½ cup unsweetened coconut water

Pinch of ground cardamom

1 scoop protein powder of your choice
(hemp, pea, rice, whey for omnivores)

Water and ice to blend

Put all the liquid and whole food ingredients into a high-speed blender first, followed by the dry ingredients, then blend everything until a fluid consistency is reached. Add more water if needed. Drink immediately.

NUTRITION INFORMATION PER SERVING

Calories	Protein (g)	Carbs (g)	Fat (g)	Sat Fat (g)	Unsat Fat (g)	Fiber (g)
320	29	45	5	0.4	0.2	7

Lunch

KALE AND MANGO SALAD WITH ALMOND SALMON *(OMNIVORE)* OR ROSEMARY-ROASTED CAULIFLOWER *(VEGAN)*
Serves 1

2 handfuls baby kale, about 3 cups

½ green apple, sliced

1 cup cubed fresh mango

FOR THE DRESSING:

4 tablespoons orange juice

1 tablespoon freshly squeezed lemon
juice

½ tablespoon extra-virgin olive oil

Dash of sea salt

Dash of ground black pepper

In a serving bowl, toss together the kale, apple, and mango. Set the mixture aside. In a small bowl, whisk together all the dressing ingredients, and pour it over the fruits and greens. Warm up yesterday's leftover Almond Salmon (omnivore) or Rosemary-Roasted Cauliflower (vegan) to serve with the salad.

NUTRITION INFORMATION PER SERVING

	Calories	Protein (g)	Carbs (g)	Fat (g)	Sat Fat (g)	Unsat Fat (g)	Fiber (g)
Omnivore	769	43	74	39	5	25	13
Vegan	576	15	87	26	3	21	17

Snack

TOASTED NORI
Serves 1

3 sheets pressed nori

1 tablespoon sesame oil

Sea salt

Dash of turmeric powder

Preheat the oven to 250°F.

Cut each nori sheet into wide strips using clean scissors. Place the nori strips on a baking sheet. Lightly brush them front and back with sesame oil, then sprinkle them with sea salt and turmeric.

Bake the nori for 10 to 15 minutes, watching to be sure they do not burn. Let them cool before serving.

NUTRITION INFORMATION PER SERVING

Calories	Protein (g)	Carbs (g)	Fat (g)	Sat Fat (g)	Unsat Fat (g)	Fiber (g)
149	3	4	14	2	12	0

Dinner

THAI COCONUT CHICKEN *(OMNIVORE)* OR CHICKPEAS *(VEGAN)*
Serves 2

FOR OMNIVORES:

8 ounces organic, free-range, boneless chicken breasts, cut into 1-inch-thick strips

FOR VEGANS:

1½ cups cooked chickpeas

FOR BOTH:

1 tablespoon coconut oil

2 garlic cloves, minced

1-inch piece fresh ginger, minced

¼ cup diced yellow onion

2 tablespoons curry powder

⅛ teaspoon ground black pepper

1 teaspoon sea salt

1 cup unsweetened, full-fat coconut
   milk

1 small zucchini, cubed

2 small red potatoes, cubed

In a large skillet set over medium-high heat, warm the coconut oil, then add the garlic, ginger, and onion, sautéing until the onion becomes soft and translucent. Stir in the curry powder, pepper, and salt. Cook the mixture for about 1 minute. Add the coconut milk, zucchini, and potatoes, coating everything well, then add the chicken (*omnivore*) or the chickpeas (*vegan*). Stir the ingredients consistently until everything is cooked through.

Serve half the mixture warm. (Save the other half for tomorrow's lunch.)

NUTRITION INFORMATION PER SERVING

	Calories	Protein (g)	Carbs (g)	Fat (g)	Sat Fat (g)	Unsat Fat (g)	Fiber (g)
Omnivore	439	32	34	21	17	2	4
Vegan	390	9	47	21	17	2	7

DAY 14: THE TRUTH—AFFIRMATIONS

Words mean more than what is set down on paper. It takes the human voice to infuse them with deeper meaning.

—MAYA ANGELOU

Meal Plan

	Omnivore	Vegan
Breakfast	Mango-Mint Smoothie	Mango-Mint Smoothie
Lunch	Bitters-Sweet Salad Thai Coconut Chicken	Bitters-Sweet Salad Thai Coconut Chickpeas
Snack	Rainbow Fruit and Nut Salad	Rainbow Fruit and Nut Salad
Dinner	Halibut Stew	Mung Bean Stew

Whole Detox Emotion Log
At the end of the day, track any emotions that you had on the Whole Detox Emotion Log.

Thought Pattern Activity
The following are some limiting thoughts that relate to the TRUTH:

I've been taught that it's impolite to disagree.
I am at a loss for words.
I am afraid to say what I really want to say.

Pick the limiting thought that seems to ring most true for you. If none of the examples feel true, write down your own limiting thought as it relates to the TRUTH.

Next, set your timer for five minutes. Spend that time journaling on that thought, how it has affected your life, and how you feel when you have that thought.

Movement
Do five rounds of gentle neck rolls in both counterclockwise and clockwise directions. Feel where there is tenderness and gently massage that area. Also, take five minutes to lightly massage your jaw, mouth, and throat area.

Affirmation
Spend three minutes saying aloud the following affirmation:
My words are crafted with honesty, integrity, and truth.

Feel how your body responds to these words. You can also create your own statement. Feel free to write it on a beautiful notecard or a plain Post-it note and put it in your immediate environment for the day.

Visualization
Set a timer for three minutes. During that time, close your eyes and visualize your mouth as a spinning wheel of words. See your mouth as a moving wheel that can generate words of your choice. Allow certain words to come forward that speak to your inner truth, perhaps something you would like to

say but haven't said. Let them spin on the wheel until they have been shaped with honesty and integrity. Say them out loud at the end of the visualization.

Meditation

Sit still for five minutes and observe any and all sounds in your environment. Notice each of them without engagement.

DAY 14 RECIPES

Breakfast

MANGO-MINT SMOOTHIE
Serves 1

- 1 cup cubed fresh mango
- 1½ cups unsweetened coconut water
- 2 tablespoons freshly chopped mint leaves (about 4–6 whole mint leaves)
- 1 scoop protein powder of your choice (hemp, pea, rice, whey for omnivores)
- Water and ice to blend

Put all the liquid and whole food ingredients into a high-speed blender first, followed by the dry protein powder, then blend everything until a fluid consistency is reached. Add more water if needed. Drink immediately.

NUTRITION INFORMATION PER SERVING

Calories	Protein (g)	Carbs (g)	Fat (g)	Sat Fat (g)	Unsat Fat (g)	Fiber (g)
308	28	46	3	0.6	0	8

Lunch

BITTERS-SWEET SALAD WITH THAI COCONUT CHICKEN *(OMNIVORE)* OR CHICKPEAS *(VEGAN)*
Serves 1

- 1 cup arugula
- 1 cup dandelion greens
- ¼ cup shredded carrots
- 2 radishes, sliced

FOR THE DRESSING:

1 tablespoon honey

1 tablespoon sesame oil

½ teaspoon mustard seeds

In a serving bowl, toss together the arugula, dandelion greens, carrots, and radishes. In a small mixing bowl, whisk together all the dressing ingredients, then pour the dressing over the salad.

Warm up yesterday's leftover Thai Coconut Chicken (*omnivore*) or Chickpeas (*vegan*) to serve with the salad.

NUTRITION INFORMATION PER SERVING

	Calories	Protein (g)	Carbs (g)	Fat (g)	Sat Fat (g)	Unsat Fat (g)	Fiber (g)
Omnivore	674	35	61	36	19	15	8
Vegan	625	12	79	36	19	15	11

Snack

RAINBOW FRUIT AND NUT SALAD

Serves 1

1 kiwi fruit, peeled and sliced

1 cup cubed honeydew melon

2 strawberries, sliced

5–6 blueberries

½ small banana, sliced

3 to 4 fresh mint leaves, chopped

3 tablespoons pecan pieces

1 tablespoon unsweetened, shredded coconut

1 teaspoon honey

1 tablespoon freshly squeezed lime juice

In a small bowl, combine all the ingredients and serve immediately.

NUTRITION INFORMATION PER SERVING

Calories	Protein (g)	Carbs (g)	Fat (g)	Sat Fat (g)	Unsat Fat (g)	Fiber (g)
353	4	50	18	4	12	8

Dinner

HALIBUT *(OMNIVORE)* OR MUNG BEAN *(VEGAN)* STEW
Serves 2

FOR OMNIVORES:

    8 ounces wild-caught halibut, skin removed, cut into 1-inch pieces

FOR VEGANS:

    1½ cups cooked mung beans

FOR BOTH:

    ⅔ cup unsweetened, full-fat coconut milk

    3 cups organic vegetable broth

    1 tablespoon freshly squeezed lime juice

    2 teaspoons grated or minced fresh ginger

    2 carrots, sliced into bite-size strips

    3-inch piece fresh lemongrass

    2 cups chopped cauliflower

    ½ teaspoon Thai green curry paste

    4 fresh basil leaves, chopped

    Sea salt and freshly ground black pepper to taste

In a large saucepan set over medium-high heat, combine the halibut (*omnivore*) or mung beans (*vegan*) with the coconut milk, broth, lime juice, ginger, carrots, lemongrass, cauliflower, and curry paste. Bring the mixture to a quick boil, then reduce the heat, gently simmering for about 10 to 15 minutes, or until the fish or beans are cooked through.

Top the soup with the chopped basil, and season it with salt and pepper to taste.

NUTRITION INFORMATION PER SERVING

	Calories	Protein (g)	Carbs (g)	Fat (g)	Sat Fat (g)	Unsat Fat (g)	Fiber (g)
Omnivore	370	29	21	20	15	3	6
Vegan	405	16	50	18	14	1	17

DAY 15: THE TRUTH—LIQUID FOODS

A first-rate soup is more creative than a second-rate painting.

—ABRAHAM MASLOW

Meal Plan

	Omnivore	Vegan
Breakfast	Pomegranate-Apple Smoothie	Pomegranate-Apple Smoothie
Lunch	Rainbow Salad Halibut Stew	Rainbow Salad Mung Bean Stew
Snack	Dates and Almonds	Dates and Almonds
Dinner	Shiitake–Sea Plant Soup	Shiitake–Sea Plant Soup

Whole Detox Emotion Log

At the end of the day, track any emotions that you had on the Whole Detox Emotion Log.

Thought Pattern Activity

The following are some limiting thoughts that relate to the TRUTH:

I feel closed off.
I am not free to be me.
My true self feels shut down.

Pick the limiting thought that seems to ring most true for you. If none of the examples feel true, write down your own limiting thought as it relates to the TRUTH.

Next, set your timer for five minutes. Spend that time journaling on that thought, how it has affected your life, and how you feel when you have that thought.

Movement

PLOW POSE (HALASANA)

This exercise lengthens the back of your neck and can aid in balancing the throat. As with all yoga poses, go to your comfortable limit. If this pose seems too daunting for you, modify it accordingly, or simply spend the time doing gentle neck rolls. Nothing should be painful.

1. Fold two blankets into firm rectangles about one to two feet across and stack them together on the floor.
2. Lie down on your back with your shoulders and torso on the blankets, with your head extending beyond the folded edges.
3. Bend your knees, keeping your feet flat on the floor. Your arms should be parallel at your sides.
4. On an exhale, push your feet off the floor, lifting your bent legs, and bring your hands to your mid-back, just above your waist, to support your body.
5. Straighten your legs and allow them to extend back over your head. Your toes will touch the floor behind you. You may let your hands go and extend the arms to lie along the floor.
6. Keep your neck long.
7. Remain in the pose for one to three minutes, then roll back down on an exhale.

Affirmation

Spend three minutes saying aloud the following affirmation:

My throat is open and moist to release my authentic voice.

Feel how your body responds to these words. You can also create your own statement. Feel free to write it on a beautiful notecard or a plain Post-it note and put it in your immediate environment for the day.

Visualization

Set a timer for three minutes. During that time, close your eyes and visualize your throat as an open canal. Fill it with healing aquamarine light. Let this light cast out any stuck words, dryness, or scratchy patches. Imagine your throat as smooth, soft, and open to your deepest truths.

Meditation

Meditate using a conscious "sipping" exercise, using either water, tea, or broth, in which you take a sip and envision that the liquid carries healing for your throat, thyroid, and authentic voice. Meditate for as long as it takes to empty a glass of water, or a cup of tea or broth. It may take as long as five minutes.

DAY 15 RECIPES

Breakfast

POMEGRANATE-APPLE SMOOTHIE
Serves 1

1 cup pomegranate juice
½ green apple, sliced
1 handful spinach, about 1½ cups

1 scoop protein powder of your choice
(hemp, pea, rice, whey for omnivores)
Water and ice to blend

Put all the liquid and whole food ingredients into a high-speed blender first, followed by the dry protein powder, then blend everything until a fluid consistency is reached. Add more water if needed. Drink immediately.

NUTRITION INFORMATION PER SERVING

Calories	Protein (g)	Carbs (g)	Fat (g)	Sat Fat (g)	Unsat Fat (g)	Fiber (g)
315	26	51	2	0	0	4

Lunch

RAINBOW SALAD WITH HALIBUT *(OMNIVORE)* OR MUNG BEAN *(VEGAN)* STEW
Serves 1

½ red bell pepper, diced
1 carrot, sliced in rounds
½ small yellow squash, sliced
1 cup baby kale

¼ cup finely sliced red cabbage
5 walnut halves, chopped
1 teaspoon unhulled sesame seeds
Freshly ground black pepper to taste

FOR THE DRESSING:

2 tablespoons freshly squeezed lemon
juice

1½ tablespoons extra-virgin olive oil

¼ teaspoon minced fresh ginger

¾ teaspoon honey

Pinch of ground cayenne pepper

Pinch of sea salt

In a serving bowl, toss together the bell pepper, carrot, squash, kale, cabbage, walnuts, and sesame seeds, and season with black pepper to taste. In a small bowl, whisk together all the dressing ingredients, then pour the dressing over the salad.

Warm up yesterday's leftover Halibut (*Omnivore*) or Mung Bean (*Vegan*) Stew to serve with the salad.

NUTRITION INFORMATION PER SERVING

	Calories	Protein (g)	Carbs (g)	Fat (g)	Sat Fat (g)	Unsat Fat (g)	Fiber (g)
Omnivore	750	35	47	50	19	27	12
Vegan	785	22	76	48	18	25	23

Snack

DATES AND ALMONDS
Serves 1

2 Medjool dates

1 handful raw almonds, about 12

Calories	Protein (g)	Carbs (g)	Fat (g)	Sat Fat (g)	Unsat Fat (g)	Fiber (g)
123	3	14	7	0.5	6	3

Dinner

SHIITAKE–SEA PLANT SOUP
Serves 2

FOR OMNIVORES:

6 ounces organic, free-range, boneless chicken breasts, cubed

FOR VEGANS:

1 cup cooked adzuki beans

FOR BOTH:

4 cups organic vegetable broth	1 cup dulse flakes
1½ cups shredded bok choy	1 tablespoon coconut aminos
5 large shiitake mushrooms, sliced	1 teaspoon sea salt
1 green onion, finely chopped	½ cup cooked brown rice

In a large saucepan set over medium-low heat, combine the chicken (*omnivore*) or beans (*vegan*) with the broth, bok choy, mushrooms, onion, dulse, coconut aminos, and salt, and allow the mixture to simmer for about 15 to 20 minutes. Stir in the rice, and serve half the soup warm. (Save the other half for tomorrow's lunch.)

NUTRITION INFORMATION PER SERVING

	Calories	Protein (g)	Carbs (g)	Fat (g)	Sat Fat (g)	Unsat Fat (g)	Fiber (g)
Omnivore	243	26	27	3	0.4	1	5
Vegan	297	15	56	2	0.2	0.4	13

DAY 16: THE INSIGHT—MOODS AND COGNITION

Be curious always! For knowledge will not acquire you; you must acquire it.

—BERTRAND RUSSELL

Meal Plan

	Omnivore	Vegan
Breakfast	Pomegranate-Berry Smoothie	Pomegranate-Berry Smoothie
Lunch	Purple Kale and Cabbage Salad Shiitake-Seaplant Soup (with chicken)	Purple Kale and Cabbage Salad Shiitake-Seaplant Soup (with beans)
Snack	Berry and Nut Cobbler	Berry and Nut Cobbler
Dinner	Wild Salmon with Blackberry-Basil Sauce Super Spinach	Purple Rice and Vegetables with Blackberry-Cashew Cream

Whole Detox Emotion Log

At the end of the day, track any emotions that you had on the Whole Detox Emotion Log.

Thought Pattern Activity

The following are some limiting thoughts that relate to the INSIGHT:

I'm not good at learning new things.
I am not intuitive.
I can't focus my attention.

Pick the limiting thought that seems to ring most true for you. If none of the examples feel true, write down your own limiting thought as it relates to the INSIGHT.

Next, set your timer for five minutes. Spend that time journaling on that thought, how it has affected your life, and how you feel when you have that thought.

Movement

Allow yourself to do some gentle neck rolls to loosen up your neck and head area. Lift your chin and let your eyes gaze up toward your forehead for a couple of seconds, then return to facing straight ahead. After a couple of seconds, tilt your chin down and let your gaze fall on your chest, then return to facing straight ahead. Repeat a few times, to the level of comfort.

Affirmation

Spend three minutes saying aloud the following affirmation:
My moods are balanced and my thinking is clear and precise.

Feel how your body responds to these words. You can also create your own statement. Feel free to write it on a beautiful notecard or a plain Post-it note and put it in your immediate environment for the day.

Visualization

Set a timer for three minutes. During that time, close your eyes and visualize your mind as being clear and bright. The light transforms any blocks or barriers to clear your thinking. Your neurons communicate rapidly back and forth, transmitting information seamlessly. Your mood is brightened by the light, and you feel balanced.

Meditation

For six minutes, envision your mind as a suitcase, tightly packed with excessive thoughts, stress, and unrealized ideas and dreams. Now see your mind let go of all the excesses, one by one, emptying itself out. After the meditation, make a conscious effort to scrutinize everything you put into the suitcase of your mind.

DAY 16 RECIPES

Breakfast

POMEGRANATE-BERRY SMOOTHIE
Serves 1

1 cup pomegranate juice
½ cup fresh blackberries
½ cup hibiscus tea, cooled
½ small banana, sliced

⅛ teaspoon ground cardamom
1 scoop protein powder of your choice
   (hemp, pea, rice, whey for omnivores)
Water and ice to blend

Put all the liquid and whole food ingredients into a high-speed blender first, followed by the dry protein powder, then blend everything until a fluid consistency is reached. Add more water if needed. Drink immediately.

NUTRITION INFORMATION PER SERVING

Calories	Protein (g)	Carbs (g)	Fat (g)	Sat Fat (g)	Unsat Fat (g)	Fiber (g)
336	27	54	3	0	0.3	5

Lunch

PURPLE KALE AND CABBAGE SALAD WITH SHIITAKE–SEA PLANT SOUP
Serves 1

1 cup chopped purple kale
½ cup chopped red cabbage

⅓ cup thinly sliced red apple
2 tablespoons chopped walnuts

FOR THE DRESSING:

1 tablespoon freshly squeezed lemon
juice
½ tablespoon Dijon mustard
1 teaspoon honey

1 tablespoon extra-virgin olive oil
Sea salt and ground black pepper to
taste

In a serving bowl, combine the kale, cabbage, apple, and walnuts. In a small bowl, whisk together all the dressing ingredients, then pour the dressing over the salad.

Warm up yesterday's leftover Shiitake–Sea Plant Soup to serve with the salad.

NUTRITION INFORMATION PER SERVING

	Calories	Protein (g)	Carbs (g)	Fat (g)	Sat Fat (g)	Unsat Fat (g)	Fiber (g)
Omnivore	563	31	53	27	3	25	9
Vegan	617	20	82	26	3	21	17

Snack

BERRY AND NUT COBBLER
Serves 4

1 teaspoon plus 2 tablespoons coconut
oil
1 cup blueberries, frozen or fresh
1 cup blackberries
1 cup raspberries
½ cup chopped pecans

½ cup chopped walnuts
1 cup gluten-free oats
1 tablespoon flaxseed meal
1 tablespoon honey

Preheat the oven to 375°F.

Grease a 9 × 9 glass baking dish with 1 teaspoon of the coconut oil.

In a medium bowl, combine the blueberries, blackberries, and raspberries. In another bowl, combine the pecans, walnuts, oats, flaxseed meal, and honey with the remaining 2 tablespoons of coconut oil.

Spread the berry mixture evenly in the greased baking dish. Sprinkle the nut and oat mixture on top. Bake the cobbler for 20 to 25 minutes, or until the berries are gently bubbling. Remove it from the oven and allow it to cool.

Spoon a quarter of the cobbler onto a dish and eat it mindfully. (Save the remaining cobbler for tomorrow's snack plus future additional snacks.)

NUTRITION INFORMATION PER SERVING

Calories	Protein (g)	Carbs (g)	Fat (g)	Sat Fat (g)	Unsat Fat (g)	Fiber (g)
206	4	18	15	4	9	4

Dinner

WILD SALMON WITH BLACKBERRY-BASIL SAUCE *(OMNIVORE)*
Serves 2

¼ cup freshly squeezed lime juice
1 tablespoon extra-virgin olive oil
Dash of sea salt
1 garlic clove, minced
2 4-ounce wild-caught salmon fillets

1 tablespoon coconut oil
2 cups fresh blackberries
5 fresh basil leaves (purple basil preferred)
1 cup purified water

In a large bowl, combine the lime juice, olive oil, sea salt, and garlic. Dip each salmon fillet into the bowl, coating both well.

In a skillet set over low heat, melt the coconut oil, and add the coated salmon fillets. Cover the skillet and let the salmon cook for 7 to 10 minutes, turning them halfway through to cook on their other sides.

In a saucepan set over medium heat, combine the blackberries, basil, and water. Allow the berries to reach a boil, then reduce the heat to gently simmer them until they take on the consistency of a thick sauce, about 8 to 10 minutes. Add more water if needed.

On a serving plate, place 1 salmon fillet. Season it with black pepper to taste, and spoon half the sauce over the top. Serve it with Super Spinach (recipe on page 301). (Save the other salmon fillet for tomorrow's lunch.)

NUTRITION INFORMATION PER SERVING

Calories	Protein (g)	Carbs (g)	Fat (g)	Sat Fat (g)	Unsat Fat (g)	Fiber (g)
398	25	17	27	11	16	7

PURPLE RICE AND VEGETABLES WITH BLACKBERRY-CASHEW CREAM *(VEGAN)*
Serves 2

¼ cup uncooked purple/black rice

2 cups stemmed, chopped purple kale

2 cups shredded red cabbage

2 cups chopped cauliflower

FOR THE CREAM:

¾ cup raw cashews

¾ cup fresh blackberries

1 tablespoon freshly squeezed lemon juice

1 tablespoon walnut oil

¼ cup water, or as needed for blending

Sea salt to taste

Cook the purple rice in a rice cooker if available. If not, cook it on the stovetop according to the package instructions.

Meanwhile, in a vegetable steamer, heat about 1 cup of water. Steam the kale, cabbage, and cauliflower, allowing the vegetables to cook lightly yet not lose color.

In a high-speed blender or food processor, blend together all the ingredients for the cream.

On a serving plate, arrange a bed of half the cooked rice topped with half the vegetables, then drizzle everything with half the blackberry-cashew cream. (Save the remaining half-portions for tomorrow's lunch.)

NUTRITION INFORMATION PER SERVING

Calories	Protein (g)	Carbs (g)	Fat (g)	Sat Fat (g)	Unsat Fat (g)	Fiber (g)
547	16	58	32	5	24	10

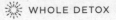

DAY 17: THE INSIGHT—VISUALIZATIONS

Your vision will become clear only when you can look into your own heart.
Who looks outside, dreams; who looks inside, awakens.

—CARL JUNG

Meal Plan

	Omnivore	Vegan
Breakfast	Berryananda Smoothie	Berryananda Smoothie
Lunch	Cool Blue Salad Wild Salmon with Blackberry-Basil Sauce	Cool Blue Salad Purple Rice and Vegetables with Blackberry-Cashew Cream
Snack	Berry and Nut Cobbler	Berry and Nut Cobbler
Dinner	Coconut Cod Fillet with Plum-Lavender Sauce Steamed Broccoli	Purple Buddha Bowl

Whole Detox Emotion Log

At the end of the day, track any emotions that you had on the Whole Detox Emotion Log.

Thought Pattern Activity

The following are some limiting thoughts that relate to the INSIGHT:

I have difficulty seeing the big picture.
I lack vision about where my life is going.
It's difficult for me to zoom out of my everyday view and have perspective on the larger whole of my life.

Pick the limiting thought that seems to ring most true for you. If none of the examples feel true, write down your own limiting thought as it relates to the INSIGHT.

Next, set your timer for five minutes. Spend that time journaling on that thought, how it has affected your life, and how you feel when you have that thought.

Movement

Strengthen your eyes by doing a simple three-minute eye-stretching activity in which you look up with both eyes, then to the right, down, and to the left. Repeat the pattern three times. Do the series again but in the opposite direction.

Affirmation

Spend three minutes saying aloud the following affirmation:

My inner vision is aligned with my outer sight.

Feel how your body responds to these words. You can also create your own statement. Feel free to write it on a beautiful notecard or a plain Post-it note and put it in your immediate environment for the day.

Visualization

Set a timer for three minutes. During that time, close your eyes and visualize not your outer eyes but an inner eye at your forehead. Allow this inner, wise eye to look into your future. Visualize your next couple of years. Imagine the best vision possible for yourself. Bring that vision back with you after the three minutes end, and jot a couple of notes about what you discovered.

Meditation

Close your eyes and fix your gaze toward your forehead, especially at the end of the day before bedtime. After three minutes, with your fingertips, gently tap the area around the eyes.

DAY 17 RECIPES

Breakfast

BERRYANANDA SMOOTHIE

Serves 1

1 small banana
1 cup frozen blueberries
1 cup unsweetened almond milk
¼ teaspoon ground cardamom
¼ teaspoon ground cinnamon

1 teaspoon bee pollen granules
(optional)
1 scoop protein powder of your choice
(hemp, pea, rice, whey for omnivores)
Water and ice to blend

Put all the liquid and whole food ingredients into a high-speed blender first, followed by the dry protein powder, then blend everything until a fluid consistency is reached. Add more water if needed. Drink immediately.

NUTRITION INFORMATION PER SERVING

Calories	Protein (g)	Carbs (g)	Fat (g)	Sat Fat (g)	Unsat Fat (g)	Fiber (g)
334	27	48	6	0.1	0.4	7

Lunch

COOL BLUE SALAD WITH WILD SALMON *(OMNIVORE)* OR PURPLE RICE AND VEGETABLES *(VEGAN)*

Serves 1

2 cups baby kale
½ cup fresh blueberries

¼ cup cubed cucumber

FOR THE DRESSING:

1 tablespoon hempseed oil
1 tablespoon freshly squeezed lemon
  juice
¼ teaspoon lemon zest
2 fresh purple basil leaves, chopped

finely
Sea salt and ground black pepper to
  taste

In a serving bowl, combine the kale, blueberries, and cucumber. In a separate bowl, whisk together all the dressing ingredients, and drizzle the dressing over the salad.

Warm up yesterday's leftover Wild Salmon (*omnivore*) or Purple Rice and Vegetables (*vegan*) to serve with the salad.

NUTRITION INFORMATION PER SERVING

	Calories	Protein (g)	Carbs (g)	Fat (g)	Sat Fat (g)	Unsat Fat (g)	Fiber (g)
Omnivore	635	30	43	41	12	28	12
Vegan	784	21	85	47	7	37	15

Snack

BERRY AND NUT COBBLER (LEFTOVER FROM YESTERDAY'S SNACK)

NUTRITION INFORMATION PER SERVING

Calories	Protein (g)	Carbs (g)	Fat (g)	Sat Fat (g)	Unsat Fat (g)	Fiber (g)
206	4	18	15	4	9	4

Dinner

COCONUT COD FILLET WITH PLUM-LAVENDER SAUCE *(OMNIVORE)*
Serves 2

2 tablespoons coconut oil, melted

2 tablespoons unsweetened shredded coconut

⅛ teaspoon ground cardamom

Pinch of sea salt

⅛ teaspoon freshly ground black pepper

2 4-ounce wild-caught cod fillets

FOR THE PLUM-LAVENDER SAUCE:

2 plums, pitted and sliced

2 tablespoons extra-virgin olive oil

1¼ tablespoons freshly squeezed lemon juice

2 teaspoons lavender buds, ground in a mortar and pestle

½ teaspoon sea salt

In a large bowl, whisk together the coconut oil, shredded coconut, cardamom, salt, and pepper. Set the mixture aside.

Set a large skillet over low heat. Dip each cod fillet into the oil and spice mixture, then lay both fillets in the heated skillet. Cover the skillet and let the cod cook, flipping the fillets to cook their other sides after about 5 minutes for a total cooking time of 10 minutes.

Meanwhile, make the sauce. In a small saucepan, warm the plums in about ¼ cup water. When they have softened, after about 1 minute, add the olive oil, lemon juice, lavender, and salt. Heat the mixture for about 2 minutes, stirring constantly.

Place 1 cooked cod fillet on a serving plate and drizzle it with half the sauce. Serve the cod with Steamed Broccoli (recipe follows). (Save the remaining fillet for tomorrow's lunch.)

NUTRITION INFORMATION PER SERVING

Calories	Protein (g)	Carbs (g)	Fat (g)	Sat Fat (g)	Unsat Fat (g)	Fiber (g)
349	21	12	25	11	14	2

STEAMED BROCCOLI *(OMNIVORE)*

Serves 1

1½ cups chopped broccoli   1 teaspoon chia seeds
1 teaspoon extra-virgin olive oil

In a saucepan or pot fitted with a steamer basket, bring about ¼ cup water to a boil. Add the broccoli to the steamer basket, cover the pot, and let the broccoli steam for about 1 minute, or until the pieces turn bright green.

Transfer the broccoli to a serving dish. Drizzle the broccoli with the olive oil, and sprinkle the chia seeds on top as desired. Serve warm.

NUTRITION INFORMATION PER SERVING

Calories	Protein (g)	Carbs (g)	Fat (g)	Sat Fat (g)	Unsat Fat (g)	Fiber (g)
87	4	7	6	1	5	4

PURPLE BUDDHA BOWL *(VEGAN)*
Serves 2

¼ cup uncooked purple/black rice

1 tablespoon coconut oil

½ cup diced red onion

1 garlic clove, minced

2½ cups chopped broccoli

1 cup cooked adzuki beans (you may
want to cook them with the rice)

2 purple carrots, diced

2 tablespoons hemp seeds

½ red bell pepper, sliced

½ avocado, cubed

1 tablespoon flaxseed oil

Sea salt and ground black pepper to
taste

Dash of ground cayenne pepper

Cook the rice in a rice cooker if available. If not, cook it in a saucepan on the stovetop according to the package instructions.

In a large skillet set over medium heat, melt the coconut oil, then sauté the onion and garlic in the oil for about 2 minutes, or until the onion becomes soft. Add the broccoli, cooked beans, carrots, hemp seeds, and bell pepper. (If you opt to cook the beans with the rice, omit them in this step.) Stir and heat the mixture until the colors of the broccoli and carrots are bright, about 1 to 2 minutes.

Into a large, wide serving bowl, spoon half the cooked rice (or half the rice and beans), then half the cooked vegetables, then half the avocado cubes. Drizzle everything with half the flaxseed oil, and season it with salt, black pepper, and cayenne. (Save the other half-portions of everything for tomorrow's lunch.)

NUTRITION INFORMATION PER SERVING

Calories	Protein (g)	Carbs (g)	Fat (g)	Sat Fat (g)	Unsat Fat (g)	Fiber (g)
568	19	70	26	8	13	18

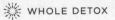
DAY 18: THE INSIGHT—SPICES

Variety is the spice of life.

—WILLIAM COWPER

Meal Plan

	Omnivore	Vegan
Breakfast	Cacao-Coconut Smoothie	Cacao-Coconut Smoothie
Lunch	Zesty Purple Spiral Salad Coconut Cod Fillet	Zesty Purple Spiral Salad Purple Buddha Bowl
Snack	Blueberries and Pecans	Blueberries and Pecans
Dinner	Ginger Chicken with Blackberry Sauce Purple Potatoes	Spiced Eggplant Purple Potatoes

Whole Detox Emotion Log

At the end of the day, track any emotions that you had on the Whole Detox Emotion Log.

Thought Pattern Activity

The following are some limiting thoughts that relate to the INSIGHT:

To feel alive, I need to feel like I'm living on the edge.
I am too spicy for most people.
My life lacks spice and intensity.

Pick the limiting thought that seems to ring most true for you. If none of the examples feel true, write down your own limiting thought as it relates to the INSIGHT.

Next, set your timer for five minutes. Spend that time journaling on that thought, how it has affected your life, and how you feel when you have that thought.

Movement

DOWNWARD FACING DOG (ADHO MUKHA SVANASANA)

This pose increases blood flow to your head while calming and energizing the entire body. As with all yoga poses, go to your comfortable limit. Nothing should be painful.

1. Kneel on all fours on the floor, a mat, or a blanket with your back flat.
2. Walk your hands farther forward, keeping your palms flat on the floor.
3. Spread your fingers and establish solid contact with the floor, mat, or blanket.
4. Exhale as you lift your tailbone and straighten your legs.
5. Keep your feet flat on the floor, and lengthen your spine. Keep lifting your tailbone toward the ceiling while keeping your heels as close to the floor as you can. Do not lock your knees but keep them activated.
6. Maintain straight arms, keeping contact with the floor with your hands. Your palms should press firmly into the mat.
7. After holding this pose for up to three minutes, lower your tailbone, bend your knees, walk your hands back, and return to your original position to rest. You may repeat the activity a few more times, stretching each time just a little bit deeper than the previous time, to the level of comfort.

Affirmation

Spend three minutes saying aloud the following affirmation:

My life is filled with healthy intensity and flavorful moments.

Feel how your body responds to these words. You can also create your own statement. Feel free to write it on a beautiful notecard or a plain Post-it note and put it in your immediate environment for the day.

Visualization

Set a timer for three minutes. During that time, close your eyes and visualize yourself as a kaleidoscope of colors on the inside. See yourself as a brightly colored mosaic. Feel the intensity of your inner artwork. Let it invigorate every cell of your being.

Meditation

Watch your thoughts intently in a six-minute meditation. Adjust their speed, allowing them to move in slow motion and then speeding them up as fast as you'd like them to go. See how you feel when you look attentively and carefully at your thoughts versus letting them whiz by you in a whirlwind. While you do this activity, remain detached and free from their influence.

DAY 18 RECIPES

Breakfast

CACAO-COCONUT SMOOTHIE
Serves 1

1 cup unsweetened coconut milk
  (boxed variety)
1 teaspoon honey
1 tablespoon raw cacao nibs
1 tablespoon unsweetened cocoa
  powder
1 teaspoon flaxseed meal
1 scoop protein powder of your choice
  (hemp, pea, rice, whey for omnivores)
Water and ice to blend

Put all the liquid and whole food ingredients into a high-speed blender first, followed by the dry ingredients, then blend everything until a fluid consistency is reached. Add more water if needed. Drink immediately.

NUTRITION INFORMATION PER SERVING

Calories	Protein (g)	Carbs (g)	Fat (g)	Sat Fat (g)	Unsat Fat (g)	Fiber (g)
259	27	13	12	8	0.3	3

Lunch

ZESTY PURPLE SPIRAL SALAD WITH COCONUT COD FILLET *(OMNIVORE)* OR PURPLE BUDDHA BOWL *(VEGAN)*
Serves 1

2 large red cabbage leaves

¼ red cabbage, sliced lengthwise

1 large shallot, sliced into ringlets

1 tablespoon grated carrot

2 tablespoons raw pine nuts

1 tablespoon flaxseed oil

1 tablespoon freshly squeezed lemon juice

½ teaspoon lemon zest

1 teaspoon honey

Sea salt and ground black pepper to taste

Lay the 2 cabbage leaves inside a serving bowl, overlapping to cover the bottom surface.

In a small mixing bowl, combine the sliced cabbage, shallot, carrot, and pine nuts. Add the flaxseed oil, lemon juice, lemon zest, and honey. Combine the mixture well, seasoning with salt and pepper to taste. Then spoon it into the middle of the cabbage leaves in the serving bowl.

Either eat the salad taco style (rolled up in the cabbage leaves) or dig into the salad with a fork.

Warm up yesterday's leftover Coconut Cod Fillet (omnivore) or Purple Buddha Bowl (vegan) to serve with the salad.

NUTRITION INFORMATION PER SERVING

	Calories	Protein (g)	Carbs (g)	Fat (g)	Sat Fat (g)	Unsat Fat (g)	Fiber (g)
Omnivore	655	27	44	45	13	30	10
Vegan	873	25	102	46	10	29	26

Snack

BLUEBERRIES AND PECANS
Serves 1

1 cup fresh blueberries   1 handful pecans, about 8 halves

NUTRITION INFORMATION PER SERVING

Calories	Protein (g)	Carbs (g)	Fat (g)	Sat Fat (g)	Unsat Fat (g)	Fiber (g)
167	2	23	9	1	8	5

Dinner

GINGER CHICKEN WITH BLACKBERRY SAUCE *(OMNIVORE)*
Serves 1

1 tablespoon extra-virgin olive oil   1 teaspoon sea salt
2 tablespoons coconut aminos   1 4-ounce organic, free-range, boneless
1-inch piece fresh ginger, thinly sliced   chicken breast, cut into strips

FOR THE SAUCE:

¼ cup fresh blackberries   ½ teaspoon sea salt
1 tablespoon apple cider vinegar   1 teaspoon minced fresh mint leaves
1 teaspoon grated fresh ginger

In a skillet set over medium heat, warm the olive oil, then add the coconut aminos, ginger, salt, and chicken strips, stir-frying until the chicken is cooked through, about 7 to 10 minutes.

In a small saucepan set over medium heat, combine all the sauce ingredients, mashing the berries with a fork to release their juices. Let the mixture simmer, stirring it constantly, until it thickens slightly, approximately 2 minutes.

Arrange the chicken on a serving plate and drizzle it with the sauce. Serve immediately with Purple Potatoes (recipe follows).

NUTRITION INFORMATION PER SERVING

Calories	Protein (g)	Carbs (g)	Fat (g)	Sat Fat (g)	Unsat Fat (g)	Fiber (g)
301	27	11	16	2	13	2

SPICED EGGPLANT *(VEGAN)*
Serves 1

1 tablespoon extra-virgin olive oil

1 small red onion, finely chopped

1 garlic clove, minced

⅛ teaspoon ground cinnamon

⅛ teaspoon ground cardamom

1 teaspoon sea salt

1 small eggplant, peeled and cubed

½ medium tomato, chopped

3 shiitake mushrooms, diced

2 tablespoons raw pine nuts

1 teaspoon freshly squeezed lemon juice

Ground black pepper to taste

In a skillet set over medium heat, warm the olive oil, then add the onion, garlic, cinnamon, cardamom, and salt, sautéing the mixture until the onions are translucent, about 2 minutes. Add the eggplant and cook it until it's soft, about 5 to 7 minutes. Lower the heat, then stir in the tomato, mushrooms, and pine nuts and let warm for about 30 seconds. Drizzle the ingredients with lemon juice and add black pepper to taste.

Serve the eggplant with Purple Potatoes (recipe follows).

NUTRITION INFORMATION PER SERVING

Calories	Protein (g)	Carbs (g)	Fat (g)	Sat Fat (g)	Unsat Fat (g)	Fiber (g)
388	9	36	27	3	21	15

PURPLE POTATOES
Serves 1

2 small purple potatoes, cubed

½ tablespoon coconut oil

½ teaspoon dried rosemary

½ teaspoon turmeric powder

½ teaspoon sea salt

In a large skillet, boil the potatoes in just enough water to cover them. Cook them for about 7 to 10 minutes, until they are soft yet still firm in texture. Rinse the potatoes in a colander.

Drain any excess water from the skillet, and set it over medium heat. Melt the coconut oil in the skillet, then add the rosemary, turmeric, and salt, and transfer the potatoes into the spiced oil. Stir to coat the potatoes well. After about 1 minute, remove the skillet from the heat.

Serve the potatoes warm, with either the Ginger Chicken (*omnivore*) or the Spiced Eggplant (*vegan*).

NUTRITION INFORMATION PER SERVING

Calories	Protein (g)	Carbs (g)	Fat (g)	Sat Fat (g)	Unsat Fat (g)	Fiber (g)
298	6	54	7	6	1	6

DAY 19: THE SPIRIT—CONNECTION

The true way to be humble is not to stoop until you are smaller than yourself but to stand at your real height against some higher nature that will show you what the real smallness of your greatness is.

—PHILLIPS BROOKS

Meal Plan

	Omnivore	Vegan
Breakfast	Pear-Coconut Smoothie	Pear-Coconut Smoothie
Lunch	Arugula with Seed Medley	Arugula with Seed Medley
Snack	Divine Cleansing Broth	Divine Cleansing Broth
Dinner	Lemony Sole (Soul) with Turnips and Carrots	Enlightenment (Raw) Soup

Whole Detox Emotion Log

At the end of the day, track any emotions that you had on the Whole Detox Emotion Log.

Thought Pattern Activity

The following are some limiting thoughts that relate to the SPIRIT:

It is difficult for me to feel connected to a greater whole.

I don't feel inspired by my life.

I feel alone and disconnected from my everyday life.

Pick the limiting thought that seems to ring most true for you. If none of the examples feel true, write down your own limiting thought as it relates to the SPIRIT.

Next, set your timer for five minutes. Spend that time journaling on that thought, how it has affected your life, and how you feel when you have that thought.

Movement

Let your nervous system experience the contracting strength and relaxation of doing a whole-body progressive relaxation activity. Lie flat on your back, and insert a cushion under your knees if you need some lower-back support. Start the exercise by closing your eyes and tensing up all your muscles, starting with your feet and moving into your legs, torso, hands and arms, and face. Once your body is fully contracted, imagine what you want to let go of . . . and with a deep exhale, slowly let go of each part of your body, starting with where you tensed up first, your feet, and at the same time, release what you no longer need in your mind (maybe "stress" or "difficulty with my job"). Let the relaxation wash through your being, and feel your nervous system relax and calm down. Repeat this process three times and feel your body being connected throughout.

Affirmation

Spend three minutes saying aloud the following affirmation:

I am united with all of life.

Feel how your body responds to these words. You can also create your own statement. Feel free to write it on a beautiful notecard or a plain Post-it note and put it in your immediate environment for the day.

Visualization

Set a timer for three minutes. During that time, close your eyes and visualize a white, glitter-like coating over your entire being. Imagine that this coating represents your highest potential and purpose in life. Spend time basking in this glow of your illuminated self, feeling connection with all life within you and in your environment.

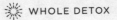
Meditation

For three minutes, meditate on the color white as you sit quietly on a cushion or chair.

DAY 19 RECIPES

Breakfast

PEAR-COCONUT SMOOTHIE

Serves 1

1 pear, sliced

1 cup unsweetened coconut water

1 scoop protein powder of your choice
(hemp, pea, rice, whey for omnivores)

Water and ice to blend

Put all the liquid and whole food ingredients into a high-speed blender first,
followed by the dry protein powder, then blend everything until a fluid consistency is reached. Add more water if needed. Drink immediately.

NUTRITION INFORMATION PER SERVING

Calories	Protein (g)	Carbs (g)	Fat (g)	Sat Fat (g)	Unsat Fat (g)	Fiber (g)
269	26	37	3	0.4	0.1	8

Lunch

ARUGULA WITH SEED MEDLEY

Serves 1

2 cups arugula

½ cup diced cucumber

1 tablespoon chia seeds

1 tablespoon hemp seeds

FOR THE DRESSING:

1 tablespoon freshly squeezed lemon
juice

1 tablespoon tahini

⅛ teaspoon turmeric powder

⅛ teaspoon ground black pepper

Pinch of sea salt

In a serving bowl, combine the arugula, cucumber, chia seeds, and hemp seeds. In a separate small bowl, whisk together all the dressing ingredients and drizzle the dressing over the salad.

NUTRITION INFORMATION PER SERVING

Calories	Protein (g)	Carbs (g)	Fat (g)	Sat Fat (g)	Unsat Fat (g)	Fiber (g)
205	8	12	15	2	9	5

Snack

DIVINE CLEANSING BROTH
Serves 3

7 cups purified water

2 carrots, sliced

3 celery stalks, diced

¼ cup chopped fresh parsley

¼ cup finely sliced green onions

¼ cup chopped leeks

5-inch piece burdock root, finely diced

7 shiitake mushrooms, sliced

1½ teaspoons freshly squeezed lemon juice

1 teaspoon sea salt

Ground black pepper to taste

In a large saucepan or soup pot, bring all the ingredients to a boil, then lower the heat and gently simmer the soup for 30 minutes. Serve the soup warm, spooning up one-third of it for today's snack. (Save the remaining two-thirds for the next two days' snacks.)

NUTRITION INFORMATION PER SERVING

Calories	Protein (g)	Carbs (g)	Fat (g)	Sat Fat (g)	Unsat Fat (g)	Fiber (g)
60	2	13	0.2	0	0.1	3

Dinner

LEMONY SOLE (SOUL) WITH TURNIPS AND CARROTS *(OMNIVORE)*
Serves 1

1 tablespoon freshly squeezed lemon juice

1 cup unsweetened coconut milk (boxed variety)

1 teaspoon dried thyme

1 teaspoon ground oregano

Pinch of sea salt

Freshly ground pepper to taste

1 5-ounce wild-caught sole fillet

2 medium turnips, cut into bite-size pieces

1 large carrot, cut into bite-size pieces

In a large skillet set over medium heat, combine the lemon juice, coconut milk, thyme, oregano, and salt, and season with pepper to taste. Gently add the sole fillet and let each side cook for 3 to 5 minutes, or until thoroughly cooked.

In a saucepan fitted with a steamer basket, boil ¼ to ½ cup water. Add the turnips and carrots to the steamer basket, and steam them until they are soft yet still colorful and firm, about 7 to 10 minutes.

Serve the sole alongside the steamed vegetables while they're still warm.

NUTRITION INFORMATION PER SERVING

Calories	Protein (g)	Carbs (g)	Fat (g)	Sat Fat (g)	Unsat Fat (g)	Fiber (g)
291	30	25	7	5	1	6

ENLIGHTENMENT (RAW) SOUP (VEGAN)

Serves 1

3 celery stalks

1 red bell pepper

2 cups spinach

½ avocado

1 green onion, diced

1 garlic clove

¼ cup raw cashews

2 tablespoons unhulled sesame seeds

1 teaspoon dulse flakes

3 fresh basil leaves

½ teaspoon dried dill

¼ teaspoon turmeric powder

Dash of ground cayenne pepper

1 teaspoon sea salt

Blend all the ingredients together in a high-speed blender or food processor. Thin the soup with purified water as desired. Serve it in a soup bowl, unheated.

NUTRITION INFORMATION PER SERVING

Calories	Protein (g)	Carbs (g)	Fat (g)	Sat Fat (g)	Unsat Fat (g)	Fiber (g)
544	14	42	39	5	24	18

DAY 20: THE SPIRIT—MEDITATION

Meditation is to dive all the way within, beyond thought, to the source of thought and pure consciousness. It enlarges the container, every time you transcend. When you come out, you come out refreshed, filled with energy and enthusiasm for life.

—DAVID LYNCH

Meal Plan

	Omnivore	Vegan
Breakfast	Mango-Coconut Smoothie	Mango-Coconut Smoothie
Lunch	Sweet-Sour Slaw	Sweet-Sour Slaw
Snack	Divine Cleansing Broth	Divine Cleansing Broth
Dinner	Creamy Spiced Cauliflower Soup with Lamb	Creamy Spiced Cauliflower Soup

Whole Detox Emotion Log

At the end of the day, track any emotions that you had on the Whole Detox Emotion Log.

Thought Pattern Activity

The following are some limiting thoughts that relate to the SPIRIT:

I can't meditate.
Sitting still is a waste of time.
I need to be always going somewhere or doing something.

Pick the limiting thought that seems to ring most true for you. If none of the examples feel true, write down your own limiting thought as it relates to the SPIRIT.

Next, set your timer for five minutes. Spend that time journaling on that thought, how it has affected your life, and how you feel when you have that thought.

Movement
HALF LOTUS (ARDHA PADMASANA)
As with all yoga poses, go to your comfortable limit. Nothing should be painful. Be careful with this pose if you have knee issues. Go with a modified pose if you are unable to complete the pose in its description below.

1. Sit on a mat or cushion.
2. Place one foot on the opposite thigh and the other foot on the floor beneath the opposite thigh.
3. Ideally both knees are on the floor; however, do not be discouraged if you cannot achieve this. Honor where your body is.

Alternatively, you can modify the pose by sitting with both feet on the floor, one in front of the other.

Once you have established your comfort in this pose, spend a couple of minutes here breathing deeply and fully.

Now, alternate your legs and repeat the same pose.

Affirmation
Spend three minutes saying aloud the following affirmation:

I move into the mystery of life with grace and ease.

Feel how your body responds to these words. You can also create your own statement. Feel free to write it on a beautiful notecard or a plain Post-it note and put it in your immediate environment for the day.

Visualization
Set a timer for three minutes. During that time, close your eyes and visualize rays of sunlight beaming down into every cell of your body, cleansing and purifying you of all toxins. Take your time to let the sunbeams radiate fully and completely from the outside to the inside.

Meditation
Meditate for seven minutes while basking in sunlight or while imagining that you are engulfed by a glow of purifying sunlight.

DAY 20 RECIPES

Breakfast

MANGO-COCONUT SMOOTHIE
Serves 1

1 cup diced mango

1 cup unsweetened coconut milk
(boxed variety)

¼ cup unsweetened coconut water

1 scoop protein powder of your choice
(hemp, pea, rice, whey for omnivores)

Water and ice to blend

Put all the liquid and whole food ingredients into a high-speed blender first, followed by the dry protein powder, then blend everything until a fluid consistency is reached. Add more water if needed. Drink immediately.

NUTRITION INFORMATION PER SERVING

Calories	Protein (g)	Carbs (g)	Fat (g)	Sat Fat (g)	Unsat Fat (g)	Fiber (g)
325	25	39	8	5	0.3	4

Lunch

SWEET-SOUR SLAW
Serves 1

1 cup diced green cabbage

½ cup diced red cabbage

1 pear, sliced

1 tablespoon diced white onion

2 tablespoons chopped walnuts

2 tablespoons golden raisins

FOR THE DRESSING:

1 tablespoon Dijon mustard

1 teaspoon honey

1 tablespoon apple cider vinegar

1 tablespoon flaxseed oil

½ teaspoon fennel seeds

Pinch of ground cayenne pepper

Pinch of sea salt

In a serving bowl, combine the cabbages, pear, onion, walnuts, and raisins. In a separate small bowl, whisk together all the dressing ingredients and drizzle the dressing over the salad.

NUTRITION INFORMATION PER SERVING

Calories	Protein (g)	Carbs (g)	Fat (g)	Sat Fat (g)	Unsat Fat (g)	Fiber (g)
468	5	65	24	2	20	11

Snack

DIVINE CLEANSING BROTH

Enjoy one serving—half—of yesterday's leftovers

NUTRITION INFORMATION PER SERVING

Calories	Protein (g)	Carbs (g)	Fat (g)	Sat Fat (g)	Unsat Fat (g)	Fiber (g)
60	2	13	0.2	0	0.1	3

Dinner

CREAMY SPICED CAULIFLOWER SOUP *(VEGAN)* WITH LAMB *(OMNIVORE)*
Serves 2

FOR OMNIVORES:

½ pound organic, grass-fed, boneless lamb, cubed

FOR BOTH:

2 teaspoons coconut oil
½ medium yellow onion, diced
2 garlic cloves, minced
Pinch of crushed red pepper flakes
1 teaspoon ground cumin
1 teaspoon turmeric powder
Pinch of ground coriander
Pinch of ground cardamom
Pinch of sea salt

Dash of ground black pepper
½ large head cauliflower, roughly chopped
1 cup unsweetened, full-fat coconut milk
2 cups organic vegetable broth
1 bay leaf
1 tablespoon cashew nut butter

In a large soup pot set over medium heat, warm the coconut oil.

Omnivores, add the lamb and sauté it for several minutes before adding the onion and garlic.

Both omnivores and vegans, sauté the onion and garlic, stirring occasionally, until the onions become translucent, about 3 minutes. Add the red pepper flakes, cumin, turmeric, coriander, cardamom, salt, and black pepper, and stir the mixture well for about 1 minute. Then add the cauliflower, coconut milk, broth, bay leaf, and cashew nut butter. Bring the soup to a boil, then reduce the heat and let it simmer gently for about 15 minutes, until the cauliflower is tender and, for omnivores, the lamb is cooked.

Ladle half the soup into a serving bowl and serve it warm. (Save the remaining half for tomorrow's lunch.)

NUTRITION INFORMATION PER SERVING

	Calories	Protein (g)	Carbs (g)	Fat (g)	Sat Fat (g)	Unsat Fat (g)	Fiber (g)
Omnivore	550	32	23	40	29	5	6
Vegan	390	9	23	33	26	2	6

DAY 21: THE SPIRIT—FASTING

I continue to be drawn to clarity and simplicity. "Less is more" remains my mantra.

—STÉPHANE ROLLAND

Meal Plan

	Omnivore	Vegan
Breakfast	Pear-Ginger Smoothie	Pear-Ginger Smoothie
Lunch	Pure and Simple Detox Salad Creamy Spiced Cauliflower Soup with Lamb	Pure and Simple Detox Salad Creamy Spiced Cauliflower Soup
Snack	Divine Cleansing Broth	Divine Cleansing Broth
Dinner	Coconut-Flaked Halibut with White Onion	Divine Rainbow Noodles with Heavenly Basil-Cauliflower Pesto

Whole Detox Emotion Log

At the end of the day, track any emotions that you had on the Whole Detox Emotion Log.

Thought Pattern Activity

The following are some limiting thoughts that relate to the SPIRIT:

I never have enough.
I need to eat to feel secure and fulfilled.
I feel scared when I "go without."

Pick the limiting thought that seems to ring most true for you. If none of the examples feel true, write down your own limiting thought as it relates to the SPIRIT.

Next, set your timer for five minutes. Spend that time journaling on that thought, how it has affected your life, and how you feel when you have that thought.

Movement

Gentle bouncing is excellent stimulation for the lymphatic system. You can jump on a trampoline, jump rope, or just jump in place. The up-and-down rhythmic gravitational force causes the lymph system's one-way valves to open and close. This motion increases the flow of lymphatic fluid and oxygen uptake, and promotes detoxification through the lungs, skin, and lymph.

Affirmation

Spend three minutes saying aloud the following affirmation:

I am filled with the abundance of life.

Feel how your body responds to these words. You can also create your own statement. Feel free to write it on a beautiful notecard or a plain Post-it note and put it in your immediate environment for the day.

Visualization

Set a timer for three minutes. During that time, close your eyes and visualize yourself as a vast universe. See your inner self filled with planets, stars, and galaxies. Imagine that your being is the expanse of all that lives and exists. Feel nourished and abundant by seeing this interconnection within you.

Meditation

What is your favorite food to eat? Meditate for seven minutes on that food; see it as a symbol or a metaphor for what you are really experiencing by eating that food on the level of your soul. In the meditation, what comes forth from your thought patterns, childhood, and the sensation of eating that food?

DAY 21 RECIPES

Breakfast

PEAR-GINGER SMOOTHIE
Serves 1

1 small ripe pear, cored
1-inch piece fresh ginger, minced
¼ teaspoon ground ginger
½ cup water

1 scoop protein powder of your choice
   (hemp, pea, rice, whey for omnivores)
Water and ice to blend

Put all the liquid and whole food ingredients into a high-speed blender first, followed by the dry protein powder, then blend everything until a fluid consistency is reached. Add more water if needed. Drink immediately.

NUTRITION INFORMATION PER SERVING

Calories	Protein (g)	Carbs (g)	Fat (g)	Sat Fat (g)	Unsat Fat (g)	Fiber (g)
223	25	29	2	0	0.1	6

Lunch

PURE AND SIMPLE DETOX SALAD WITH CREAMY SPICED CAULIFLOWER SOUP (VEGAN) WITH LAMB (OMNIVORE)

Serves 1

1 cup chopped romaine lettuce
½ cup chopped cucumber
1 tablespoon chia seeds

1 tablespoon freshly squeezed lemon juice
1 tablespoon hempseed oil

Simply combine everything in a serving bowl, coating all the ingredients with lemon juice and hempseed oil.

Warm up yesterday's Creamy Spiced Cauliflower Soup (*vegan*) with Lamb (*omnivore*) to serve with the salad.

NUTRITION INFORMATION PER SERVING

	Calories	Protein (g)	Carbs (g)	Fat (g)	Sat Fat (g)	Unsat Fat (g)	Fiber (g)
Omnivore	733	34	31	56	30	19	11
Vegan	573	11	31	49	27	16	11

Snack

DIVINE CLEANSING BROTH

Enjoy the remaining serving of leftovers from Day 19

NUTRITION INFORMATION PER SERVING

Calories	Protein (g)	Carbs (g)	Fat (g)	Sat Fat (g)	Unsat Fat (g)	Fiber (g)
60	2	13	0.2	0	0.1	3

Dinner

COCONUT-FLAKED HALIBUT WITH WHITE ONION *(OMNIVORE)*
Serves 1

1 teaspoon coconut oil

1 small white onion, sliced thinly

2 tablespoons coconut flour

2 tablespoons unsweetened coconut flakes

2 tablespoons flaxseed meal

2 tablespoons coconut oil, melted, divided

¼ cup unsweetened, full-fat coconut milk

1 5-ounce halibut fillet

1 tablespoon finely chopped green onion, for garnish

In a small skillet set over low heat, warm the 1 teaspoon coconut oil, then add the onion, sautéing it until it is lightly browned.

While the onion is cooking, prepare the fish. In a shallow bowl or plate, combine the coconut flour, coconut flakes, and flaxseed meal. In a separate shallow bowl, combine 1 tablespoon of the melted coconut oil with the coconut milk. Dip both sides of the halibut fillet first into the oil and milk mixture, then into the flour and meal mixture, completely coating the fillet.

In a skillet set over medium heat, add the remaining 1 tablespoon of melted coconut oil, then gently place the fillet into the pan, and cook it about 5 minutes on each side, depending on its thickness.

Serve the fillet topped with a sprinkle of chopped green onion and alongside the sautéed onions.

NUTRITION INFORMATION PER SERVING

Calories	Protein (g)	Carbs (g)	Fat (g)	Sat Fat (g)	Unsat Fat (g)	Fiber (g)
559	34	13	42	33	6	7

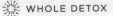

DIVINE RAINBOW NOODLES WITH HEAVENLY BASIL-CAULIFLOWER PESTO *(VEGAN)*

Serves 1

- 1 red bell pepper, sliced thinly
- 1 carrot, sliced into "noodles" with a vegetable peeler
- 1 small zucchini, sliced into "noodles" with a vegetable peeler or spiralizer
- 1 small yellow squash, sliced into "noodles" with a vegetable peeler or spiralizer
- 2 tablespoons Heavenly Basil-Cauliflower Pesto (recipe follows)
- Sliced green onions, for garnish

On a serving plate, gently combine the bell pepper, carrot, zucchini, and yellow squash with the pesto, and garnish the dish with the green onions.

NUTRITION INFORMATION PER SERVING

Calories	Protein (g)	Carbs (g)	Fat (g)	Sat Fat (g)	Unsat Fat (g)	Fiber (g)
96	4	20	1	0.1	0.3	6

HEAVENLY BASIL-CAULIFLOWER PESTO *(VEGAN)*

Makes about ½ cup, or about four servings

- 1 cup tightly packed fresh basil leaves (purple basil preferred)
- 1 cup chopped cauliflower
- 2 garlic cloves
- 1 teaspoon sea salt
- ½ cup raw pine nuts
- ½ cup extra-virgin olive oil

Place all the ingredients in a high-speed blender or food processor, and blend the mixture until it's smooth. Add more oil if needed for a better flow. Save any leftover pesto in a glass jar for future use.

NUTRITION INFORMATION PER SERVING

Calories	Protein (g)	Carbs (g)	Fat (g)	Sat Fat (g)	Unsat Fat (g)	Fiber (g)
131	2	3	13	1	11	1

CHAPTER 12

∴⁄∴

WHOLE DETOX FOR LIFE

Congratulations! You've completed your twenty-one-day Whole Detox and brought a whole new rainbow of possibilities into your life. You've taken some exciting steps toward clearing up symptoms, losing weight, boosting your vitality, and tapping into new reserves of purpose and meaning. You've learned something about which foods sap your energy and discovered some new foods that have brought more color, flavor, and sparkle into your life. You've found out more about the toxic barriers that are holding you back, and you've found some new ways to break through them and move on to a new level of inspiration.

I'm excited for the new possibilities you have unlocked, and I want to help you make the most of them. So let's talk about what comes next.

WHOLE DETOX: WHAT COMES NEXT?

Right after the program: Reintroduce foods you have eliminated while enjoying a daily rainbow of good food.

One month later: Complete the Whole Detox Spectrum Quiz again and identify which system of full-spectrum health is most out of balance now. Focus on bringing that system back into balance through food, lifestyle, color, or any combination of the three.

Six months later: Complete another entire Whole Detox. After the twenty-one days, you can try reintroducing foods that didn't work for you the last time. Then continue to do your monthly check-in with your systems of health through the Whole Detox Spectrum Quiz.

Going forward: Every six months, complete another Whole Detox. If you like, you can try reintroducing foods that you haven't yet been able to tolerate. Use the Whole Detox Food Reintroduction Symptoms Tracker to track your progress.

RIGHT AFTER THE PROGRAM:
REINTRODUCE FOODS AND CONSUME THE RAINBOW

You've just spent twenty-one days finding out what it's like when your body isn't burdened by problem foods. You've also found out how great it feels to eat from the full spectrum of the rainbow. Now it's time to figure out which foods you can bring back into your daily diet while also continuing to eat a rainbow-colored diet.

What is Reintroduction?

As we saw in chapter 1, Whole Detox begins at the ROOT, pulling out any food that might trigger inflammation. Inflammation is a response from your immune system that can be healing when it is acute and specific but becomes highly problematic when it is chronic.

The following foods frequently trigger inflammation, which is why we pulled them from our twenty-one-day detox:

- Alcohol
- Caffeine (chocolate, coffee, soft drinks, tea)
- Dairy products (cheese, milk, yogurt)
- Eggs
- Gluten (barley, spelt, wheat, and, in some cases, oats)
- Peanuts
- Processed carbohydrates
- Processed meats
- Shellfish
- Sugar and sweeteners (includes artificial ones)
- Soy

However, after a twenty-one-day Whole Detox, your immune system has become healthier without the daily interference of foods you had before you started the program. Using the following protocol, you can find whether you can now eat foods that formerly gave you trouble.

The Reintroduction Protocol

Make a list of the foods and beverages you have omitted and would like to add back into your diet.

For example:

- Caffeine (coffee, soda, tea)
- Chocolate
- Corn (chips, fresh corn, tortillas)
- Dairy products (cheese, milk, yogurt)
- Eggs
- Shellfish (lobster, shrimp)
- Soy (miso, soy sauce, tofu)

1. *Find a simple version of the first food you want to test.* Ensure that the food you test is simple enough in composition and not a complex food with multiple ingredients. For example, if you are testing corn, you will want to test a pure corn product in multiple forms that you typically eat, like organic corn on the cob or a straightforward corn chip or a simple-ingredient corn tortilla, not a corn chip with gluten-containing spices or a high-fructose corn syrup sweetener. If you try the food in a complex version with multiple ingredients and you have a problematic reaction, you won't know whether you're reacting to the problem food or to one of the other ingredients.
2. *While maintaining your baseline diet, add in two daily servings of the test food.* For example, if you are reintroducing cheese, you might have one slice of cheese with your daily smoothie and another with your salad at lunch.
3. *Allow four to six hours after you consume a new food before eating any more of it.* If you notice symptoms at any point, stop eating the food and pull it from your diet for at least six months. If you're okay, continue on to the next serving.

4. *Observe your symptoms the day after the food challenge.* If you notice symptoms, stop eating it immediately. If you manage two successful symptom-free days (one of those days is the day you challenged the food), you can now add the food back into your diet. Don't overdo it, though; you might provoke another bad reaction. Stick to two to five times a week for any formerly problematic food. Rotating foods is always a good idea.

5. *Reintroduce the next food.* If you have successfully introduced the first food, you can reintroduce the next food. If you had problematic symptoms from the first food, wait for those symptoms to fully subside. Then, after two symptom-free days, introduce the next food.

You can use the Food Reintroduction Symptoms Tracker (see page 384) to keep a record of the process.

If a food gives you problems, don't despair. You can try to reintroduce it again in another six to twelve months, after your immune system has become stronger. You may be able to enjoy it in small amounts or at times when you're not too stressed. Listen to your intuition and let your body tell you what you are able to handle. You might also consult a functional medicine practitioner to work with you more closely to figure out which foods are right for you through laboratory testing.

COMMON REACTIONS FROM PROBLEM FOODS

- Digestion difficulties, such as gas or bloating
- Changes in bowel movements, such as diarrhea or constipation
- Skin rashes, itching, acne, rosacea, and/or hives
- Extreme fatigue
- Chills or temperature shifts, such as flushing and atypical body heat
- Pain in the joints or throughout the body

Consuming the Rainbow

As you have seen, Whole Detox isn't just about taking foods out. It's also about making sure you get the right foods to fortify your system. The more you support your system with healthy, colorful, whole foods, the more you will be able to tolerate life's stresses and perhaps also some of the foods that gave you problems before.

Remember is to get the full rainbow every day. Make sure you eat at least one food from each of the seven colors on a daily basis. You can use the Rainbow Tracker (see page 385) to help ensure you're covering the entire rainbow. I suggest using the tracker for twenty-one days, which is typically how long it takes to create a new habit.

BECOMING AWARE OF COLOR

One of the most transformative results of Whole Detox is how much your awareness of color grows. You will find yourself noticing how different colored foods affect you, and also how color affects you in other domains: the clothes you wear, the colors you choose for your home, the objects you bring in to brighten up your work space. I encourage you to remain open to the healing, energizing, and inspiring properties of color!

ONE MONTH LATER: START YOUR MONTHLY CHECK-IN

Once you've finished the process of reintroducing problem foods, give yourself a month to process the results of your Whole Detox. Then check in by retaking the entire Whole Detox Spectrum Quiz (see pages 35–41). Use your score to determine which of your seven systems is most out of balance. Then focus on that system for the next month. You can restore balance with food, lifestyle, color, or any combination of the three.

SIX MONTHS LATER: COMPLETE ANOTHER WHOLE DETOX

The exciting thing about this approach is that each time you conduct a Whole Detox, your experience will be profoundly different. Barriers that existed before may now have disappeared; new challenges, perhaps in different systems, will have emerged. As long as we are alive, we will face some barriers to health and fulfillment. Learning how to remove each new barrier as it appears offers us a continual process of discovery and growth—and an ongoing opportunity to deepen our relationship with ourselves.

GOING FORWARD

• Continue your monthly check-in
• Repeat Whole Detox every six months

As I tell my patients, we can learn more about ourselves, breaking through barriers and accessing new potential. Accordingly, each time you complete a Whole Detox, your experience will teach you something you didn't expect. You might find yourself working on different systems of health or returning again and again to the same one or two systems, but each time the issues that arise will seem slightly different and the possibilities you unlock will take you to new places.

Throughout your journey, however, you can count on the Whole Detox Spectrum Quiz to guide you, helping you identify where your strengths lie and your toxic barriers appear. Clarifying and healing one set of issues makes room for some new issues to come to the surface, in an ongoing process of detoxification and renewal.

This is why I'd like you also to use the Whole Detox Food Reintroduction Systems Tracker (see page 384) to track your progress from one week to the next. As "happy," "energized," and "symptom-free" become your new normal, you might forget how far you've come. And even if some of the same issues recur—as they do for most of us—your Systems Tracker will help you realize that they are returning in new forms. Often we are making progress even when it doesn't feel like it, and the Systems Tracker can help you see that.

THE POWER OF SYSTEMS

One of the extraordinary things about Whole Detox is how work on one system of health profoundly affects all the other systems. Even tiny, incremental adjustments—starting to eat a colorful food, adding in a few minutes of daily exercise, taking five minutes to meditate or do a yoga stretch—can, over time, be transformative, because one small change leads to another, and then another, and then another. Likewise, a modification in the ROOT can quickly produce changes in one of the other systems, which can lead to a change in yet another system, and then another, and then another.

Although Whole Detox moves through the systems of health in a linear fashion, the systems are less a straight line than a web, a dynamic interconnected network. Some people feel overwhelmed by the idea that we are truly a web and that anything we do is going to have an impact: from teeny tiny actions to great big huge actions. Don't get stuck or stagnated on trying to figure out how to be perfect; just move through your colors, go where you feel drawn, and you will be on the path of healing. Let yourself be guided by the inspiration of color and the information you now have about food and lifestyle as you continue to live a full-spectrum life!

UNIVERSAL CONVERSION CHART

OVEN TEMPERATURE EQUIVALENTS

250°F = 120°C   400°F = 200°C

275°F = 135°C   425°F = 220°C

300°F = 150°C   450°F = 230°C

325°F = 160°C   475°F = 240°C

350°F = 180°C   500°F = 260°C

375°F = 190°C

MEASUREMENT EQUIVALENTS

Measurements should always be level unless directed otherwise.

⅛ teaspoon = 0.5 mL

¼ teaspoon = 1 mL

½ teaspoon = 2 mL

1 teaspoon = 5 mL

1 tablespoon = 3 teaspoons = ½ fluid ounce = 15 mL

2 tablespoons = ⅓ cup = 1 fluid ounce = 30 mL

4 tablespoons = ½ cup = 2 fluid ounces = 60 mL

5⅓ tablespoons = ⅓ cup = 3 fluid ounces = 80 mL

8 tablespoons = ½ cup = 4 fluid ounces = 120 mL

10⅔ tablespoons = ⅔ cup = 5 fluid ounces = 160 mL

12 tablespoons = ½ cup = 6 fluid ounces = 180 mL

16 tablespoons = 1 cup = 8 fluid ounces = 240 mL

OMNIVORE SHOPPING LISTS
THE ROOT

PRODUCE

Apples, red	2 (1 small, 1 medium)
Avocado	1 medium
Beets with their greens	2 medium
Bell pepper, red	2 small
Broccoli	1 cup, chopped
Carrots	3 (1 small, 2 medium)
Cauliflower	1 cup, chopped
Grapefruit	1
Grapes, red	7
Kale	4 medium to large leaves
Lettuce, red- or green-leaf	2 cups roughly chopped
Mushroom, portobello	1
Mushrooms, shiitake	6
Onion, red	2 medium
Radishes	4
Raspberries	About 1 ½ cups
Strawberries	About 1 cup
Swiss chard	2 medium to large leaves
Tomatoes	2 medium
Turnip	1 medium

GROCERY

Almond butter	2 tablespoons
Bee pollen granules (optional)	1 tablespoon
Hummus	½ cup
Quinoa (red variety preferred)	¼ cup uncooked (½ cup cooked)
Sesame seeds, unhulled	1 tablespoon
Sunflower seeds, raw	1 tablespoon
Tomato juice, low-sodium, bottled	2 cups
Walnut halves (red variety preferred)	8

MEAT AND FISH

Chicken breasts, organic, free-range, boneless, skinless	2 breasts, 4 ounces each
Flank steak, organic, grass-fed	4 to 6 ounces
Ground beef, organic, grass-fed	⅓ pound
Ground turkey, organic, free-range, lean	½ pound

THE FLOW

PRODUCE

Apricots	3
Arugula or other leafy greens	2 cups
Avocado	1 medium
Banana	1 small
Bell pepper, orange	1 large
Cabbage, red	1 small head (need ½ cup shredded)
Carrots	3 medium
Fennel bulb with fronds	1
Green onions	3
Kale	2 large leaves
Leek	1 medium
Mangoes	2
Mixed greens	1 cup

Nectarine (or orange, if you prefer)	1
Onion, yellow	1 small (need 2 tablespoons diced)
Oranges (save the zest)	2
Peach	2 small
Shallot	1 medium

FRESH HERBS

| Basil | 1 cup leaves |
| Mint | 2 tablespoons chopped |

GROCERY

Brown rice flour	¼ cup
Cashews, raw (or other nuts of choice; optional)	2 tablespoons
Coconut flakes, unsweetened	1 tablespoon
Dates, Medjool	2
Macadamia nuts, lightly salted	10 whole nuts plus ¼ cup finely chopped
Orange juice	2¼ cups
Pine nuts, raw	½ cup
Pumpkin seeds, roasted	2 tablespoons
Quinoa	¼ cup uncooked (½ cup cooked)
Raisins, golden	2 tablespoons
Sunflower oil, high oleic, or extra-virgin olive oil	1 tablespoon
Vegetable broth, organic	1¼ cups
Walnut halves	2 cups plus 2 tablespoons

MEAT AND FISH

Cod, wild-caught	3 ounces
Ground lamb, organic, grass-fed	10 ounces
Halibut, wild-caught	2 fillets, 5 ounces each
Salmon, wild-caught	1 8- to 10-ounce fillet (with its skin)

THE FIRE

PRODUCE

Apple, Golden Delicious	1
Arugula	2 cups
Bananas	2 small
Bell peppers, yellow	1½
Cauliflower	2 cups chopped
Celery	1 to 2 stalks (need ¼ cup finely chopped)
Cucumber	¼ medium
Green onions	1 to 2 (need 3 tablespoons chopped)
Kale	1 to 2 leaves (need ¾ cup finely chopped)
Onion, yellow	1 large
Pineapple chunks, frozen or fresh	½ cup
Shallots	2 medium to large
Spaghetti squash	1 small
Spinach	2 cups
Summer squash, yellow	1 small plus ¼ cup cubed

FRESH HERBS

Basil	¼ cup chopped
Cilantro	5 tablespoons chopped
Parsley	¼ cup finely chopped

GROCERY

Almonds, raw	¼ cup
Amaranth	3 tablespoons uncooked (½ cup cooked)
Date, Medjool	1
Lentils, French green	¼ cup uncooked (½ cup cooked)
Mustard, Dijon	1 tablespoon
Pineapple juice	1 cup
Pine nuts, raw	2 tablespoons
Quinoa	¾ cup uncooked (1½ cups cooked)
Rice, brown, long grain	¼ cup uncooked

Rice vinegar	½ tablespoon
Sesame seeds, unhulled	½ tablespoon
Sunflower oil, high-oleic, or extra-virgin olive oil	1 tablespoon
Sunflower seed butter	2 tablespoons
Tahini	1 tablespoon
Tapioca flour	1 teaspoon
Vegetable broth, organic (optional)	½ cup

MEAT AND FISH

Chicken breasts, organic, free-range, boneless, skinless	4 breasts, 4 ounces each
Ground turkey, organic, free-range	8 ounces

THE LOVE

PRODUCE

Apple, green	1
Asparagus stalks	5
Avocado	1 large
Broccoli	1½ cups chopped
Broccoli sprouts	¼ cup
Cabbage, green	½ head or 1 small (need ½ cup shredded)
Cucumber	1½ small
Green onions	1 bunch
Honeydew melon	1 cup cubed
Kale, green curly-leaf	2½ to 3 bunches
Kiwi fruits	2
Microgreens	About 1 cup
Mushrooms, shiitake	¼ cup chopped
Spinach	8½ to 9 cups
Strawberries	About 2 (need ¼ cup sliced)
Swiss chard	1 bunch (about 5 large leaves)

FRESH HERBS

Dill	¼ teaspoon
Mint	4 to 5 leaves
Parsley	2 tablespoons minced

GROCERY

Almond meal	2 tablespoons
Almonds, raw	¼ cup
Almonds, toasted, slivered	2 tablespoons
Apple juice	¼ cup
Avocado oil	4 tablespoons
Cacao nibs, raw	1 tablespoon
Green tea, decaffeinated	⅔ cup
Olives, green	5
Pine nuts, raw	2 tablespoons
Pistachios, unsalted, raw, shelled	5 tablespoons
Walnut halves	4 to 5
White beans (Great Northern)	3 tablespoons uncooked (½ cup cooked)
Other	Parchment paper, kitchen string

MEAT AND FISH

Anchovies (Vital Choice brand preferred)	4
Lox	4 ounces
Salmon, wild-caught	2 fillets, 3 to 4 ounces each
Turkey breasts, organic, free-range, boneless	2 breasts, 4 to 5 ounces each

THE TRUTH

PRODUCE

Apple, green	1
Arugula	1 cup
Banana	1 medium
Bell pepper, red	½

Bok choy	1 to 2 heads (need 1½ cups chopped)
Cabbage, red	Less than ¼ head (need ¼ cup finely sliced)
Cantaloupe	½ cup cubed
Carrots	4
Cauliflower	2 cups chopped
Dandelion greens	1 cup
Green onion	1
Honeydew melon	1½ cups cubed
Kale, baby	4 cups
Kiwi fruit	1
Mango	2 cups cubed
Mushrooms, shiitake	5 large
Onion, yellow	¼ cup diced
Potatoes, red	2 small
Radishes	2
Spinach	1½ cups
Squash, yellow	½ small
Strawberries	2
Zucchini	1 small

FRESH HERBS

Basil	4 leaves
Lemongrass	3-inch piece
Mint	7 or 8 leaves

GROCERY

Almonds, raw	12
Coconut, unsweetened, shredded	1 tablespoon
Dates, Medjool	2
Dulse flakes	1 cup
Nori, pressed	3 sheets
Orange juice	4 tablespoons
Pecan pieces	½ cup
Pomegranate juice	1 cup

Rice, brown	½ cup cooked
Sesame seeds, unhulled	1 teaspoon
Thai green curry paste	½ teaspoon
Vegetable broth, organic	7 cups
Walnut halves	5

MEAT AND FISH

Chicken breasts, organic, free-range, boneless	14 ounces total
Halibut, wild-caught	8 ounces

THE INSIGHT

PRODUCE

Apple, red	⅓ cup sliced
Banana	1 medium
Blackberries	3¾ cups
Blueberries, frozen or fresh	3½ cups
Broccoli	1½ cups chopped
Cabbage, red	1 large
Carrot	1 tablespoon shredded
Cucumber	¼ cup cubed
Kale, baby	2 cups
Kale, purple	3 cups chopped
Plums	2
Potatoes, purple	2 small
Raspberries	1 cup
Shallot	1 large
Spinach	3 cups

FRESH HERBS

Basil, purple	7 leaves
Mint	1 teaspoon minced

GROCERY

Bee pollen granules (optional)	1 teaspoon
Cacao nibs, raw	1 tablespoon
Cocoa powder, unsweetened	1 tablespoon
Coconut, unsweetened, shredded	2 tablespoons
Hempseed oil	1 tablespoon
Hibiscus tea	½ cup
Mustard, Dijon	½ tablespoon
Oats, gluten-free	1 cup
Pecan halves	8
Pecans	½ cup chopped
Pine nuts, raw	2 tablespoons
Pomegranate juice	1 cup
Walnuts	¾ cup chopped

MEAT AND FISH

Chicken breast, organic, free-range, boneless	1 breast, 4 ounces
Cod, wild-caught	2 fillets, 4 ounces each
Salmon, wild-caught	2 fillets, 4 ounces each

THE SPIRIT

PRODUCE

Arugula	2 cups
Burdock root	5-inch piece
Cabbage, green	¼ to ½ head (need 1 cup diced)
Cabbage, red	¼ head (need ½ cup diced)
Carrots	3
Cauliflower	½ large head
Celery	3 stalks
Cucumber	1 cup diced
Green onions	1 small bunch

Leeks	¼ cup chopped
Mango, frozen or fresh	1 cup diced
Mushrooms, shiitake	7
Onion, white	1 medium or 2 small
Onion, yellow	½ medium
Pears	3
Romaine lettuce	1 cup chopped
Turnips	2 medium

FRESH HERBS

Parsley	¼ cup chopped

GROCERY

Cashew nut butter	1 tablespoon
Coconut flakes, unsweetened	2 tablespoons
Coconut flour	2 tablespoons
Hempseed oil	1 tablespoon
Mustard, Dijon	1 tablespoon
Raisins, golden	2 tablespoons
Tahini	1 tablespoon
Vegetable broth, organic	2 cups
Walnuts	2 tablespoons chopped

MEAT AND FISH

Halibut, wild-caught	1 fillet, 5 ounces
Lamb, organic, grass-fed, boneless	8 ounces
Sole, wild-caught	1 fillet, 5 ounces

VEGAN SHOPPING LISTS
THE ROOT

PRODUCE

Apples, red	2 (1 small, 1 medium)
Avocado	1 medium
Beets with their greens	2 medium
Bell pepper, red	2 small
Broccoli	1 cup chopped
Carrots	3 (1 small, 2 medium)
Cauliflower	1 cup, chopped
Grapefruit	1
Grapes, red	7
Kale	4 large leaves
Lettuce, red- or green-leaf	2 cups roughly chopped
Mushroom, portobello	1
Mushrooms, shiitake	6
Onion, red	2 medium
Radishes	4
Raspberries	About 1½ cups
Strawberries	About 1 cup
Swiss chard	2 medium to large leaves
Tomatoes	2 medium
Turnip	1 medium

GROCERY

Adzuki beans	½ cup uncooked (1½ cups cooked)
Almond butter	2 tablespoons
Bee pollen granules (optional)	1 tablespoon
Black beans	¼ cup uncooked (¾ cup cooked)
Chickpeas	½ cup uncooked (1½ cups cooked)
Hummus	½ cup
Kidney beans	¼ cup uncooked (¾ cup cooked)

Quinoa (red variety preferred)	¼ cup uncooked (½ cup cooked) plus 2 tablespoons uncooked
Sesame seeds, unhulled	1 tablespoon
Sunflower seeds, raw	1 tablespoon
Tomato juice, low-sodium, bottled	2 cups
Walnut halves (red variety preferred)	8

THE FLOW

PRODUCE

Avocado	1 medium
Banana	1 small
Bell peppers, orange	3 large
Cabbage, red	1 small head (need ½ cup shredded)
Carrots	12 medium to large
Celery	1 to 2 stalks (need ¼ cup diced)
Fennel bulb with fronds	1
Kale	2 large leaves
Leek	1 small to medium
Mangoes	2
Mixed greens	1 cup
Nectarine (or orange, if you prefer)	1
Onion, yellow	1 small to medium
Oranges (save the zest)	2
Peach	2 small
Shallot	1 medium

FRESH HERBS

Basil	1 cup leaves
Mint	2 tablespoons chopped

GROCERY

Almond butter	3 tablespoons
Almonds, slivered	2 tablespoons
Cashews, raw	6 tablespoons
Coconut flakes, unsweetened	1 tablespoon
Dates, Medjool	2
Lentils, dried, sprouted	½ cup uncooked
Lentils, orange/red	¾ cup uncooked (1½ cups cooked)
Macadamia nuts, lightly salted	10
Orange juice	¾ cup
Pine nuts, raw	¾ cup
Pumpkin seeds, roasted	2 tablespoons
Quinoa	¼ cup uncooked (½ cup cooked)
Raisins, golden	2 tablespoons
Sunflower oil, high oleic	1 tablespoon
Sunflower seeds, raw	¼ cup
Tahini	2 tablespoons
Vegetable broth, organic	3 cups
Walnut halves	2 cups plus 2 tablespoons
Wild rice	½ cup uncooked

THE FIRE

PRODUCE

Apple, Golden Delicious	1
Arugula	2 cups
Avocado	1 small
Bananas	2 small
Bell pepper, yellow	1
Carrots	2
Cucumber	½ small
Onion, red	1 small
Onion, yellow	1 small
Pineapple chunks, frozen or fresh	½ cup

Potato, yellow	1 large
Romaine lettuce heart	1 large
Shallots	3 medium to large
Spinach	2 cups
Summer squash, yellow	1 small

FRESH HERBS

Basil	¼ cup chopped
Cilantro	5 tablespoons chopped
Parsley	2 tablespoons chopped
Thyme	2 tablespoons chopped

GROCERY

Almonds, raw	¼ cup
Amaranth	3 tablespoons uncooked (½ cup cooked)
Black beans	½ cup uncooked (1½ cups cooked)
Chickpeas	½ cup uncooked (1½ cups cooked)
Date, Medjool	1
Lentils, yellow	½ cup uncooked
Pineapple juice	1 cup
Pine nuts, raw	2 tablespoons
Quinoa	¼ cup uncooked (½ cup cooked)
Sunflower seed butter	2 tablespoons
Tahini	2 tablespoons
Vegetable broth, organic	4 cups

THE LOVE

PRODUCE

Apple, green	1
Asparagus stalks	1 large bunch
Avocados	2 large
Broccoli	1½ cups chopped

Broccoli sprouts	¼ cup
Brussels sprouts	6 or 7
Cabbage, green	½ head or 1 small (need ½ cup shredded)
Cauliflower	3 cups chopped
Cucumber	1 medium
Green onions	2
Honeydew melon	1 cup cubed
Kale, green curly-leaf	2½ to 3 bunches
Kiwi fruits	2
Microgreens	About 1 cup
Spinach	7½ cups
Strawberries	About 2 (need ¼ cup sliced)

FRESH HERBS

Cilantro	2 tablespoons chopped
Dill	¼ teaspoon
Mint	4 to 5 leaves
Parsley	2 tablespoons minced

GROCERY

Almonds, raw	¼ cup
Almonds, toasted, slivered	2 tablespoons
Apple juice	¼ cup
Avocado oil	5 tablespoons
Cacao nibs, raw	1 tablespoon
Cannellini beans	2 tablespoons uncooked (¼ cup cooked)
Green tea, decaffeinated	⅔ cup
Lima beans	2 tablespoons uncooked (¼ cup cooked)
Olives, green	5
Pine nuts, raw	4 tablespoons
Pistachios, unsalted, raw, shelled	5 tablespoons
Rice, brown	¼ cup uncooked (¾ cup cooked)
Tahini	1 tablespoon
Walnut halves	4 to 5
White beans, Great Northern	¼ cup uncooked (¾ cup cooked)

THE TRUTH

PRODUCE

Apple, green	1
Arugula	1 cup
Banana	1 medium
Bell pepper, red	½
Bok choy	1 to 2 heads (need 1½ cups chopped)
Cabbage, red	Less than ¼ head (need ¼ cup finely sliced)
Cantaloupe	½ cup cubed
Carrots	4
Cauliflower	2 cups chopped
Dandelion greens	1 cup
Green onion	1
Honeydew melon	1½ cups cubed
Kale, baby	4 cups
Kiwi fruit	1
Mango	2 cups cubed
Mushrooms, shiitake	5 large
Onion, yellow	¼ cup diced
Potatoes, red	2 small
Radishes	2
Spinach	1½ cups
Squash, yellow	½ small
Strawberries	2
Zucchini	1 small

FRESH HERBS

Basil	4 leaves
Lemongrass	3-inch piece
Mint	7 or 8 leaves

GROCERY

Adzuki beans	⅓ cup uncooked (1 cup cooked)
Almonds, raw	12
Chickpeas	½ cup uncooked (1½ cups cooked)
Coconut, unsweetened, shredded	1 tablespoon
Dates, Medjool	2
Dulse flakes	1 cup
Mung beans	½ cup uncooked (1½ cups cooked)
Nori, pressed	3 sheets
Orange juice	4 tablespoons
Pecan pieces	½ cup
Pomegranate juice	1 cup
Rice, brown	½ cup cooked
Sesame seeds, unhulled	1 teaspoon
Thai green curry paste	½ teaspoon
Vegetable broth, organic	7 cups
Walnut halves	5

THE INSIGHT

PRODUCE

Apple, red	⅓ cup sliced
Avocado	½
Bananas	1½ small
Bell pepper, red	½
Blackberries	2¼ cups
Blueberries, frozen or fresh	3½ cups
Broccoli	2½ cups chopped
Cabbage, red	1 large
Carrots	1 tablespoon shredded
Carrots, purple	2
Cauliflower	2 cups chopped
Cucumber	¼ cup cubed
Eggplant	1 small

Kale, baby	2 cups
Kale, purple	1 cup chopped
Mushrooms, shiitake	3
Onions, red	2 small
Potatoes, purple	2 small
Raspberries	1 cup
Shallot	1 large
Tomato	½ medium

FRESH HERBS

| Basil (purple preferred) | 2 leaves |

GROCERY

Adzuki beans	⅓ cup uncooked (1 cup cooked)
Bee pollen granules (optional)	1 teaspoon
Cacao nibs, raw	1 tablespoon
Cashews, raw	¾ cup
Cocoa powder, unsweetened	1 tablespoon
Hempseed oil	1 tablespoon
Hibiscus tea	½ cup
Mustard, Dijon	½ tablespoon
Oats, gluten-free	1 cup
Pecan halves	8
Pecans	½ cup chopped
Pine nuts, raw	4 tablespoons
Pomegranate juice	1 cup
Rice, purple/black	½ cup uncooked
Walnut oil	1 tablespoon
Walnuts	¾ cup chopped

THE SPIRIT

PRODUCE

Arugula	2 cups
Avocado	1 small
Bell peppers, red	2
Burdock root	5-inch piece
Cabbage, green	¼ to ½ head (need 1 cup diced)
Cabbage, red	¼ head (need ½ cup diced)
Carrots	3
Cauliflower	1 large head
Celery	3 stalks
Cucumber	1 cup diced
Green onions	1 bunch
Leeks	¼ cup chopped
Mango, frozen or fresh	1 cup diced
Onion, white	1 medium or 2 small
Onion, yellow	1 small
Mushrooms, shiitake	7
Pears	3
Romaine lettuce	1 cup chopped
Spinach	2 cups
Squash, yellow	1 small
Zucchini	1 small

FRESH HERBS

Basil (purple variety preferred for most of it)	2 cups leaves
Parsley	¼ cup chopped

GROCERY

Cashew nut butter	1 tablespoon
Cashews, raw	¼ cup
Dulse flakes	1 teaspoon
Hempseed oil	1 tablespoon

Mustard, Dijon	1 tablespoon
Pine nuts, raw	½ cup
Raisins, golden	2 tablespoons
Sesame seeds, unhulled	2 tablespoons
Tahini	1 tablespoon
Vegetable broth, organic	2 cups
Walnuts	2 tablespoons chopped

WHOLE DETOX TRACKING CHARTS

WHOLE DETOX EMOTION LOG

The Whole Detox Emotion Log is designed to help you track and see patterns in your emotions over time. At the end of each day, simply go through each of the emotions listed and put an X in boxes that correspond to the emotions you felt that day. After you've completed one week of this activity, look at any patterns that may be obvious, such as a predominance of one emotion (e.g., fear) or a pattern of emotions that feel uplifting or nonserving. You can match this information to your food intake to see how your daily emotions might be driving your food choices. Additionally, you may want to use the results of your Whole Detox Emotion Log to fuel your journaling process or your engagement in other therapies with a qualified practitioner.

	ROOT			FLOW			FIRE		
	1	2	3	4	5	6	7	8	9
Able to express self									
Angry									
Appreciative									
Authentic									
Aware									
Balanced									
Compassionate									
Courageous									
Creative									
Daring									
Energetic									
Fearful									
Forgiving									
Frustrated									
Grateful									
Grieving									
Happy									
Helpful									
Honest									
Interested									
Joyful									
Loving									
Optimistic									
Peaceful									
Playful									
Relaxed									
Sad									
Self-accepting									
Solutions-oriented									
Upset									
Worried									
Other (please list):									

LOVE			TRUTH			INSIGHT			SPIRIT		
10	11	12	13	14	15	16	17	18	19	20	21

WHOLE DETOX FOOD REINTRODUCTION
SYMPTOMS TRACKER

The Food Reintroduction Symptoms Tracker is a tool you use to help you gauge your reactions to the foods that you eliminated as part of the twenty-one-day Whole Detox. See the instructions for reintroducing foods on pages 354–56.

WHOLE DETOX FOOD REINTRODUCTION SYMPTOMS TRACKER

Date	Time	Food	Symptoms (e.g., rash, bloating, loss of energy, joint pain)
	____:____ A.M. / P.M.		
	____:____ A.M. / P.M.		
	____:____ A.M. / P.M.		
	____:____ A.M. / P.M.		
	____:____ A.M. / P.M.		
	____:____ A.M. / P.M.		
	____:____ A.M. / P.M.		
	____:____ A.M. / P.M.		
	____:____ A.M. / P.M.		
	____:____ A.M. / P.M.		

RAINBOW TRACKER

Use the Rainbow Tracker after you have completed your twenty-one-day Whole Detox. It is intended to help you continue to focus on getting the rainbow variety of colors on a daily basis, so your seven systems feel nourished and complete. Each time you have natural, whole foods (not anything artificially dyed or colored) that correspond to the colors listed, just put an X in the box of that color. By the end of the day, check to see if you have the full spectrum of your rainbow!

RAINBOW TRACKER

Date	Red: ROOT	Orange: FLOW	Yellow: FIRE	Green: LOVE	Aqua-marine: TRUTH	Indigo: INSIGHT	White: SPIRIT

WHOLE DETOX SYSTEMS TRACKER

The Whole Detox Systems Tracker will help you track the progress of your seven systems of health over time, after you have completed your twenty-one-day Whole Detox, so you can see the subtle changes and improvements. Use this form to log your no responses from the Whole Detox Spectrum Quiz (see pages 35–41) and plot your scores in the corresponding system sections. What you are looking for is to have lower no scores over time. You can compare your no scores among all the systems at a specific time point. You can also look at your scores within a particular system over time to see if the numbers go down, indicating an improvement.

WHOLE DETOX SYSTEMS TRACKER

Date	The ROOT	The FLOW	The FIRE	The LOVE	The TRUTH	The INSIGHT	The SPIRIT

RESOURCES

WHOLE DETOX PROGRAMS

To find out about further participation in online Whole Detox programs, visit my websites:

Dr. Deanna Minich: www.drdeannaminich.com

Whole Detox: www.whole-detox.com

The online Whole Detox program is also twenty-one days in duration and is available throughout the year. You would follow the program as outlined in the book but with a larger community through social media. Additional benefits are live webinars with Dr. Deanna Minich.

HEALTH PROFESSIONALS

If you want to work with a Certified Food & Spirit Practitioner, who has been trained in the Seven Systems of Full-Spectrum Health, see the website: www.foodandspiritprofessional.com

To learn more about becoming a Certified Food & Spirit Practitioner, visit the program website for information: www.foodandspiritprofessional.com.

To learn more about functional medicine and finding a Certified Functional Medicine Practitioner, visit the Institute for Functional Medicine website: www.functionalmedicine.org.

If you have dental amalgams, consider getting them removed and replaced with a functional or biological dentist who takes the necessary precautions. Check out the International Academy of Biological Dentistry and Medicine to find a practitioner: https://iabdm.org.

THE DETOX SUMMIT

If you are interested in listening to more cutting-edge information about detox, everything from nutrition to emotions to spiritual health, you will want to listen to The Detox Summit, a virtual online summit of thirty leaders in Whole Detox organized and led by Dr. Deanna Minich: http://thedetoxsummit.com.

SOCIAL MEDIA

Whole Detox Fan Page: www.facebook.com/wholedetox

Whole Detox Community Page: www.facebook.com/groups/FullSpectrum DetoxCommunity

Deanna Minich, Ph.D.: www.facebook.com/deanna.minich

Certified Food & Spirit Practitioner Program: www.facebook.com/Certified -Food-Spirit-Practitioner-Program-703507403030620

Twitter: www.twitter.com/drdeannaminich

Pinterest: www.pinterest.com/foodandspirit

YouTube: www.youtube.com/foodandspirit

OTHER BOOKS AND MATERIALS BY DR. DEANNA MINICH TO SUPPORT YOU THROUGH THE WHOLE DETOX PROGRAM

All of these are available at www.amazon.com:

An A–Z Guide to Food Additives: Never Eat What You Can't Pronounce (Conari Press, 2009)—A pocketbook listing the important food additives in foods. What's good and what's not? This book will rate ingredients and foods using a simple scoring system of A through F. It is concise and targeted for the busy consumer. Make sure you have this in your purse, backpack, or pocket while shopping!

The Complete Handbook of Quantum Healing: An A–Z Self-Healing Guide for Over 100 Common Ailments (Red Wheel / Weiser, 2010)—A reference book full of Whole Detox nutrition and lifestyle suggestions for specific ailments. You may want to review it for specific ailments you have so you can fine-tune your detox modalities to fit you specifically.

Nourish Your Whole Self Cards—A creative, inspirational deck of 56 cards, each with an affirmation and visual to add greater nourishment to your eating experience throughout Whole Detox. Pick a card before, during, or after a meal, or even at the start of the day to see what eating message is waiting for you. Read more about the card you chose in the accompanying booklet.

WHERE TO GET FOODS, EQUIPMENT, AND PRODUCTS FOR THE WHOLE DETOX PROGRAM

Seafood
Get quality seafood at Vital Choice: www.vitalchoice.com.

Seaweeds
Make sure your edible seaweeds are organically certified and carefully harvested. Maine Coast Sea Vegetables specializes in sustainably harvested seaweeds from the North Atlantic: www.seaveg.com/shop.

Spices
For single spices or simple blends, a great choice is Frontier Natural Products Co-op brands, including Simply Organic: www.simplyorganic.com.

Teeny Tiny Spice Company has a wide variety of mixed spices (tandoori masala, vindaloo, etc.): www.teenytinyspice.com. (Use coupon code "FOOD+SPIRIT" to receive 10% off.)

Teas
Pukka Herbs: www.pukkaherbs.com

Rishi Tea: www.rishi-tea.com

Teeccino gluten-free herbal teas: www.teeccino.com (Use coupon code "FOOD&SPIRIT" to receive 15% off.)

Yogi teas: www.yogiproducts.com

Green Food Powders

Whole-food, green food powder—pHresh Greens: www.phreshproducts .com/food-spirit (Use coupon code "foodspirit" to receive 10% off.)

Professional-Grade Dietary Supplements

Allergy Research Group: www.allergyresearchgroup.com

Biotics Research: www.bioticsresearch.com

Designs for Health: www.designsforhealth.com

Douglas Laboratories: www.douglaslabs.com

Innate Response: www.innateresponse.com

Metagenics: www.metagenics.com; Food & Spirit: www.foodandspirit.com /shop/metagenics-food-spirit-store (Receive 20% off your first order and 10% off every subsequent order.)

MicroNourish: www.micronutrients.com

Nature's Sunshine Products: www.naturessunshine.com/us/shop

Nordic Naturals: www.nordicnaturals.com/consumers.php

Nutrilite: www.nutrilite.com

ProThera/Klaire Labs: www.protherainc.com

Pure Encapsulations: www.pureencapsulations.com

Thorne Research: www.thorne.com

Vital Nutrients: www.vitalnutrients.net

Xymogen: www.xymogen.com

Blenders
Buy yourself a high-speed blender—any of the different brands available on the market, including Blendtec, Ninja, NutriBullet, or Vitamix. They all work well for making morning smoothies.

Water Filters
Here is the best, most thorough guide to finding a good water filter: www .ewg.org/tap-water/getawaterfilter.php.

Personal Care Products
General

Dr. Bronner's soap and toothpaste products: www.drbronner.com

Desert Essence personal care items: www.desertessence.com

Seventh Generation toilet paper, tampons, and other household goods: www.seventhgeneration.com

Hair

Morrocco Method, especially Sapphire Volumizer Mist, which is a combination of ionized water with essential oils: http://tinyurl.com/fsmorrocco method

Skin

Aubrey Organics: www.aubrey-organics.com

MyChelle: www.mychelle.com

Simply Divine Botanicals, especially the Black Velvet Fabulous Foaming Facial Cleanser and Skincredible Revitalizing Sandalwood Elixir: www .simplydivinebotanicals.com

INFORMATIONAL WEBSITES

These websites provide information on lifestyle medicine, nutrition, and personal growth that may be useful to you:

American College of Nutrition, for research into nutrition science and the prevention and treatment of disease: www.americancollegeofnutrition.org

Environmental Working Group (EWG), for the "Dirty Dozen Plus" list of the most pesticide-laden fruits and vegetables, updates on mercury levels in fish, and many other resources on the quality of foods, household products, and our environment: www.ewg.org

Green Med Info, for the latest research into the use of natural substances in disease prevention and treatment: www.greenmedinfo.com

The Grief Recovery Institute, for assistance with grief counseling: www.griefrecoverymethod.com

HeartMath Institute, for biofeedback and heart rate variability devices: www.heartmath.com and www.heartmath.org

MindBodyGreen, for blogs, videos, and information on mind and body: www.mindbodygreen.com

Natural Resources Defense Council (NRDC), for mercury levels in fish: www.nrdc.org/health/effects/mercury/guide.asp

Dr. Jeffrey Bland's Personalized Lifestyle Medicine Institute: www.plm institute.org

The World's Healthiest Foods, a website with practical nutrition information: http://whfoods.com

Yoga Alliance, to find a yoga teacher: www.yogaalliance.org

ACKNOWLEDGMENTS

At times our own light goes out and is rekindled by a spark from another person.
Each of us has cause to think with deep gratitude of those who have lighted the
flame within us.

—ALBERT SCHWEITZER

Just as a human being comprises a spectrum of systems, so too does a book. A book is an artful synthesis of thoughts, experience, and people, which is what makes it so satisfying to write. One of my favorite parts of creating the tapestry is giving gratitude to all the people whose beautiful threads I had the opportunity to weave together.

The ROOT: There is nothing more grounding than a solid, supportive family who help you to feel safe and protected in all you do. I thank my generous, loving parents, John and Sharon, who have been incredible and wonderful at every step of my life journey, all while teaching me through their examples. I am deeply grateful for the gift of having them both in my life in the present day and for showing me the power of choice on the spectrum of health and disease. A huge thanks to my sister, Brenda, who has always been my advocate.

The FLOW: I am flowing with boundless thanks to all the creative people in my life and to those who have inspired me to create and to go with the organic flow of my emotions through art, including my aunt Kim and my brother Ian. I thank Wendy Alfaro for providing me with the creative inspiration for colorful, whole-foods-based recipes and for helping me to think more expansively about food combinations. I am indebted to Barb Schiltz's creative culinary eye as she put the finishing touches on the recipes in this book.

The FIRE: So many people have allowed me to ignite the Food & Spirit message to the world by supporting the business, including team members Kimberlee, Marchel, and Laura. Kimberlee, a special hug to you for your fiery loyalty and dedication in working with me for several years. You have all been amazing to work with—thank you for keeping your flame burning bright for this work. Sean Bonsell, thanks for stepping in with your creative flair to get ideas into motion. Thanks to all the Certified Food & Spirit Practitioners who have committed to the Food & Spirit full-spectrum approach of whole-self healing. I am still burning bright with the experience of doing the Detox Summit in August 2014, and I thank everyone for being part of that event, including the experts and the team behind the scenes making it all happen. I appreciate all the people who have taken part in the many detox programs I've offered over the years. A huge thanks to Dhrumil Purohit for his laser-like leadership and business coaching. Thanks to all the wonderful colleagues who have helped me grow within the business realm, giving me guidance to make my dream a reality, including Aviva Romm, Pilar Gerasimo, Amy Myers, Howard Hoffman, and Alejandro Junger.

The LOVE: I bow to my life partner and love, Mark, for being my teacher, friend, and supporter. You encourage my passion, dreams, and heartfelt wishes to come forth in the highest and most meaningful way. I thank my dear friends and healers, including Scott Whittaker, Char Sundust, Patrice Connelly, Alan Pritz, Barbara Maddoux, Barb Schiltz, Mark Houston, Lyra Heller, Kristi Hughes, Caroline Myss, Mink Fire, Gay McCray, Lorraine Leas, Janet Ridgeway, Joel Kahn, Michael Stone, John Principe, Sayer Ji, Annie Basu, Andy Maxwell, Hong and Mike Curley, Anthony William, and Anna Kong.

The TRUTH: I can still remember the initial phone call with my soon-to-be literary agent, Stephanie Tade. I am so grateful for her initial enthusiasm and eventual guidance through the publishing "birth canal" and for assisting me with pivotal decisions. If it weren't for her, I might not have met the utterly brilliant and lovely soul Rachel Kranz, who helped me shift into my authentic truth through choosing the right words and expressions. Rachel, thank you for being a master of words and for bridging the spectrum between the grounding of facts and the flowing art of people's lives. Gideon Weil, my amazing editor at HarperCollins, you have been outstanding in seeing the vision of this work very early on and providing gentle coaching and steering when needed. So many people sing your praises, and you can now count me as one of the choir! Finally, I want to thank my mom a second time, for teaching me the importance of being in my truth and the necessity of honesty in one's life. I now realize how precious it was to learn from her that it's perfectly fine to be different and to revel in the uniqueness of who I am. Thanks, Mom, for being my truth-shining star.

The INSIGHT: Several people have illuminated my neurons with an understanding of systems thinking and through inspiring the depth of scientific intellect needed to write this book, including all my teachers in nutritional and functional medicine. My biggest thanks goes to Dr. Jeffrey Bland, who has a multitude of titles. His best known is probably the Father of Functional Medicine, but now I add to the list Father of Nutritional Detoxification. It was Dr. Bland who forged the early path in detoxification, doing studies, publishing papers, and paving the way for "detox" to become what it is today. I also want to thank my many other teachers in biochemistry, nutrition, and functional medicine, including Drs. Phyllis Bowen, Maria Sapuntzakis, Clare Hasler, Henkjan Verkade, Folkert Kuipers, and Roel Vonk; everyone at the Institute for Functional Medicine, especially Laurie Hofmann; Drs. Patrick Hanaway, Mark Hyman, Kristi Hughes, and Dan Lukaczer; the Detox Module Team, including Bob Rountree, Rick Mayfield, Mary Ellen Chalmers, and T. R. Morris; all my wise physician teachers at the Functional Medicine Research Center, Jack Kornberg, Joe Lamb, and Bob Lerman.

The SPIRIT: For the soul and spirit of all I do, I give humble, immense thanks to God; in all the divine forms I feel the oneness and grace of life.

BIBLIOGRAPHY

NOTE: Entries are listed in order of their reference in the text.

INTRODUCTION: WHY WHOLE DETOX?

Chan, S. Y., and J. Loscalzo. "The Emerging Paradigm of Network Medicine in the Study of Human Disease." *Circulation Research* 111, no. 3 (2012): 359–74. doi:10.1161/CIRCRES AHA.111.258541.

Westerhoff, H. V., and B. O. Palsson. "The Evolution of Molecular Biology into Systems Biology." *Nature Biotechnology* 22, no. 10 (2004): 1249–52.

Edmondson, D., J. D. Newman, W. Whang, and K. W. Davidson. "Emotional Triggers in Myocardial Infarction: Do They Matter?" *European Heart Journal* 34, no. 4 (2013): 300–6. doi:10.1093/eurheartj/ehs398.

Strike, P. C., and A. Steptoe. "Behavioral and Emotional Triggers of Acute Coronary Syndromes: A Systematic Review and Critique." *Psychosomatic Medicine* 67, no. 2 (2005): 179–86.

Buckley, T., D. Sunari, A. Marshall, R. Bartrop, S. McKinley, and G. Tofler. "Physiological Correlates of Bereavement and the Impact of Bereavement Interventions." *Dialogues in Clinical Neuroscience* 14, no. 2 (2012): 129–39.

Steptoe, A., A. Shankar, P. Demakakos, and J. Wardle. "Social Isolation, Loneliness, and All-Cause Mortality in Older Men and Women." *PNAS* 110, no. 15 (2013): 5797–801. doi:10.1073/pnas.1219686110.

Luo, Y., L. C. Hawkley, L. J. Waite, and J. T. Cacioppo. "Loneliness, Health, and Mortality in Old Age: A National Longitudinal Study." *Social Science and Medicine* 74, no. 6 (2012): 907–14. doi:10.1016/j.socscimed.2011.11.028.

CHAPTER 1: WHOLE DETOX FOR YOUR WHOLE SELF

Dickerson, S. S. and M. E. Kemeny. "Acute Stressors and Cortisol Responses: A Theoretical Integration and Synthesis of Laboratory Research." *Psychological Bulletin* 130, no. 3 (2004): 355–91.

Khalfa, S., S. D. Bella, M. Roy, I. Peretz, and S. J. Lupien. "Effects of Relaxing Music on Salivary Cortisol Level After Psychological Stress." *Annals of the New York Academy of Sciences* no. 999 (2003): 374–76.

Maslow, A. H. "A Theory of Human Motivation." *Psychological Review* 50, no. 4 (1943): 370–96. psychclassics.yorku.ca.

Csikszentmihalyi, Mihaly. Flow: The Psychology of Optimal Experience. New York: Harper and Row, 1990.

Cantin, M., and J. Genest. "The Heart as an Endocrine Gland." Pharmacological Research Communications 20, suppl. 3 (1988): 1–22.

CHAPTER 3: THE ROOT

Segerstrom, S. C., and G. E. Miller. "Psychological Stress and the Human Immune System: A Meta-Analytic Study of 30 Years of Inquiry." Psychological Bulletin 130, no. 4 (2004): 601–30.

Avitsur, R., S. Levy, N. Goren, and R. Grinshpahet. "Early Adversity, Immunity and Infectious Disease." Stress 18, no. 3 (2015): 289–96.

Carlsson, E., A. Frostell, J. Ludvigsson, and M. Faresjö. "Psychological Stress in Children May Alter the Immune Response." Journal of Immunology 192, no. 5 (2014): 2071–81. doi:10.4049/jimmunol.1301713.

Dube, S. R., D. Fairweather, W. S. Pearson, V. J. Felitti, R. F. Anda, and J. B. Croft. "Cumulative Childhood Stress and Autoimmune Diseases in Adults." Psychosomatic Medicine 71, no. 2 (2009): 243–50. doi:10.1097/PSY.0b013e3181907888.

Tian, R., G. Hou, D. Li, and T.-F. Yuan. "A Possible Change Process of Inflammatory Cytokines in the Prolonged Chronic Stress and Its Ultimate Implications for Health." Scientific World Journal 2014 (2014): 780616. doi:10.1155/2014/780616.

Rutledge, T., S. E. Reis, M. Olson, J. Owens, S. F. Kelsey, C. J. Pepine, S. Mankad, et al. "Social Networks Are Associated with Lower Mortality Rates Among Women with Suspected Coronary Disease: The National Heart, Lung, and Blood Institute–Sponsored Women's Ischemia Syndrome Evaluation Study." Psychosomatic Medicine 66, no. 6 (2004): 882–88.

Cohen, S., W. J. Doyle, R. Turner, C. M. Alper, and D. P. Skoner. "Sociability and Susceptibility to the Common Cold." Psychological Science 14, no. 5 (2003): 389–95.

Pinquart, M., and P. R. Duberstein. "Associations of Social Networks with Cancer Mortality: A Meta-Analysis." Critical Reviews in Oncology/Hematology 75, no. 2 (2010): 122–37. doi:10.1016/j.critrevonc.2009.06.003.

Pressman, S. D., S. Cohen, G. E. Miller, A. Barkin, B. S. Rabin, and J. J. Treanor. "Loneliness, Social Network Size, and Immune Response to Influenza Vaccination in College Freshmen." Health Psychology 24, no. 3 (2005): 297–306.

Sroykham, W., J. Wongsathikun, and Y. Wongsawat. "The Effects of Perceiving Color in Living Environment on QEEG, Oxygen Saturation, Pulse Rate, and Emotion Regulation in Humans." Conference Proceedings: IEEE Engineering in Medicine and Biology Society 2014 (2014): 6226–29. doi:10.1109/EMBC.2014.6945051.

Bertrams, A., R. F. Baumeister, C. Englert, and P. Furley. "Ego Depletion in Color Priming Research: Self-Control Strength Moderates the Detrimental Effect of Red on Cognitive Test Performance." Personal and Social Psychology Bulletin 41, no. 3 (2015): 311–22. doi:10.1177/0146167214564968.

Buechner, V. L., M. A. Maier, S. Lichtenfeld, and S. Schwarz. "Red—Take a Closer Look." PLoS ONE 9, no. 9 (2014): e108111. doi:10.1371/journal.pone.0108111.

Young, S. G., A. J. Elliot, R. Feltman, and N. Ambady. "Red Enhances the Processing of Facial Expressions of Anger." Emotion 13, no. 3 (2013): 380–84. doi:10.1037/a0032471.

Genschow, O., L. Reutner, and M. Wänke. "The Color Red Reduces Snack Food and Soft Drink Intake." Appetite 58, no. 2 (2012): 699–702. doi:10.1016/j.appet.2011.12.023.

Ley, S. H., Q. Sun, W. C. Willett, A. H. Eliassen, K. Wu, A. Pan, F. Grodstein, and F. B. Hu. "Associations Between Red Meat Intake and Biomarkers of Inflammation and Glucose Metabolism in Women." *American Journal of Clinical Nutrition* 99, no. 2 (2014): 352–60. doi:10.3945/ajcn.113.075663.

Montonen, J., H. Boeing, A. Fritsche, E. Schleicher, H. G. Joost, M. B. Schulze, A. Steffen, and T. Pischon. "Consumption of Red Meat and Whole-Grain Bread in Relation to Biomarkers of Obesity, Inflammation, Glucose Metabolism and Oxidative Stress." *European Journal of Nutrition* 52, no. 1 (2013): 337–45. doi:10.1007/s00394-012-0340-6.

Sinha, R., M. Kulldorff, W. H. Chow, J. Denobile, and N. Rothman. "Dietary Intake of Heterocyclic Amines, Meat-Derived Mutagenic Activity, and Risk of Colorectal Adenomas." *Cancer Epidemiology, Biomarkers and Prevention* 10, no. 5 (2001): 559–62.

Li, Z., A. Wong, S. M. Henning, Y. Zhang, A. Jones, A. Zerlin, G. Thames, S. Bowerman, C. H. Tseng, and D. Heber. "Hass Avocado Modulates Postprandial Vascular Reactivity and Postprandial Inflammatory Responses to a Hamburger Meal in Healthy Volunteers." *Food and Function* 4, no. 3 (2013): 384–91. doi:10.1039/c2fo30226h.

Shaughnessy, D. T., L. M. Gangarosa, B. Schliebe, D. M. Umbach, Z. Xu, B. MacIntosh, M. G. Knize, et al. "Inhibition of Fried Meat–Induced Colorectal DNA Damage and Altered Systemic Genotoxicity in Humans by Crucifera, Chlorophyllin, and Yogurt." *PLoS ONE* 6, no. 4 (2011): e18707. doi:10.1371/journal.pone.0018707.

Dashwood, R. "Chlorophylls as Anticarcinogens (Review)." *International Journal of Oncology* 10, no. 4 (1997): 721–27.

United States Department of Agriculture, Agricultural Research Service. "National Nutrient Database for Standard Reference Release 28." http://ndb.nal.usda.gov/ndb/foods.

Houston, M. C. "The Role of Mercury and Cadmium Heavy Metals in Vascular Disease, Hypertension, Coronary Heart Disease, and Myocardial Infarction." *Alternative Therapies in Health and Medicine* 13, no. 2 (2007): S128–33.

Driscoll, C.T., R. P. Mason, H. M. Chan, D. J. Jacob, and N. Pirrone. "Mercury as a Global Pollutant: Sources, Pathways, and Effects." *Environmental Science and Technology* 47, no. 10 (2013): 4967–83. doi:10.1021/es305071v.

Zwicker, J. D., D. J. Dutton, and J. C. H. Emery. "Longitudinal Analysis of the Association Between Removal of Dental Amalgam, Urine Mercury and 14 Self-Reported Health Symptoms." *Environmental Health* 13 (2014): 95. doi:10.1186/1476-069X-13-95.

Cech, I., M. H. Smolensky, M. Afshar, G. Broyles, M. Barczyk, K. Burau, and R. Emery. "Lead and Copper in Drinking Water Fountains—Information for Physicians." *Southern Medical Journal* 99, no. 2 (2006): 137–42.

James, S. C. "Metals in Municipal Landfill Leachate and Their Health Effects." *American Journal of Public Health* 65, no. 5 (1977): 429–32.

Olmedo, P., A. Pla, A. F. Hernández, F. Barbier, L. Ayouni, and F. Gil. "Determination of Toxic Elements (Mercury, Cadmium, Lead, Tin and Arsenic) in Fish and Shellfish Samples. Risk Assessment for the Consumers." *Environment International* 59 (2013): 63–72. doi:10.1016/j.envint.2013.05.005.

Consumer Reports. "How Much Arsenic Is in Your Rice? Consumer Reports' New Data and Guidelines Are Important for Everyone but Especially for Gluten Avoiders." November 2014. Accessed September 7, 2015. http://www.consumerreports.org/cro/magazine/2015/01/how-much-arsenic-is-in-your-rice/index.htm.

Yoshinaga, J., K. Yamasaki, A. Yonemura, Y. Ishibashi, T. Kaido, K. Mizuno, M. Takagi, and A. Tanaka. "Lead and Other Elements in House Dust of Japanese Residences—Source of Lead and Health Risks Due to Metal Exposure." *Environmental Pollution* 189 (2014): 223–28. doi:10.1016/j.envpol.2014.03.003.

Butte, W., and B. Heinzow. "Pollutants in House Dust as Indicators of Indoor Contamination." *Reviews of Environmental Contamination and Toxicology* 175 (2002): 1–46.

Fergusson, J. E., and N. D. Kim. "Trace Elements in Street and House Dusts: Sources and Speciation." *Science of the Total Environment* 100 (1991): 125–50. doi:10.1016/0048-9697 (91)90376-P.

Zakaria, A., and Y. B. Ho. "Heavy Metals Contamination in Lipsticks and Their Associated Health Risks to Lipstick Consumers." *Regulatory Toxicology and Pharmacology* 73, no. 1 (2015): 191–95. doi:10.1016/j.yrtph.2015.07.005.

Hepp, N. M. "Determination of Total Lead in 400 Lipsticks on the U.S. Market Using a Validated Microwave-Assisted Digestion, Inductively Coupled Plasma-Mass Spectrometric Method." *Journal of Cosmetic Science* 63, no. 3 (2012): 159–76.

Associated Press. "FDA to Examine Claim That Lipstick Lead Levels Unsafe." *Seattle Times.* October 13, 2007. Accessed September 7, 2015. http://www.seattletimes.com/nation-world /fda-to-examine-claim-that-lipstick-lead-levels-unsafe/.

Yokoi, K., and A. Konomi. "Toxicity of So-Called Edible Hijiki Seaweed (*Sargassum fusiforme*) Containing Inorganic Arsenic." *Regulatory Toxicology and Pharmacology* 63, no. 2 (2012): 291–97. doi:10.1016/j.yrtph.2012.04.006.

Hong, Y. S., K. H. Song, and J. Y. Chung. "Health Effects of Chronic Arsenic Exposure." *Journal of Preventative Medicine and Public Health* 47, no. 5 (2014): 245–52. doi:10.3961/jpmph .14.035.

Nash, R. A. "Metals in Medicine." *Alternative Therapies in Health and Medicine* 11, no. 4 (2005): 18–25.

Adal, A. "Heavy Metal Toxicity." *Medscape.* Last modified March 24, 2015. Accessed September 7, 2015. http://emedicine.medscape.com/article/814960-overview.

Peters, J. L., M. P. Fabian, and J. I. Levy. "Combined Impact of Lead, Cadmium, Polychlorinated Biphenyls and Non-Chemical Risk Factors on Blood Pressure in NHANES." *Environmental Research* 132 (2014): 93–99. doi:10.1016/j.envres.2014.03.038.

Hara, A., L. Thijs, K. Asayama, Y. M. Gu, L. Jacobs, Z. Y. Zhang, Y. P. Liu, T. S. Nawrot, and J. A. Staessen. "Blood Pressure in Relation to Environmental Lead Exposure in the National Health and Nutrition Examination Survey 2003 to 2010." *Hypertension* 65, no. 1 (2015): 62–69. doi:10.1161/HYPERTENSIONAHA.114.04023.

Zalewska, M., J. Trefon, and H. Milnerowicz. "The Role of Metallothionein Interactions with Other Proteins." *Proteomics* 14, no. 11 (2014): 1343–56. doi:10.1002/pmic.201300496.

Rotruck, J. T., A. L. Pope, H. E. Ganther, A. B. Swanson, D. G. Hafeman, and W. G. Hoekstra. "Selenium: Biochemical Role as a Component of Glutathione Peroxidase." *Science* 179, no. 4073 (1973): 588–90.

The World's Healthiest Foods. "Selenium." Accessed September 7, 2015. http://www .whfoods.com/genpage.php?tname=nutrient&dbid=95.

The World's Healthiest Foods. "Zinc." Accessed September 7, 2015. http://www.whfoods .com/genpage.php?tname=nutrient&dbid=115.

Kodama, M., T. Kodama, M. Murakami, and M. Kodama. "Vitamin C Infusion Treatment Enhances Cortisol Production of the Adrenal via the Pituitary ACTH Route." *InVivo* (Athens, Greece) 8, no. 6 (1994): 1079–85.

Peters, E. M., R. Anderson, D. C. Nieman, H. Fickl, and V. Jogessar. "Vitamin C Supplementation Attenuates the Increases in Circulating Cortisol, Adrenaline and Anti-Inflammatory Polypeptides Following Ultramarathon Running." *International Journal of Sports Medicine* 22, no. 7 (2001): 537–43.

Peters, E. M., R. Anderson, and A. J. Theron. "Attenuation of Increase in Circulating Cortisol and Enhancement of the Acute Phase Protein Response in Vitamin C–Supplemented Ultra-marathoners." *International Journal of Sports Medicine* 22, no. 2 (2001): 120–26.

Sorice, A., E. Guerriero, F. Capone, G. Colonna, G. Castello, and S. Costantini. "Ascorbic Acid: Its Role in Immune System and Chronic Inflammation Diseases." *Mini Reviews in Medicinal Chemistry* 14, no. 5 (2014): 444–52.

Mann, D. "Red Foods: The New Health Powerhouses?" WebMD. Last modified April 1, 2008. Accessed September 7, 2015. http://www.webmd.com/food-recipes/red-foods-the-new-health-powerhouses.

Nutrition Data. "Foods Highest in Vitamin C." Accessed September 7, 2015. http://nutrition data.self.com/foods-011101000000000000000-w.html?mbid=enews_nd0823.

Boyer, J., and R. H. Liu. "Apple Phytochemicals and Their Health Benefits." *Nutrition Journal* 3 (2004): 5.

Min, Y. D., C. H. Choi, H. Bark, H. Y. Son, H. H. Park, S. Lee, J. W. Park, et al. "Quercetin Inhibits Expression of Inflammatory Cytokines Through Attenuation of NF-kappaB and p38 MAPK in HMC–1 Human Mast Cell Line." *Inflammation Research* 56, no. 5 (2007): 210–15.

Park, H. J., C. M. Lee, I. D. Jung, J. S. Lee, Y. I. Jeong, J. H. Chang, S. H. Chun, et al. "Quercetin Regulates Th1/Th2 Balance in a Murine Model of Asthma." *International Immunopharmacology* 9, no. 3 (2009): 261–67. doi:10.1016/j.intimp.2008.10.021.

Chung, S., H. Yao, S. Caito, J. W. Hwang, G. Arunachalam, and I. Rahman. "Regulation of SIRT1 in Cellular Functions: Role of Polyphenols." *Archives of Biochemistry and Biophysics* 501, no. 1 (2010): 79–90. doi:10.1016/j.abb.2010.05.003.

Environmental Working Group. "Apples Top Dirty Dozen List for Fifth Year in a Row." News release. February 25, 2015. Accessed September 7, 2015. http://www.ewg.org/release /apples-top-dirty-dozen-list-fifth-year-row.

Hodges, R. E., and D. M. Minich. "Modulation of Metabolic Detoxification Pathways Using Foods and Food-Derived Components: A Scientific Review with Clinical Application." *Journal of Nutrition and Metabolism* 2015 (2015): 760689. doi:10.1155/2015/760689.

Gajowik, A., and M. M. Dobrzyńska. "Lycopene—Antioxidant with Radioprotective and Anticancer Properties. A Review." *Roczniki Państwowego Zakładu Higieny* 65, no. 4 (2014): 263–71.

Rao, A. V., M. R. Ray, and L. G. Rao. "Lycopene." *Advances in Food and Nutrition Research* 51 (2006): 99–164.

Agarwal, A., H. Shen, S. Agarwal, and A. V. Rao. "Lycopene Content of Tomato Products: Its Stability, Bioavailability and In Vivo Antioxidant Properties." *Journal of Medicinal Food* 4, no. 1 (Spring 2001): 9–15.

Unlu, N. Z., T. Bohn, D. M. Francis, H. N. Nagaraja, S. K. Clinton, and S. J. Schwartz. "Lycopene from Heat-Induced Cis-Isomer-Rich Tomato Sauce Is More Bioavailable than from All-Trans-Rich Tomato Sauce in Human Subjects." *British Journal of Nutrition* 98, no. 1 (2007): 140–46.

Vallverdú-Queralt, A., J. Regueiro, J. F. Rinaldi de Alvarenga, X. Torrado, and R. M. Lamuela-Raventos. "Carotenoid Profile of Tomato Sauces: Effect of Cooking Time and Content of Extra Virgin Olive Oil." *International Journal of Molecular Sciences* 16, no. 5 (2015): 9588–99. doi:10.3390/ijms16059588.

Bugianesi, R., M. Salucci, C. Leonardi, R. Ferracane, G. Catasta, E. Azzini, and G. Maiani. "Effect of Domestic Cooking on Human Bioavailability of Naringenin, Chlorogenic Acid, Lycopene and Beta-Carotene in Cherry Tomatoes." *European Journal of Nutrition* 43, no. 6 (2004): 360–66.

Casas-Grajales, S., and P. Muriel. "Antioxidants in Liver Health." *World Journal of Gastrointestinal Pharmacology and Therapeutics* 6, no. 3 (2015): 59–72. doi:10.4292/wjgpt.v6.i3.59.

Meng, S., J. Cao, Q. Feng, J. Peng, and Y. Hu. "Roles of Chlorogenic Acid on Regulating Glucose and Lipids Metabolism: A Review." *Evidence-Based Complementary and Alternative Medicine* 2013 (2013): 801457. doi:10.1155/2013/801457.

Oschman, J. L., G. Chevalier, and R. Brown. "The Effects of Grounding (Earthing) on Inflammation, the Immune Response, Wound Healing, and Prevention and Treatment of Chronic Inflammatory and Autoimmune Diseases." *Journal of Inflammation Research* 8 (2015): 83–96. doi:10.2147/JIR.S69656.

Chevalier, G. "The Effect of Grounding the Human Body on Mood." *Psychological Reports* 116, no. 2 (2015): 534–43. doi:10.2466/06.PR0.116k21w5.

Chevalier, G., S. T. Sinatra, J. L. Oschman, and R. M. Delany. "Earthing (Grounding) the Human Body Reduces Blood Viscosity—A Major Factor in Cardiovascular Disease." *Journal of Alternative and Complementary Medicine* 19, no. 2 (2013): 102–10. doi:10.1089/acm .2011.0820.

Sokal, K., and P. Sokal. "Earthing the Human Organism Influences Bioelectrical Processes." *Journal of Alternative and Complementary Medicine* 18, no. 3 (2012): 229–34. doi:10.1089/acm .2010.0683.

Chevalier, G., S. T. Sinatra, J. L. Oschman, K. Sokal, and P. Sokal. "Earthing: Health Implications of Reconnecting the Human Body to the Earth's Surface Electrons." *Journal of Environmental and Public Health* 2012 (2012): 291541. doi:10.1155/2012/291541.

CHAPTER 4: THE FLOW

Denton, D. A., M. J. McKinley, and R. S. Weisinger. "Hypothalamic Integration of Body Fluid Regulation." *PNAS* 93, no. 14 (1996): 7397–404.

Schug, T. T., A. Janesick, B. Blumberg, and J. J. Heindel. "Endocrine Disrupting Chemicals and Disease Susceptibility." *Journal of Steroid Biochemistry and Molecular Biology* 127, nos. 3–5 (2011): 204–15. doi:10.1016/j.jsbmb.2011.08.007.

Győrffy, Z., D. Dweik, and E. Girasek. "Reproductive Health and Burn-Out Among Female Physicians: Nationwide, Representative Study from Hungary." *BMC Women's Health* 14 (2014): 121. doi:10.1186/1472-6874-14-121.

Liu, F., W. N. Liu, Q. X. Zhao, and M. M. Han. "Study on Environmental and Psychological Risk Factors for Female Infertility." [Article in Chinese; abstract in English.] *Zhonghua Lao Dong Wei Sheng Zhi Ye Bing Za Zhi* 31, no. 12 (2013): 922–23.

Fido, A. "Emotional Distress in Infertile Women in Kuwait." *International Journal of Fertility and Women's Medicine* 49, no. 1 (2004): 24–28.

Peterson, B. D, C. S. Sejbaek, M. Pirritano, and L. Schmidt. "Are Severe Depressive Symptoms Associated with Infertility-Related Distress in Individuals and Their Partners?" *Human Reproduction* 29, no. 1 (2014): 76–82. doi:10.1093/humrep/det412.

Lynch, C. D., R. Sundaram, J. M. Maisog, A. M. Sweeney, and G. M. Buck Louis. "Preconception Stress Increases the Risk of Infertility: Results from a Couple-Based Prospective Cohort Study—The Life Study." *Human Reproduction* 29, no. 5 (2014): 1067–75. doi:10.1093 /humrep/deu032.

Pauli, S. A., and S. L. Berga. "Athletic Amenorrhea: Energy Deficit or Psychogenic Challenge?" *Annals of the New York Academy of Sciences* 1205 (2010): 33–38. doi:10.1111/j.1749 -6632.2010.05663.x.

Podfigurna-Stopa, A., S. Luisi, C. Regini, K. Katulski, G. Centini, B. Meczekalski, and F. Petraglia. "Mood Disorders and Quality of Life in Polycystic Ovary Syndrome." *Gynecological Endocrinology* 31, no. 6 (2015): 431–34. doi:10.3109/09513590.2015.1009437.

Sköld, H. N., T. Amundsen, P. A. Svensson, I. Mayer, J. Bjelvenmark, and E. Forsgren. "Hormonal Regulation of Female Nuptial Coloration in a Fish." *Hormones and Behavior* 54, no. 4 (2008): 549–56. doi:10.1016/j.yhbeh.2008.05.018.

De Serrano, A. R., C. J. Weadick, A. C. Price, and F. H. Rodd. "Seeing Orange: Prawns Tap Into a Pre-Existing Sensory Bias of the Trinidadian Guppy." *Proceedings of the Royal Society B: Biological Sciences* 279, no. 1741 (2012): 3321–28. doi:10.1098/rspb.2012.0633.

Locatello, L., M. B. Rasotto, J. P. Evans, and A. Pilastro. "Colourful Male Guppies Produce Faster and More Viable Sperm." *Journal of Evolutionary Biology* 19, no. 5 (2006): 1595–602.

Helfenstein, F., S. Losdat, A. P. Møller, J. D. Blount, and H. Richner. "Sperm of Colourful Males Are Better Protected Against Oxidative Stress." *Ecology Letters* 13, no. 2 (2010): 213–22. doi:10.1111/j.1461-0248.2009.01419.x.

O'Fallon, J. V., and B. P. Chew. "The Subcellular Distribution of Beta-Carotene in Bovine Corpus Luteum." *Proceedings of the Society for Experimental Biology and Medicine* 177, no. 3 (1984): 406–11.

Arellano-Rodriguez, G., C. A. Meza-Herrera, R. Rodriguez-Martinez, R. Dionisio-Tapia, D. M. Hallford, M. Mellado, and A. Gonzalez-Bulnes. "Short-Term Intake of Beta-Carotene-Supplemented Diets Enhances Ovarian Function and Progesterone Synthesis in Goats." *Journal of Animal Physiology and Animal Nutrition* (Berlin) 93, no. 6 (2009): 710–15. doi:10.1111/j.1439-0396.2008.00859.x.

Meza-Herrera, C. A., F. Vargas-Beltran, H. P. Vergara-Hernandez, U. Macias-Cruz, L. Avendaño-Reyes, R. Rodriguez-Martinez, G. Arellano-Rodriguez, and F. G. Veliz-Deras. "Betacarotene Supplementation Increases Ovulation Rate Without an Increment in LH Secretion in Cyclic Goats." *Reproductive Biology* 13, no. 1 (2013): 51–57. doi:10.1016/j.repbio.2013.01.171.

Czeczuga-Semeniuk, E., and S. Wołczyński. "Dietary Carotenoids in Normal and Pathological Tissues of Corpus Uteri." *Folia Histochemica et Cytobiologica* 46, no. 3 (2008): 283–90. doi:10.2478/v10042-008-0040-5.

Ruder, E. H., T. J. Hartman, R. H. Reindollar, and M. B. Goldman. "Female Dietary Antioxidant Intake and Time to Pregnancy Among Couples Treated for Unexplained Infertility." *Fertility and Sterility* 101, no. 3 (2014): 759–66. doi:10.1016/j.fertnstert.2013.11.008.

Miles, E. A., P. S. Noakes, L. S. Kremmyda, M. Vlachava, N. D. Diaper, G. Rosenlund, H. Urwin, et al. "The Salmon in Pregnancy Study: Study Design, Subject Characteristics, Maternal Fish and Marine n–3 Fatty Acid Intake, and Marine n–3 Fatty Acid Status in Maternal and Umbilical Cord Blood." *American Journal of Clinical Nutrition* 94, no. 6 suppl. (2011): 1986S–1992S. doi:10.3945/ajcn.110.001636.

Imhoff-Kunsch, B., V. Briggs, T. Goldenberg, and U. Ramakrishnan. "Effect of n–3 Long-Chain Polyunsaturated Fatty Acid Intake During Pregnancy on Maternal, Infant, and Child Health Outcomes: A Systematic Review." *Paediatric and Perinatal Epidemiology* 26, no. 1, suppl. 1 (2012): 91–107. doi:10.1111/j.1365-3016.2012.01292.x.

Klebanoff, M. A., M. Harper, Y. Lai, J. Thorp Jr., Y. Sorokin, M. W. Varner, R. J. Wapner, et al. "Fish Consumption, Erythrocyte Fatty Acids, and Preterm Birth." *Obstetrics and Gynecology* 117, no. 5 (2011): 1071–77. doi:10.1097/AOG.0b013e31821645dc.

Furuhjelm, C., K. Warstedt, J. Larsson, M. Fredriksson, M. F. Böttcher, K. Fälth-Magnusson, and K. Duchén. "Fish Oil Supplementation in Pregnancy and Lactation May Decrease the Risk of Infant Allergy." *Acta Paediatrica* 98, no. 9 (2009): 1461–67. doi:10.1111/j.1651-2227.2009.01355.x.

Feng, Y., Y. Ding, J. Liu, Y. Tian, Y. Yang, S. Guan, and C. Zhang. "Effects of Dietary Omega-3/Omega-6 Fatty Acid Ratios on Reproduction in the Young Breeder Rooster." *BMC Veterinary Research* 11 (2015): 73. doi:10.1186/s12917-015-0394-9.

Wathes, D. C., D. R. Abayasekara, and R. J. Aitken. "Polyunsaturated Fatty Acids in Male and Female Reproduction." *Biology of Reproduction* 77, no. 2 (2007): 190–201.

Rahman, M. M., C. Gasparini, G. M. Turchini, and J. P. Evans. "Experimental Reduction in Dietary Omega-3 Polyunsaturated Fatty Acids Depresses Sperm Competitiveness." *Biology Letters* 10, no. 9 (2014): 20140623. doi:10.1098/rsbl.2014.0623.

Wabner, C. L., and C. Y. Pak. "Effect of Orange Juice Consumption on Urinary Stone Risk Factors." *Journal of Urology* 149, no. 6 (1993): 1405–8.

Ishii, H., M. Nagashima, M. Tanno, A. Nakajima, and S. Yoshino. "Does Being Easily Moved to Tears as a Response to Psychological Stress Reflect Response to Treatment and the General Prognosis in Patients with Rheumatoid Arthritis?" *Clinical and Experimental Rheumatology* 21, no. 5 (2003): 611–16.

Benito, M. J., M. J. González-García, M. Tesón, N. García, I. Fernández, M. Calonge, and A. Enríquez-de-Salamanca. "Intra- and Inter-Day Variation of Cytokines and Chemokines in Tears of Healthy Subjects." *Experimental Eye Research* 120 (2014): 43–49. doi:10.1016/j.exer.2013.12.017.

Sawada, T., K. Matsuo, and I. Hashimoto. "Psychological Effects of Emotional Crying in Adults: Events That Elicit Crying and Social Reactions to Crying." [Article in Japanese; abstract in English.] *Shinrigaku Kenkyu* 82, no. 6 (2012): 514–22.

Pinazo-Durán, M. D., C. Galbis-Estrada, S. Pons-Vázquez, J. Cantú-Dibildox, C. Marco-Ramírez, and J. Benítez-del-Castillo. "Effects of a Nutraceutical Formulation Based on the Combination of Antioxidants and ω–3 Essential Fatty Acids in the Expression of Inflammation and Immune Response Mediators in Tears from Patients with Dry Eye Disorders." *Clinical Interventions in Aging* 8 (2013): 139–48. doi:10.2147/CIA.S40640.

Liu, A., and J. Ji. "Omega-3 Essential Fatty Acids Therapy for Dry Eye Syndrome: A Meta-Analysis of Randomized Controlled Studies." *Medical Science Monitor* 20 (2014): 1583–89. doi:10.12659/MSM.891364.

Genuis, S. J., S. Beesoon, and D. Birkholz. "Biomonitoring and Elimination of Perfluorinated Compounds and Polychlorinated Biphenyls Through Perspiration: Blood, Urine, and Sweat Study." *ISRN Toxicology* 2013 (2013): 483832. doi:10.1155/2013/483832.

Genuis, S. J., S. Beesoon, R. A. Lobo, and D. Birkholz. "Human Elimination of Phthalate Compounds: Blood, Urine, and Sweat (BUS) Study." *Scientific World Journal* 2012 (2012): 615068. doi:10.1100/2012/615068.

Genuis, S. J., S. Beesoon, D. Birkholz, and R. A. Lobo. "Human Excretion of Bisphenol A: Blood, Urine, and Sweat (BUS) Study." *Journal of Environmental and Public Health* 2012 (2012): 185731. doi:10.1155/2012/185731.

James, J. W., and R. Friedman. *The Grief Recovery Handbook, 20th Anniversary Expanded Edition: The Action Program for Moving Beyond Death, Divorce, and Other Losses Including Health, Career, and Faith.* New York: William Morrow, 2009.

Minich, D. M. "Essential Fatty Acid Absorption and Metabolism." Ph.D. thesis, Rijksuniversiteit Groningen, 1999. Accessed September 7, 2015. http://www.direct-ms.org/pdf/NutritionFats/EFA%20metabolism.pdf.

Lavialle, M., I. Denis, P. Guesnet, and S. Vancassel. "Involvement of Omega-3 Fatty Acids in Emotional Responses and Hyperactive Symptoms." *Journal of Nutritional Biochemistry* 21, no. 10 (2010): 899–905. doi:10.1016/j.jnutbio.2009.12.005.

Grosso, G., A. Pajak, S. Marventano, S. Castellano, F. Galvano, C. Bucolo, F. Drago, and F. Caraci. "Role of Omega-3 Fatty Acids in the Treatment of Depressive Disorders: A Comprehensive Meta-Analysis of Randomized Clinical Trials." *PLoS ONE* 9, no. 5 (2014): e96905. doi:10.1371/journal.pone.0096905.

Spector, A. A., and H. Y. Kim. "Discovery of Essential Fatty Acids." *Journal of Lipid Research* 56, no. 1 (2015): 11–21. doi:10.1194/jlr.R055095.

Perica, M. M., and I. Delas. "Essential Fatty Acids and Psychiatric Disorders." *Nutrition in Clinical Practice* 26, no. 4 (2011): 409–25. doi:10.1177/0884533611411306.

Haag, M. "Essential Fatty Acids and the Brain." *Canadian Journal of Psychiatry* 48, no. 3 (2003): 195–203.

Gehrig, K. A., and J. G. Dinulos. "Acrodermatitis Due to Nutritional Deficiency." *Current Opinion in Pediatrics* 22, no. 1 (2010): 107–12. doi:10.1097/MOP.0b013e328335107f.

Finner, A. M. "Nutrition and Hair: Deficiencies and Supplements." *Dermatologic Clinics* 31, no. 1 (2013): 167–72. doi:10.1016/j.det.2012.08.015.

Das, U. N. "Essential Fatty Acids and Their Metabolites as Modulators of Stem Cell Biology with Reference to Inflammation, Cancer, and Metastasis." *Cancer Metastasis Reviews* 30, nos. 3–4 (2011): 311–24. doi:10.1007/s10555-011-9316-x.

The World's Healthiest Foods. "Omega-3 Fatty Acids." Accessed September 7, 2015. http://www.whfoods.com/genpage.php?tname=nutrient&dbid=84.

United States Department of Agriculture, Agricultural Research Service. "National Nutrient Database for Standard Reference Release 28." http://ndb.nal.usda.gov/ndb/foods.

Daley, C. A., A. Abbott, P. S. Doyle, G. A. Nader, and S. Larson. "A Review of Fatty Acid Profiles and Antioxidant Content in Grass-Fed and Grain-Fed Beef." *Nutrition Journal* 9 (2010): 10. doi:10.1186/1475-2891-9-10.

Bourre, J. M. "Where to Find Omega-3 Fatty Acids and How Feeding Animals with Diet Enriched in Omega-3 Fatty Acids to Increase Nutritional Value of Derived Products for Human: What Is Actually Useful?" *Journal of Nutrition, Health, and Aging* 9, no. 4 (2005): 232–42.

Simopoulos, A. P. "Evolutionary Aspects of Diet, the Omega-6/Omega-3 Ratio and Genetic Variation: Nutritional Implications for Chronic Diseases." *Biomedicine and Pharmacotherapy* 60, no. 9 (2006): 502–7.

Jandacek, R. J., and P. Tso. "Factors Affecting the Storage and Excretion of Toxic Lipophilic Xenobiotics." *Lipids* 36, no. 12 (2001): 1289–305.

Moreira, A. P., T. F. Texeira, A. B. Ferreira, C. Peluzio Mdo, and C. Alfenas Rde. "Influence of a High-Fat Diet on Gut Microbiota, Intestinal Permeability and Metabolic Endotoxaemia." *British Journal of Nutrition* 108, no. 5 (2012): 801–9. doi:10.1017/S0007114512001213.

Fukui, H. "Gut-Liver Axis in Liver Cirrhosis: How to Manage Leaky Gut and Endotoxemia." *World Journal of Hepatology* 7, no. 3 (2015): 425–42. doi:10.4254/wjh.v7.i3.425.

Pendyala, S., J. M. Walker, and P. R. Holt. "A High-Fat Diet Is Associated with Endotoxemia That Originates from the Gut." *Gastroenterology* 142, no. 5 (2012): 1100–101.e2. doi:10.1053/j.gastro.2012.01.034.

United States Department of Agriculture, Agricultural Research Service. "National Nutrient Database for Standard Reference Release 28." http://ndb.nal.usda.gov/ndb/foods.

Sirato-Yasumoto, S., M. Katsuta, Y. Okuyama, Y. Takahashi, and T. Ide. "Effect of Sesame Seeds Rich in Sesamin and Sesamolin on Fatty Acid Oxidation in Rat Liver." *Journal of Agricultural and Food Chemistry* 49, no. 5 (2001): 2647–51.

Ide, T., Y. Nakashima, H. Iida, S. Yasumoto, and M. Katsuta. "Lipid Metabolism and Nutrigenomics—Impact of Sesame Lignans on Gene Expression Profiles and Fatty Acid Oxidation in Rat Liver." *Forum of Nutrition* 61 (2009): 10–24. doi:10.1159/000212735.

Callaway, J. C. "Hempseed as a Nutritional Resource: An Overview." *Euphytica* 140 (2004): 65–72. doi:10.1007/s10681-004-4811-6.

Goyal, A., V. Sharma, N. Upadhyay, S. Gill, and M. Sihag. "Flax and Flaxseed Oil: An Ancient

Medicine and Modern Functional Food." *Journal of Food Science and Technology* 51, no. 9 (2014): 1633–53. doi:10.1007/s13197-013-1247-9.

Tur, J. A., M. M. Bibiloni, A. Sureda, and A. Pons. "Dietary Sources of Omega-3 Fatty Acids: Public Health Risks and Benefits." *British Journal of Nutrition* 107, suppl. 2 (2012): S23–52. doi:10.1017/S0007114512001456.

DebMandal, M., and S. Mandal. "Coconut (*Cocos nucifera* L.: *Arecaceae*): In Health Promotion and Disease Prevention." *Asian Pacific Journal of Tropical Medicine* 4, no. 3 (2011): 241–47. doi:10.1016/S1995-7645(11)60078-3.

Cicerale, S., L. J. Lucas, and R. S. Keast. "Antimicrobial, Antioxidant and Anti-Inflammatory Phenolic Activities in Extra-Virgin Olive Oil." *Current Opinion in Biotechnology* 23, no. 2 (2012): 129–35. doi:10.1016/j.copbio.2011.09.006.

Ortiz-Avila, O., M. Esquivel-Martínez, B. E. Olmos-Orizaba, A. Saavedra-Molina, A. R. Rodriguez-Orozco, and C. Cortés-Rojo. "Avocado Oil Improves Mitochondrial Function and Decreases Oxidative Stress in Brain of Diabetic Rats." *Journal of Diabetes Research* 2015 (2015): 485759. doi:10.1155/2015/485759.

Ortiz-Avila, O., M. A. Gallegos-Corona, L. A. Sánchez-Briones, E. Calderón-Cortés, R. Montoya-Pérez, A. R. Rodriguez-Orozco, J. Campos-García, et al. "Protective Effects of Dietary Avocado Oil on Impaired Electron Transport Chain Function and Exacerbated Oxidative Stress in Liver Mitochondria from Diabetic Rats." *Journal of Bioenergetics and Biomembranes* 47, no. 4 (2015): 337–53.

Alasalvar, C., and B. W. Bolling. "Review of Nut Phytochemicals, Fat-Soluble Bioactives, Antioxidant Components and Health Effects." *British Journal of Nutrition* 113, suppl. 2 (2015): S68–78. doi:10.1017/S0007114514003729.

Fardet, A. "A Shift Toward a New Holistic Paradigm Will Help to Preserve and Better Process Grain Products' Food Structure for Improving Their Health Effects." *Food and Function* 6, no. 2 (2015): 363–82. doi:10.1039/c4fo00477a.

Kaulmann, A., and T. Bohn. "Carotenoids, Inflammation, and Oxidative Stress—Implications of Cellular Signaling Pathways and Relation to Chronic Disease Prevention." *Nutrition Research* 34, no. 11 (2014): 907–29. doi:10.1016/j.nutres.2014.07.010.

Talavera, F., and B. P. Chew. "Comparative Role of Retinol, Retinoic Acid and Beta-Carotene on Progesterone Secretion by Pig Corpus Luteum In Vitro." *Journal of Reproduction and Fertility* 82, no. 2 (1988): 611–15.

Graves-Hoagland, R. L., T. A. Hoagland, and C. O. Woody. "Effect of Beta-Carotene and Vitamin A on Progesterone Production by Bovine Luteal Cells." *Journal of Dairy Science* 71, no. 4 (1988): 1058–62.

Ribaya-Mercado, J. D. "Influence of Dietary Fat on Beta-Carotene Absorption and Bioconversion into Vitamin A." *Nutrition Reviews* 60, no. 4 (2002): 104–10.

Lemmens, L., I. J. Colle, S. van Buggenhout, A. M. van Loey, and M. E. Hendrickx. "Quantifying the Influence of Thermal Process Parameters on In Vitro β-Carotene Bioaccessibility: A Case Study on Carrots." *Journal of Agriculture and Food Chemistry* 59, no. 7 (2011): 3162–67. doi:10.1021/jf104888y.

Rizza, S., R. Muniyappa, M. Iantorno, J. A. Kim, H. Chen, P. Pullikotil, N. Senese, et al. "Citrus Polyphenol Hesperidin Stimulates Production of Nitric Oxide in Endothelial Cells While Improving Endothelial Function and Reducing Inflammatory Markers in Patients with Metabolic Syndrome." *Journal of Clinical Endocrinology and Metabolism* 96, no. 5 (2011): E782–92. doi:10.1210/jc.2010-2879.

Gupta, C., and D. Prakash. "Phytonutrients as Therapeutic Agents." *Journal of Complementary and Integrative Medicine* 11, no. 3 (2014): 151–69.

CHAPTER 5: THE FIRE

Nater, U. M., R. La Marca, L. Florin, A. Moses, W. Langhans, M. M. Koller, and U. Ehlert. "Stress-Induced Changes in Human Salivary Alpha-Amylase Activity—Associations with Adrenergic Activity." *Psychoneuroendocrinology* 31, no. 1 (2006): 49–58.

Morse, D. R., G. R. Schacterle, L. Furst, M. Zaydenberg, and R. L. Pollack. "Oral Digestion of a Complex-Carbohydrate Cereal: Effects of Stress and Relaxation on Physiological and Salivary Measures." *American Journal of Clinical Nutrition* 49, no. 1 (1989): 97–105.

Moloney, R. D., L. Desbonnet, G. Clarke, T. G. Dinan, and J. F. Cryan. "The Microbiome: Stress, Health and Disease." *Mammalian Genome* 25, nos. 1–2 (2014): 49–74. doi:10.1007/s00335 -013-9488-5.

Kellman, R. *The Microbiome Diet: The Scientifically Proven Way to Restore Your Gut Health and Achieve Permanent Weight Loss*. Boston: Da Capo Lifelong, 2015.

Ishizaki, M., H. Nakagawa, Y. Morikawa, R. Honda, Y. Yamada, N. Kawakami; and Japan Work Stress and Health Cohort Study Group. "Influence of Job Strain on Changes in Body Mass Index and Waist Circumference: 6-Year Longitudinal Study." *Scandinavian Journal of Work, Environment and Health* 34, no. 4 (2008): 288–96.

Brunner, E. J., T. Chandola, and M. G. Marmot. "Prospective Effect of Job Strain on General and Central Obesity in the Whitehall II Study." *American Journal of Epidemiology* 165, no. 7 (2007): 828–37.

Steptoe, A., M. Cropley, J. Griffith, and K. Joekes. "The Influence of Abdominal Obesity and Chronic Work Stress on Ambulatory Blood Pressure in Men and Women." *International Journal of Obesity and Related Metabolic Disorders* 23, no. 11 (1999): 1184–91.

Nyberg, S. T., E. I. Fransson, K. Heikkilä, K. Ahola, L. Alfredsson, J. B. Bjorner, M. Borritz, et al. "Job Strain as a Risk Factor for Type 2 Diabetes: A Pooled Analysis of 124,808 Men and Women." *Diabetes Care* 37, no. 8 (2014): 2268–75. doi:10.2337/dc13-2936.

Huth, C., B. Thorand, J. Baumert, J. Kruse, R. T. Emeny, A. Schneider, C. Meisinger, and K. H. Ladwig. "Job Strain as a Risk Factor for the Onset of Type 2 Diabetes Mellitus: Findings from the MONICA/KORA Augsburg Cohort Study." *Psychosomatic Medicine* 76, no. 7 (2014): 562–68. doi:10.1097/PSY.0000000000000084.

Koponen, A., J. Vahtera, J. Pitkäniemi, M. Virtanen, J. Pentti, N. Simonsen-Rehn, M. Kivimäki, and S. Suominen. "Job Strain and Supervisor Support in Primary Care Health Centres and Glycaemic Control Among Patients with Type 2 Diabetes: A Cross-Sectional Study." *BMJ Open* 3, no. 5 (2013): e002297. doi:10.1136/bmjopen-2012-002297.

Eriksson, A. K., M. van den Donk, A. Hilding, and C. G. Östenson. "Work Stress, Sense of Coherence, and Risk of Type 2 Diabetes in a Prospective Study of Middle-Aged Swedish Men and Women." *Diabetes Care* 36, no. 9 (2013): 2683–89. doi:10.2337/dc12-1738.

Lett, A. M., P. S. Thondre, and A. J. Rosenthal. "Yellow Mustard Bran Attenuates Glycaemic Response of a Semi-Solid Food in Young Healthy Men." *International Journal of Food Sciences and Nutrition* 64, no. 2 (2013): 140–46. doi:10.3109/09637486.2012.728201.

Marinangeli, C. P., and P. J. Jones. "Whole and Fractionated Yellow Pea Flours Reduce Fasting Insulin and Insulin Resistance in Hypercholesterolaemic and Overweight Human Subjects." *British Journal of Nutrition* 105, no. 1 (2011): 110–17. doi:10.1017/S0007114510003156.

Kim, Y., H. Y. Yang, A. J. Kim, and Y. Lim. "Academic Stress Levels Were Positively Associated with Sweet Food Consumption Among Korean High-School Students." *Nutrition* 29, no. 1 (2013): 213–18. doi:10.1016/j.nut.2012.08.005.

Baumeister, R. F. "Self-Regulation, Ego Depletion, and Inhibition." *Neuropsychologia* 65 (2014): 313–19. doi:10.1016/j.neuropsychologia.2014.08.012.

Gröpel, P., R. F. Baumeister, and J. Beckmann. "Action Versus State Orientation and Self-Control Performance After Depletion." *Personal and Social Psychology Bulletin* 40, no. 4 (2014): 476–87. doi:10.1177/0146167213516636.

DeWall, C. N., R. F. Baumeister, N. L. Mead, and K. D. Vohs. "How Leaders Self-Regulate Their Task Performance: Evidence That Power Promotes Diligence, Depletion, and Disdain." *Journal of Personal and Social Psychology* 100, no. 1 (2011): 47–65. doi:10.1037/a0020932.

Palimeri, S., E. Palioura, and E. Diamanti-Kandarakis. "Current Perspectives on the Health Risks Associated with the Consumption of Advanced Glycation End Products: Recommendations for Dietary Management." *Diabetes, Metabolic Syndrome and Obesity* 8 (2015): 415–26. doi:10.2147/DMSO.S63089.

Bartłomiej, S., R. K. Justyna, and N. Ewa. "Bioactive Compounds in Cereal Grains—Occurrence, Structure, Technological Significance and Nutritional Benefits—A Review." *Food Sciences Technology International* 18, no. 6 (2012): 559–68. doi:10.1177/1082013211433079.

Fernie, A. R., F. Carrari, and L. J. Sweetlove. "Respiratory Metabolism: Glycolysis, the TCA Cycle and Mitochondrial Electron Transport." *Current Opinion in Plant Biology* 7, no. 3 (2004): 254–61.

Stough, C., A. Scholey, J. Lloyd, J. Spong, S. Myers, and L. A. Downey. "The Effect of 90 Day Administration of a High Dose Vitamin B-Complex on Work Stress." *Human Psychopharmacology* 26, no. 7 (2011): 470–76. doi:10.1002/hup.1229.

Kennedy, D. O., R. Veasey, A. Watson, F. Dodd, E. Jones, S. Maggini, and C. F. Haskell. "Effects of High-Dose B Vitamin Complex with Vitamin C and Minerals on Subjective Mood and Performance in Healthy Males." *Psychopharmacology* (Berlin) 211, no. 1 (2010): 55–68. doi:10.1007/s00213-010-1870-3.

Southgate, D. A. "Digestion and Metabolism of Sugars." *American Journal of Clinical Nutrition* 62, suppl. 1 (1995): 203S–10S.

Swithers, S. "Artificial Sweeteners Produce the Counterintuitive Effect of Inducing Metabolic Derangements." *Trends in Endocrinology and Metabolism* 24, no. 9 (2013): 431–41.

Suez, J., T. Korem, D. Zeevi, G. Zilberman-Schapira, C. Thaiss, O. Maza, D. Israeli, et al. "Artificial Sweeteners Induce Glucose Intolerance by Altering the Gut Microbiota." *Nature* 514, no. 7521 (2014): 181–86.

Yang, Q. "Gain Weight by 'Going Diet'? Artificial Sweeteners and the Neurobiology of Sugar Cravings: Neuroscience 2010." *Yale Journal of Biology and Medicine* 83, no. 2 (2010): 101–8.

Vazquez-Roque, M., and A. S. Oxentenko. "Nonceliac Gluten Sensitivity." *Mayo Clinic Proceedings* 90, no. 9 (2015): 1272–77. doi:10.1016/j.mayocp.2015.07.009.

Mansueto, P., A. Seidita, A. D'Alcamo, and A. Carroccio. "Non-Celiac Gluten Sensitivity: Literature Review." *Journal of the American College of Nutrition* 33, no. 1 (2014): 39–54. doi:10.1080/07315724.2014.869996.

Flood, J. E., L. S. Roe, and B. J. Rolls. "The Effect of Increased Beverage Portion Size on Energy Intake at a Meal." *Journal of the American Dietetic Association* 106, no. 12 (2006): 1984–90; discussion 1990–91.

Davy, B. M., E. A. Dennis, A. L. Dengo, K. L. Wilson, and K. P. Davy. "Water Consumption Reduces Energy Intake at a Breakfast Meal in Obese Older Adults." *Journal of the American Dietetic Association* 108, no. 7 (2008): 1236–39. doi:10.1016/j.jada.2008.04.013.

Dennis, E. A., A. L. Dengo, D. L. Comber, K. D. Flack, J. Savla, K. P. Davy, and B. M. Davy. "Water Consumption Increases Weight Loss During a Hypocaloric Diet Intervention in Middle-Aged and Older Adults." *Obesity* (Silver Spring) 18, no. 2 (2010): 300–7. doi:10.1038/oby.2009.235.

Taylor, A. G., L. E. Goehler, D. I. Galper, K. E. Innes, and C. Bourguignon. "Top-Down and Bottom-Up Mechanisms in Mind–Body Medicine: Development of an Integrative Framework for Psychophysiological Research." *Explore* (New York) 6, no. 1 (2010): 29–41. doi:10.1016/j.explore.2009.10.004.

CHAPTER 6: THE LOVE

Ogawa, T., and A. J. de Bold. "The Heart as an Endocrine Organ." *Endocrine Connections* 3, no. 2 (2014): R31–44. doi:10.1530/EC-14-0012.

McGrath, M. F., M. L. de Bold, and A. J. de Bold. "The Endocrine Function of the Heart." *Trends in Endocrinology and Metabolism* 16, no. 10 (2005): 469–77.

De Bold, A. J., K. K. Ma, Y. Zhang, M. L. de Bold, M. Bensimon, and A. Khoshbaten. "The Physiological and Pathophysiological Modulation of the Endocrine Function of the Heart." *Canadian Journal of Physiology and Pharmacology* 79, no. 8 (2001): 705–14.

Miller, S. B., L. Dolgoy, M. Friese, and A. Sita. "Dimensions of Hostility and Cardiovascular Response to Interpersonal Stress." *Journal of Psychosomatic Research* 41, no. 1 (1996): 81–95.

Suarez, E. C., E. Harlan, M. C. Peoples, and R. B. Williams Jr. "Cardiovascular and Emotional Responses in Women: The Role of Hostility and Harassment." *Health Psychology* 12, no. 6 (1993): 459–68.

Vitaliano, P. P., J. Russo, S. L. Bailey, H. M. Young, and B. S. McCann. "Psychosocial Factors Associated with Cardiovascular Reactivity in Older Adults." *Psychosomatic Medicine* 55, no. 2 (1993): 164–77.

Buckley, T., S. McKinley, G. Tofler, and R. Bartrop. "Cardiovascular Risk in Early Bereavement: A Literature Review and Proposed Mechanisms." *International Journal of Nursing Studies* 47, no. 2 (2010): 229–38. doi:10.1016/j.ijnurstu.2009.06.010.

Carey, I. M., S. M. Shah, S. DeWilde, T. Harris, C. R. Victor, and D. G. Cook. "Increased Risk of Acute Cardiovascular Events After Partner Bereavement: A Matched Cohort Study." *JAMA Internal Medicine* 174, no. 4 (2014): 598–605. doi:10.1001/jamainternmed.2013.14558.

Levin, A. "In Young Women, Depression Can Mean Literal Heartbreak." *EurekAlert!*. June 28, 2004. Accessed November 9, 2015. http://www.eurekalert.org/pub_releases/2004-06/cfta-iyw062804.php.

News Staff. "Literal Heartbreak: The Cardiovascular Impact of Rejection." *Science* 2.0 (blog). September 28, 2010. Accessed September 27, 2015. http://www.science20.com/news_articles/literal_heartbreak_cardiovascular_impact_rejection.

Crawford, C. "Why a Broken Heart Literally Hurts." Health Guidance for Better Health, Accessed November 9, 2015. http://www.healthguidance.org/entry/15607/1/Why-a-Broken-Heart-Literally-Hurts.html.

Jurkiewicz, R., and B. W. Romano. "Coronary Artery Disease and Experiences of Losses." [Article in English, Portuguese, Spanish.] *Arquivos Brasileiros de Cardiologia* 93, no. 4 (2009): 345–59.

Kaprio, J., M. Koskenvuo, and H. Rita. "Mortality After Bereavement: A Prospective Study of 95,647 Widowed Persons." *American Journal of Public Health* 77, no. 3 (1987): 283–87.

Luecken, L. J. "Childhood Attachment and Loss Experiences Affect Adult Cardiovascular and Cortisol Function." *Psychosomatic Medicine* 60, no. 6 (1998): 765–72.

Arch, J. J., K. W. Brown, D. J. Dean, L. N. Landy, K. D. Brown, and M. L. Laudenslager. "Self-Compassion Training Modulates Alpha-Amylase, Heart Rate Variability, and Subjective

Responses to Social Evaluative Threat in Women." *Psychoneuroendocrinology* 42 (2014): 49–58. doi:10.1016/j.psyneuen.2013.12.018.

Kemper, K. J., D. Powell, C. C. Helms, and D. B. Kim-Shapiro. "Loving-Kindness Meditation's Effects on Nitric Oxide and Perceived Well-Being: A Pilot Study in Experienced and Inexperienced Meditators." *Explore* (New York) 11, no. 1 (2015): 32–39. doi:10.1016/j.explore.2014.10.002.

Schäfer, A., and K. W. Kratky. "The Effect of Colored Illumination on Heart Rate Variability." *Forschende Komplementärmedizin* 13, no. 3 (2006): 167–73.

Peck, M. Scott. *The Road Less Traveled.* New York: Simon & Schuster, 1978.

Park, B. J., Y. Tsunetsugu, T. Kasetani, T. Kagawa, and Y. Miyazaki. "The Physiological Effects of Shinrin-Yoku (Taking in the Forest Atmosphere or Forest Bathing): Evidence from Field Experiments in 24 Forests Across Japan." *Environmental Health and Preventive Medicine* 15, no. 1 (2010): 18–26. doi:10.1007/s12199-009-0086-9.

Ochiai, H., H. Ikei, C. Song, M. Kobayashi, A. Takamatsu, T. Miura, T. Kagawa, et al. "Physiological and Psychological Effects of Forest Therapy on Middle-Aged Males with High-Normal Blood Pressure." *International Journal of Environmental Research and Public Health* 12, no. 3 (2015): 2532–42. doi:10.3390/ijerph120302532.

Mao, G. X., Y. B. Cao, X. G. Lan, Z. H. He, Z. M. Chen, Y. Z. Wang, X. L. Hu, et al. "Therapeutic Effect of Forest Bathing on Human Hypertension in the Elderly." *Journal of Cardiology* 60, no. 6 (2012): 495–502. doi:10.1016/j.jjcc.2012.08.003.

Lee, J., B. J. Park, Y. Tsunetsugu, T. Ohira, T. Kagawa, and Y. Miyazaki. "Effect of Forest Bathing on Physiological and Psychological Responses in Young Japanese Male Subjects." *Public Health* 125, no. 2 (2011): 93–100. doi:10.1016/j.puhe.2010.09.005.

Shaughnessy, D. T., L. M. Gangarosa, B. Schliebe, D. M. Umbach, Z. Xu, B. MacIntosh, M. G. Knize, et al. "Inhibition of Fried Meat-Induced Colorectal DNA Damage and Altered Systemic Genotoxicity in Humans by Crucifera, Chlorophyllin, and Yogurt." *PLoS ONE* 6, no. 4 (2011): e18707. doi:10.1371/journal.pone.0018707.

Dashwood, R., S. Yamane, and R. Larsen. "Study of the Forces of Stabilizing Complexes Between Chlorophylls and Heterocyclic Amine Mutagens." *Environmental and Molecular Mutagenesis* 27, no. 3 (1996): 211–18.

Walsh, M. C., L. Brennan, E. Pujos-Guillot, J. L. Sébédio, A. Scalbert, A. Fagan, D. G. Higgins, and M. J. Gibney. "Influence of Acute Phytochemical Intake on Human Urinary Metabolomic Profiles." *American Journal of Clinical Nutrition* 86, no. 6 (2007): 1687–93.

Dhonukshe-Rutten, R. A., J. H. de Vries, A. de Bree, N. van der Put, W. A. van Staveren, and L. C. de Groot. "Dietary Intake and Status of Folate and Vitamin B12 and Their Association with Homocysteine and Cardiovascular Disease in European Populations." *European Journal of Clinical Nutrition* 63, no. 1 (2009): 18–30.

Waśkiewicz, A., E. Sygnowska, and G. Broda. "Dietary Intake of Vitamins B6, B12 and Folate in Relation to Homocysteine Serum Concentration in the Adult Polish Population—WOBASZ Project." *Kardiologia Polska* 68, no. 3 (2010): 275–82.

Jones, P. J., and S. S. Abumweis. "Phytosterols as Functional Food Ingredients: Linkages to Cardiovascular Disease and Cancer." *Current Opinion in Clinical Nutrition and Metabolic Care* 12, no. 2 (2009): 147–51.

Sirotkin, A. V., and A. H. Harrath. "Phytoestrogens and Their Effects." *European Journal of Pharmacology* 741 (2014): 230–36. doi:10.1016/j.ejphar.2014.07.057.

Jenkins, D. J., C. W. Kendall, A. Marchie, D. Faulkner, E. Vidgen, K. G. Lapsley, E. A. Trautwein, et al. "The Effect of Combining Plant Sterols, Soy Protein, Viscous Fibers, and Almonds in Treating Hypercholesterolemia." *Metabolism* 52, no. 11 (2003): 1478–83.

Jenkins, D. J., C. W. Kendall, A. Marchie, A. L. Jenkins, L. S. Augustin, D. S. Ludwig, N. D. Barnard, and J. W. Anderson. "Type 2 Diabetes and the Vegetarian Diet." *American Journal of Clinical Nutrition* 78, no. 3 suppl. (2003): 610S–16S.

USDA Agricultural Research Service. National Nutrient Database "Phytosterol." Last modified December 7, 2011. Accessed September 27, 2015. http://ndb.nal.usda.gov/.

Thompson, H. J., J. Heimendinger, A. Diker, C. O'Neill, A. Haegele, B. Meinecke, P. Wolfe, et al. "Dietary Botanical Diversity Affects the Reduction of Oxidative Biomarkers in Women Due to High Vegetable and Fruit Intake." *Journal of Nutrition* 136, no. 8 (2006): 2207–12.

Liu, R. H. "Health Benefits of Fruit and Vegetables Are from Additive and Synergistic Combinations of Phytochemicals." *American Journal of Clinical Nutrition* 78, no. 3 suppl. (2003): 517S–20S.

Rylott, E. L., V. Gunning, K. Tzafestas, H. Sparrow, E. J. Johnston, A. S. Brentnall, J. R. Potts, and N. C. Bruce. "Phytodetoxification of the Environmental Pollutant and Explosive 2,4,6-Trinitrotoluene." *Plant Signaling and Behavior* 10, no. 1 (2015): e977714. doi:10.4161/15592324.2014.977714.

Hannink, N., S. J. Rosser, C. E. French, A. Basran, J. A. Murray, S. Nicklin, and N. C. Bruce. "Phytodetoxification of TNT by Transgenic Plants Expressing a Bacterial Nitroreductase." *Nature Biotechnology* 19, no. 12 (2001): 1168–72.

Khalesi, S., C. Irwin, and M. Schubert. "Flaxseed Consumption May Reduce Blood Pressure: A Systematic Review and Meta-Analysis of Controlled Trials." *Journal of Nutrition* 145, no. 4 (2015): 758–65. doi:10.3945/jn.114.205302.

Goyal, A., V. Sharma, N. Upadhyay, S. Gill, and M. Sihag. "Flax and Flaxseed Oil: An Ancient Medicine and Modern Functional Food." *Journal of Food Science and Technology* 51, no. 9 (2014): 1633–53. doi:10.1007/s13197-013-1247-9.

Peterson, J., J. Dwyer, H. Adlercreutz, A. Scalbert, P. Jacques, and M. L. McCullough. "Dietary Lignans: Physiology and Potential for Cardiovascular Disease Risk Reduction." *Nutrition Reviews* 68, no. 10 (2010): 571–603. doi:10.1111/j.1753-4887.2010.00319.x.

Adolphe, J. L., S. J. Whiting, B. H. Juurlink, L. U. Thorpe, and J. Alcorn. "Health Effects with Consumption of the Flax Lignan Secoisolariciresinol Diglucoside." *British Journal of Nutrition* 103, no. 7 (2010): 929–38. doi:10.1017/S0007114509992753.

Thompson, L. U., B. A. Boucher, Z. Lui, M. Cotterchio, and N. Kreiger. "Phytoestrogen Content of Foods Consumed in Canada, Including Isoflavones, Lignans and Coumestan." *Nutrition and Cancer* 54, no. 2 (2006): 184–201.

Feldman, E. B. "Fruits and Vegetables and the Risk of Stroke." *Nutrition Reviews* 59, no. 1, pt. 1 (2001): 24–27.

Mizrahi, A., P. Knekt, J. Montonen, M. A. Laaksonen, M. Heliövaara, and R. Järvinen. "Plant Foods and the Risk of Cerebrovascular Diseases: A Potential Protection of Fruit Consumption." *British Journal of Nutrition* 102, no. 7 (2009): 1075–83. doi:10.1017/S0007114509359097.

Virtanen, J. K., T. H. Rissanen, S. Voutilainen, and T. P. Tuomainen. "Mercury as a Risk Factor for Cardiovascular Diseases." *Journal of Nutritional Biochemistry* 18, no. 2 (2007): 75–85.

Caciari, T., A. Sancini, M. Fioravanti, A. Capozzella, T. Casale, L. Montuori, M. Fiaschetti, et al. "Cadmium and Hypertension in Exposed Workers: A Meta-Analysis." *International Journal of Occupational Medicine and Environmental Health* 26, no. 3 (2013): 440–56. doi:10.2478/s13382-013-0111-5.

Rosin, A. "The Long-Term Consequences of Exposure to Lead." *Israel Medical Association Journal* 11, no. 11 (2009): 689–94.

Uchikawa, T., I. Maruyama, S. Kumamoto, Y. Ando, and A. Yasutake. "Chlorella Suppresses Methylmercury Transfer to the Fetus in Pregnant Mice." *Journal of Toxicological Sciences* 36, no. 5 (2011): 675–80.

Rai, L. C., J. P. Gaur, and H. D. Kumar. "Protective Effects of Certain Environmental Factors on the Toxicity of Zinc, Mercury, and Methylmercury to Chlorella Vulgaris." *Environmental Research* 25, no. 2 (1981): 250–59.

Omura, Y., and S. L. Beckman. "Role of Mercury (Hg) in Resistant Infections and Effective Treatment of Chlamydia Trachomatis and Herpes Family Viral Infections (and Potential Treatment for Cancer) by Removing Localized Hg Deposits with Chinese Parsley and Delivering Effective Antibiotics Using Various Drug Uptake Enhancement Methods." *Acupuncture and Electro-Therapeutics Research* 20, nos. 3–4 (1995): 195–229.

Alcocer-Varela, J., A. Iglesias, L. Llorente, and D. Alarcón-Segovia. "Effects of L-Canavanine on T Cells May Explain the Induction of Systemic Lupus Erythematosus by Alfalfa." *Arthritis and Rheumatism* 28, no. 1 (1985): 52–57.

Malinow, M. R., E. J. Bardana Jr., B. Pirofsky, S. Craig, and P. McLaughlin. "Systemic Lupus Erythematosus-Like Syndrome in Monkeys Fed Alfalfa Sprouts: Role of a Nonprotein Amino Acid." *Science* 216, no. 4544 (1982): 415–17.

Xiao, Z., G. E. Lester, Y. Luo, and Q. Wang. "Assessment of Vitamin and Carotenoid Concentrations of Emerging Food Products: Edible Microgreens." *Journal of Agricultural and Food Chemistry* 60, no. 31 (2012): 7644–51. doi:10.1021/jf300459b.

Scholz, S., and G. Williamson. "Interactions Affecting the Bioavailability of Dietary Polyphenols In Vivo." *International Journal for Vitamin and Nutrition Research* 77, no. 3 (2007): 224–35.

Naito, Y., and T. Yoshikawa. "Green Tea and Heart Health." *Journal of Cardiovascular Pharmacology* 54, no. 5 (2009): 385–90. doi:10.1097/FJC.0b013e3181b6e7a1.

CHAPTER 7: THE TRUTH

M. L. Pelchat and S. Schaefer. "Dietary monotony and food cravings in young and elderly adults." *Physiological and Behavior* 68, no. 3 (January 2000): 353-9.

C. Noel and R. Dando. "The effect of emotional state on taste perception." *Appetite* 95 (1 December 2015): 89-95. doi: 10.1016/j.appet.2015.06.003. Epub 2015 Jun 27.

Devillier, P., E. Naline, and S. Grassin-Delyle. "The Pharmacology of Bitter Taste Receptors and Their Role in Human Airways." *Pharmacology and Therapeutics* 155 (2015): 11–12. doi:10.1016/j.pharmthera.2015.08.001.

Clark, A. A., C. D. Dotson, A. E. Elson, A. Voigt, U. Boehm, W. Meyerhof, N. I. Steinle, and S. D. Munger. "TAS2R Bitter Taste Receptors Regulate Thyroid Function." *FASEB Journal* 29, no. 1 (2015): 164–72. doi:10.1096/fj 14-262246.

Maehashi, K., and L. Huang. "Bitter Peptides and Bitter Taste Receptors." *Cellular and Molecular Life Sciences* 66, no. 10 (2009): 1661–71. doi:10.1007/s00018-009-8755-9.

Rozengurt, E. "Taste Receptors in the Gastrointestinal Tract. I. Bitter Taste Receptors and Alpha-Gustducin in the Mammalian Gut." *American Journal of Physiology: Gastrointestinal and Liver Physiology* 291, no. 2 (2006): G171–77.

Denke, C., M. Rotte, H. J. Heinze, and M. Schaefer. "Lying and the Subsequent Desire for Toothpaste: Activity in the Somatosensory Cortex Predicts Embodiment of the Moral-Purity Metaphor." *Cerebral Cortex* (September 11, 2014): bhu170.

Kreutz, G., S. Bongard, S. Rohrmann, V. Hodapp, and D. Grebe. "Effects of Choir Singing or Listening on Secretory Immunoglobulin A, Cortisol, and Emotional State." *Journal of Behavioral Medicine* 27, no. 6 (2004): 623–35.

Grape, C., M. Sandgren, L. O. Hansson, M. Ericson, and T. Theorell. "Does Singing Promote Well-Being?: An Empirical Study of Professional and Amateur Singers During a Singing Lesson." *Integrative Physiological and Behavioral Science* 38, no. 1 (2003): 65–74.

Lee, Y. Y., M. F. Chan, and E. Mok. "Effectiveness of Music Intervention on the Quality of Life of Older People." *Journal of Advanced Nursing* 66, no. 12 (2010): 2677–87. doi:10.1111 /j.1365-2648.2010.05445.x.

Coulton, S., S. Clift, A. Skingley, and J. Rodriguez. "Effectiveness and Cost-Effectiveness of Community Singing on Mental Health-Related Quality of Life of Older People: Randomised Controlled Trial." *British Journal of Psychiatry* 207, no. 3 (2015): 250–55. doi:10.1192/bjp .bp.113.129908.

MacArtain, P., C. I. Gill, M. Brooks, R. Campbell, and I. R. Rowland. "Nutritional Value of Edible Seaweeds." *Nutrition Reviews* 65, no. 12, pt. 1 (2007): 535–43.

Rajapakse, N., and S. K. Kim. "Nutritional and Digestive Health Benefits of Seaweed." *Advances in Food and Nutrition Research* 64 (2011): 17–28. doi:10.1016/B978-0-12-387669-0.00002-8.

Fitton, J. H., D. N. Stringer, and S. S. Karpiniec. "Therapies from Fucoidan: An Update." *Marine Drugs* 13, no. 9 (2015): 5920–46. doi:10.3390/md13095920.

Abuajah, C. I., A. C. Ogbonna, and C. M. Osuji. "Functional Components and Medicinal Properties of Food: A Review." *Journal of Food Science and Technology* 52, no. 5 (2015): 2522–29. doi:10.1007/s13197-014-1396-5.

Rose, M., J. Lewis, N. Langford, M. Baxter, S. Origgi, M. Barber, H. MacBain, and K. Thomas. "Arsenic in Seaweed—Forms, Concentration and Dietary Exposure." *Food and Chemical Toxicology* 45, no. 7 (2007): 1263–67.

Yokoi, K., and A. Konomi. "Toxicity of So-Called Edible Hijiki Seaweed (*Sargassum fusiforme*) Containing Inorganic Arsenic." *Regulatory Toxicology and Pharmacology* 63, no. 2 (2012): 291–97. doi:10.1016/j.yrtph.2012.04.006.

Skibola, C. F. "The Effect of *Fucus Vesiculosus*, an Edible Brown Seaweed, upon Menstrual Cycle Length and Hormonal Status in Three Pre-Menopausal Women: A Case Report." *BMC Complementary and Alternative Medicine* 4 (2004): 10.

Ramaekers, M. G., P. A. Luning, R. M. Ruijschop, C. M. Lakemond, J. H. Bult, G. Gort, and M. A. van Boekel. "Aroma Exposure Time and Aroma Concentration in Relation to Satiation." *British Journal of Nutrition* 111, no. 3 (2014): 554–62. doi:10.1017/S0007114513002729.

Carwile, J. L., X. Ye, X. Zhou, A. M. Calafat, and K. B. Michels. "Canned Soup Consumption and Urinary Bisphenol A: A Randomized Crossover Trial." *Journal of the American Medical Association* 306, no. 20 (2011): 2218–20. doi:10.1001/jama.2011.1721.

Flood, J. E., and B. J. Rolls. "Soup Preloads in a Variety of Forms Reduce Meal Energy Intake." *Appetite* 49, no. 3 (2007): 626–34.

Hord, N. G. "Dietary Nitrates, Nitrites, and Cardiovascular Disease." *Current Atherosclerosis Reports* 13, no. 6 (2011): 484–92. doi:10.1007/s11883-011-0209-9.

Hodges, R. E., and D. M. Minich. "Modulation of Metabolic Detoxification Pathways Using Foods and Food-Derived Components: A Scientific Review with Clinical Application." *Journal of Nutrition and Metabolism* 2015 (2015): 760689. doi:10.1155/2015/760689.

Llewellyn, C. H., C. H. van Jaarsveld, D. Boniface, S. Carnell, and J. Wardle. "Eating Rate Is a Heritable Phenotype Related to Weight in Children." *American Journal of Clinical Nutrition* 88, no. 6 (2008): 1560–66. doi:10.3945/ajcn.2008.26175.

Dalen, J., B. W. Smith, B. M. Shelley, A. L. Sloan, L. Leahigh, and D. Begay. "Pilot Study: Mindful Eating and Living (MEAL): Weight, Eating Behavior, and Psychological Outcomes Associated with a Mindfulness-Based Intervention for People with Obesity." *Complementary Therapies in Medicine* 18, no. 6 (2010): 260–64. doi:10.1016/j.ctim.2010.09.008.

Katterman, S. N., B. M. Kleinman, M. M. Hood, L. M. Nackers, and J. A. Corsica. "Mindfulness Meditation as an Intervention for Binge Eating, Emotional Eating, and Weight Loss: A Systematic Review." *Eating Behaviors* 15, no. 2 (2014): 197–204. doi:10.1016/j.eatbeh.2014.01.005.

Rolls, B. J., L. S. Roe, and J. S. Meengs. "Larger Portion Sizes Lead to a Sustained Increase in Energy Intake over 2 Days." *Journal of the American Dietetic Association* 106, no. 4 (2006): 543–49.

Appleton, K. M., and L. McGowan. "The Relationship Between Restrained Eating and Poor Psychological Health Is Moderated by Pleasure Normally Associated with Eating." *Eating Behaviors* 7, no. 4 (2006): 342–47.

CHAPTER 8: THE INSIGHT

Craft, S., B. Cholerton, and L. D. Baker. "Insulin and Alzheimer's Disease: Untangling the Web." *Journal of Alzheimer's Disease* 33, suppl. 1 (2013): S263–75.

Cholerton, B., L. D. Baker, and S. Craft. "Insulin, Cognition, and Dementia." *European Journal of Pharmacology* 719, nos. 1–3 (2013): 170–79. doi:10.1016/j.ejphar.2013.08.008.

Cholerton, B., L. D. Baker, and S. Craft. "Insulin Resistance and Pathological Brain Ageing." *Diabetic Medicine* 28, no. 12 (2011): 1463–75. doi:10.1111/j.1464-5491.2011.03464.x.

De la Monte, S. M. "Type 3 Diabetes Is Sporadic Alzheimer's Disease: Mini-Review." *European Neuropsychopharmacology* 24, no. 12 (2014): 1954–60. doi:10.1016/j.euroneuro.2014.06.008.

Berg, J. M., J. L. Tymoczko, and L. Stryer. "Each Organ Has a Unique Metabolic Profile." Section 30.2 in *Biochemistry*, 5th ed. New York: W. H. Freeman, 2002.

McCraty, R., M. Atkinson, and R. T. Bradley. "Electrophysiological Evidence of Intuition: Part 2. A System-Wide Process?" *Journal of Alternative and Complementary Medicine* 10, no. 2 (2004): 325–36.

Petter, M., C. T. Chambers, and J. MacLaren Chorney. "The Effects of Mindfulness-Based Attention on Cold Pressor Pain in Children." *Pain Research and Management* 18, no. 1 (2013): 39–45.

Mizrahi, M. C., R. Reicher-Atir, S. Levy, S. Haramati, D. Wengrower, E. Israeli, and E. Goldin. "Effects of Guided Imagery with Relaxation Training on Anxiety and Quality of Life Among Patients with Inflammatory Bowel Disease." *Psychology and Health* 27, no. 12 (2012): 1463–79. doi:10.1080/08870446.2012.691169.

Gedde-Dahl, M., and E. A. Fors. "Impact of Self-Administered Relaxation and Guided Imagery Techniques During Final Trimester and Birth." *Complementary Therapies in Clinical Practice* 18, no. 1 (2012): 60–65. doi:10.1016/j.ctcp.2011.08.008.

Abdoli, S., K. Rahzani, M. Safaie, and A. Sattari. "A Randomized Control Trial: The Effect of Guided Imagery with Tape and Perceived Happy Memory on Chronic Tension Type Headache." *Scandinavian Journal of Caring Sciences* 26, no. 2 (2012): 254–61. doi:10.1111/j.1471-6712.2011.00926.x.

Mannix, L. K., R. S. Chandurkar, L. A. Rybicki, D. L. Tusek, and G. D. Solomon. "Effect of Guided Imagery on Quality of Life for Patients with Chronic Tension-Type Headache." *Headache* 39, no. 5 (1999): 326–34.

Mehta, R., and R. J. Zhu. "Blue or Red? Exploring the Effect of Color on Cognitive Task Performances." *Science* 323, no. 5918 (2009): 1226–29. doi:10.1126/science.1169144.

Viola, A. U., L. M. James, L. J. Schlangen, and D. J. Dijk. "Blue-Enriched White Light in the Workplace Improves Self-Reported Alertness, Performance and Sleep Quality." *Scandinavian Journal of Work, Environment and Health* 34, no. 4 (2008): 297–306.

Phipps-Nelson, J., J. R. Redman, L. J. Schlangen, and S. M. Rajaratnam. "Blue Light Exposure Reduces Objective Measures of Sleepiness During Prolonged Nighttime Performance Testing." *Chronobiology International* 26, no. 5 (2009): 891–912. doi:10.1080
/07420520903044364.

Gabel, V., M. Maire, C. F. Reichert, S. L. Chellappa, C. Schmidt, V. Hommes, A. U. Viola, and
C. Cajochen. "Effects of Artificial Dawn and Morning Blue Light on Daytime Cognitive
Performance, Well-Being, Cortisol and Melatonin Levels." *Chronobiology International* 30, no. 8
(2013): 988–97. doi:10.3109/07420528.2013.793196.

Taillard, J., A. Capelli, P. Sagaspe, A. Anund, T. Akerstedt, and P. Philip. "In-Car Nocturnal Blue
Light Exposure Improves Motorway Driving: A Randomized Controlled Trial." *PLoS ONE* 7,
no. 10 (2012): e46750. doi:10.1371/journal.pone.0046750.

The Doc. "7 Great Examples of Scientific Discoveries Made in Dreams." *Famous Scientists* (blog).
Accessed September 28, 2015. http://www.famousscientists.org/7-great-examples-of
-scientific-discoveries-made-in-dreams/.

Whyte, A. R., and C. M. Williams. "Effects of a Single Dose of a Flavonoid-Rich Blueberry
Drink on Memory in 8 to 10 Year Old Children." *Nutrition* 31, no. 3 (2015): 531–34.
doi:10.1016/j.nut.2014.09.013.

Campbell, E. L., M. Chebib, and G. A. Johnston. "The Dietary Flavonoids Apigenin and
(-)-Epigallocatechin Gallate Enhance the Positive Modulation by Diazepam of the Activation by GABA of Recombinant GABA(A) Receptors." *Biochemical Pharmacology* 68, no. 8
(2004): 1631–38.

Cho, S., J. H. Park, A. N. Pae, D. Han, D. Kim, N. C. Cho, K. T. No, et al. "Hypnotic Effects and
GABAergic Mechanism of Licorice (*Glycyrrhiza glabra*) Ethanol Extract and Its Major Flavonoid Constituent Glabrol." *Bioorganic and Medicinal Chemistry* 20, no. 11 (2012): 3493–501.
doi:10.1016/j.bmc.2012.04.011.

Jäger, A. K., and L. Saaby. "Flavonoids and the CNS." *Molecules* 16, no. 2 (2011): 1471–85.
doi:10.3390/molecules16021471.

Kavvadias, D., V. Monschein, P. Sand, P. Riederer, and P. Schreier. "Constituents of Sage (*Salvia
Officinalis*) with In Vitro Affinity to Human Brain Benzodiazepine Receptor." *Planta Medica* 69,
no. 2 (2003): 113–17.

Nielsen, M., S. Frøkjaer, and C. Braestrup. "High Affinity of the Naturally-Occurring Biflavo-
noid, Amentoflavon, to Brain Benzodiazepine Receptors In Vitro." *Biochemical Pharmacology*
37, no. 17 (1988): 3285–87.

Medina, J. H., A. C. Paladini, C. Wolfman, M. Levi de Stein, D. Calvo, L. E. Diaz, and C. Peña.
"Chrysin (5,7-di-OH-flavone), a Naturally-Occurring Ligand for Benzodiazepine Receptors, with Anticonvulsant Properties." *Biochemical Pharmacology* 40, no. 10 (1990): 2227–31.

Salgueiro, J. B., P. Ardenghi, M. Dias, M. B. Ferreira, I. Izquierdo, and J. H. Medina. "Anxiolytic
Natural and Synthetic Flavonoid Ligands of the Central Benzodiazepine Receptor Have
No Effect on Memory Tasks in Rats." *Pharmacology, Biochemistry, and Behavior* 58, no. 4 (1997):
887–91.

Viola, H., C. Wasowski, M. Levi de Stein, C. Wolfman, R. Silveira, F. Dajas, J. H. Medina, and
A. C. Paladini. "Apigenin, a Component of Matricaria Recutita Flowers, Is a Central Benzodiazepine Receptors-Ligand with Anxiolytic Effects." *Planta Medica* 61, no. 3 (1995): 213–16.

Wolfman, C., H. Viola, A. Paladini, F. Dajas, and J. H. Medina. "Possible Anxiolytic Effects
of Chrysin, a Central Benzodiazepine Receptor Ligand Isolated from Passiflora Coerulea."
Pharmacology, Biochemistry, and Behavior 47, no. 1 (1994): 1–4.

Papanikolaou, Y., H. Palmer, M. A. Binns, D. J. Jenkins, and C. E. Greenwood. "Better Cognitive Performance Following a Low-Glycaemic-Index Compared with a High-Glycaemic-

Index Carbohydrate Meal in Adults with Type 2 Diabetes." *Diabetologia* 49, no. 5 (2006): 855–62.

Greenwood, C. E., R. J. Kaplan, S. Hebblethwaite, and D. J. Jenkins. "Carbohydrate-Induced Memory Impairment in Adults with Type 2 Diabetes." *Diabetes Care* 26, no. 7 (2003): 1961–66.

Mahoney, C. R., H. A. Taylor, R. B. Kanarek, and P. Samuel. "Effect of Breakfast Composition on Cognitive Processes in Elementary School Children." *Physiology and Behavior* 85, no. 5 (2005): 635–45.

Ciok, J., and A. Dolna. "Carbohydrates and Mental Performance—The Role of Glycemic Index of Food Products." [In Polish.] *Polski Merkuriusz Lekarski* 20, no. 117 (2006): 367–70.

Lakhan, S. E., and A. Kirchgessner. "The Emerging Role of Dietary Fructose in Obesity and Cognitive Decline." *Nutrition Journal* 12, no. 1 (2013): 114.

Abdel-Salam, O. M., N. A. Salem, M. E. El-Shamarka, J. S. Hussein, N. A. Ahmed, and M. E. El-Nagar. "Studies on the Effects of Aspartame on Memory and Oxidative Stress in Brain of Mice." *European Review for Medical and Pharmacological Sciences* 16, no. 15 (2012): 2092–101.

Collison, K. S., N. J. Makhoul, M. Z. Zaidi, S. M. Saleh, B. Andres, A. Inglis, R. Al-Rabiah, and F. A. Al-Mohanna. "Gender Dimorphism in Aspartame-Induced Impairment of Spatial Cognition and Insulin Sensitivity." *PLoS ONE* 7, no. 4 (2012): e31570. doi:10.1371/journal.pone.0031570.

Cai, W., J. Uribarri, L. Zhu, X. Chen, S. Swamy, Z. Zhao, F. Grosjean, et al. "Oral Glycotoxins Are a Modifiable Cause of Dementia and the Metabolic Syndrome in Mice and Humans." *PNAS* 111, no. 13 (2014): 4940–45. doi:10.1073/pnas.1316013111.

Györéné, K. G., A. Varga, and A. Lugasi. "A Comparison of Chemical Composition and Nutritional Value of Organically and Conventionally Grown Plant Derived Foods." [In Hungarian.] *Orvosi Hetilap* 147, no. 43 (2006): 2081–90.

Nafar, F., and K. M. Mearow. "Coconut Oil Attenuates the Effects of Amyloid-β on Cortical Neurons In Vitro." *Journal of Alzheimer's Disease* 39, no. 2 (2014): 233–37. doi:10.3233/JAD -131436.

Ford, P. A., K. Jaceldo-Siegl, J. W. Lee, W. Youngberg, and S. Tonstad. "Intake of Mediterranean Foods Associated with Positive Affect and Low Negative Affect." *Journal of Psychosomatic Research* 74, no. 2 (2013): 142–48. doi:10.1016/j.jpsychores.2012.11.002.

Conner, T. S., K. L. Brookie, A. C. Richardson, and M. A. Polak. "On Carrots and Curiosity: Eating Fruit and Vegetables Is Associated with Greater Flourishing in Daily Life." *British Journal of Health Psychology* 20, no. 2 (2015): 413–27. doi:10.1111/bjhp.12113.

Ritchie, K., I. Carrière, A. de Mendonca, F. Portet, J. F. Dartigues, O. Rouaud, P. Barberger-Gateau, and M. L. Ancelin. "The Neuroprotective Effects of Caffeine: A Prospective Population Study (the Three City Study)." *Neurology* 69, no. 6 (2007): 536–45.

Santos, C., J. Costa, J. Santos, A. Vaz-Carneiro, and N. Lunet. "Caffeine Intake and Dementia: Systematic Review and Meta-Analysis." *Journal of Alzheimer's Disease* 20, suppl. 1 (2010): S187–204. doi:10.3233/JAD-2010-091387.

Júdice, P. B., J. P. Magalhães, D. A. Santos, C. N. Matias, A. I. Carita, P. A. Armada-Da-Silva, L. B. Sardinha, and A. M. Silva. "A Moderate Dose of Caffeine Ingestion Does Not Change Energy Expenditure but Decreases Sleep Time in Physically Active Males: A Double-Blind Randomized Controlled Trial." *Applied Physiology, Nutrition, and Metabolism* 38, no. 1 (2013): 49–56. doi:10.1139/apnm-2012-0145.

Martin, F. P., N. Antille, S. Rezzi, and S. Kochhar. "Everyday Eating Experiences of Chocolate and Non-Chocolate Snacks Impact Postprandial Anxiety, Energy and Emotional States." *Nutrients* 4, no. 6 (2012): 554–67. doi:10.3390/nu4060554.

Smit, H. J., E. A. Gaffan, and P. J. Rogers. "Methylxanthines Are the Psycho-Pharmacologically Active Constituents of Chocolate." *Psychopharmacology* (Berlin) 176, nos. 3–4 (2004): 412–19.

Sudarma, V., S. Sukmaniah, and P. Siregar. "Effect of Dark Chocolate on Nitric Oxide Serum Levels and Blood Pressure in Prehypertension Subjects." *Acta Medic Indonesiana* 43, no. 4 (2011): 224–28.

Field, D. T., C. M. Williams, and L. T. Butler. "Consumption of Cocoa Flavanols Results in an Acute Improvement in Visual and Cognitive Functions." *Physiology and Behavior* 103, nos. 3–4 (2011): 255–60. doi:10.1016/j.physbeh.2011.02.013.

Radin, D., G. Hayssen, and J. Walsh. "Effects of Intentionally Enhanced Chocolate on Mood." *Explore* (New York) 3, no. 5 (2007): 485–92.

Grassi, D., G. Desideri, S. Necozione, F. Ruggieri, J. B. Blumberg, M. Stornello, and C. Ferri. "Protective Effects of Flavanol-Rich Dark Chocolate on Endothelial Function and Wave Reflection During Acute Hyperglycemia." *Hypertension* 60, no. 3 (2012): 827–32. doi:10.1161/HYPERTENSIONAHA.112.193995.

Shiah, Y. J., and D. Radin. "Metaphysics of the Tea Ceremony: A Randomized Trial Investigating the Roles of Intention and Belief on Mood While Drinking Tea." *Explore* (New York) 9, no. 6 (2013): 355–60. doi:10.1016/j.explore.2013.08.005.

Rankin, C. W., J. O. Nriagu, J. K. Aggarwal, T. A. Arowolo, K. Adebayo, and A. R. Flegal. "Lead Contamination in Cocoa and Cocoa Products: Isotopic Evidence of Global Contamination." *Environmental Health Perspectives* 113, no. 10 (2005): 1344–48. doi:10.1289/ehp.8009.

Krecisz, B., D. Chomiczewska, M. Kiec-Swierczynska, and A. Kaszuba. "Systemic Contact Dermatitis to Nickel Present in Cocoa in 14-Year-Old Boy." *Pediatric Dermatology* 28, no. 3 (2011): 335–36. doi:10.1111/j.1525-1470.2011.01235.x.

Radenahmad, N., F. Saleh, I. Sayoh, K. Sawangjaroen, P. Subhadhirasakul, P. Boonyoung, W. Rundorn, and W. Mitranun. "Young Coconut Juice Can Accelerate the Healing Process of Cutaneous Wounds." *BMC Complementary and Alternative Medicine* 12 (2012): 252. doi:10.1186/1472-6882-12-252.

Radenahmad, N., F. Saleh, K. Sawangjaroen, U. Vongvatcharanon, P. Subhadhirasakul, W. Rundorn, B. Withyachumnarnkul, and J. R. Connor. "Young Coconut Juice, a Potential Therapeutic Agent That Could Significantly Reduce Some Pathologies Associated with Alzheimer's Disease: Novel Findings." *British Journal of Nutrition* 105, no. 5 (2011): 738–46. doi:10.1017/S0007114510004241.

Yong, J. W. H., L. Ge, Y. F. Ng, and S. N. Tan. "The Chemical Composition and Biological Properties of Coconut (*Cocos Nucifera* L.) Water." *Molecules* 14, no. 12 (2009): 5144–64. doi:10.3390/molecules14125144.

Gómez-Pinilla, F. "Brain Foods: The Effects of Nutrients on Brain Function." *Nature Reviews Neuroscience* 9, no. 7 (2008): 568–78. doi:10.1038/nrn2421.

Reger, M. A., S. T. Henderson, C. Hale, B. Cholerton, L. D. Baker, G. S. Watson, K. Hyde, D. Chapman, and S. Craft. "Effects of Beta-Hydroxybutyrate on Cognition in Memory-Impaired Adults." *Neurobiology of Aging* 25, no. 3 (2004): 311–14.

Appleton, K. M., P. J. Rogers, and A. R. Ness. "Updated Systematic Review and Meta-Analysis of the Effects of n–3 Long-Chain Polyunsaturated Fatty Acids on Depressed Mood." *American Journal of Clinical Nutrition* 91, no. 3 (2010): 757–70. doi:10.3945/ajcn.2009.28313.

Kraguljac, N. V., V. M. Montori, M. Pavuluri, H. S. Chai, B. S. Wilson, and S. S. Unal. "Efficacy of Omega-3 Fatty Acids in Mood Disorders—A Systematic Review and Meta-Analysis." *Psychopharmacology Bulletin* 42, no. 3 (2009): 39–54.

Ng, T. P., P. C. Chiam, T. Lee, H. C. Chua, L. Lim, and E. H. Kua. "Curry Consumption and Cognitive Function in the Elderly." *American Journal of Epidemiology* 164, no. 9 (2006): 898–906.

Kirkham, S., R. Akilen, S. Sharma, and A. Tsiami. "The Potential of Cinnamon to Reduce Blood Glucose Levels in Patients with Type 2 Diabetes and Insulin Resistance." *Diabetes, Obesity and Metabolism* 11, no. 12 (2009): 1100–13. doi:10.1111/j.1463-1326.2009.01094.x.

Shukitt-Hale, B., D. F. Bielinski, F. C. Lau, L. M. Willis, A. N. Carey, and J. A. Joseph. "The Beneficial Effects of Berries on Cognition, Motor Behaviour and Neuronal Function in Ageing." *British Journal of Nutrition* 114, no. 10 (2015): 1542–49.

Malin, D. H., D. R. Lee, P. Goyarzu, Y. H. Chang, L. J. Ennis, E. Beckett, B. Shukitt-Hale, and J. A. Joseph. "Short-Term Blueberry-Enriched Diet Prevents and Reverses Object Recognition Memory Loss in Aging Rats." *Nutrition* 27, no. 3 (2011): 338–42. doi:10.1016/j .nut.2010.05.001.

Krikorian, R., M. D. Shidler, T. A. Nash, W. Kalt, M. R. Vinqvist-Tymchuk, B. Shukitt-Hale, and J. A. Joseph. "Blueberry Supplementation Improves Memory in Older Adults." *Journal of Agricultural and Food Chemistry* 58, no. 7 (2010): 3996–4000. doi:10.1021/jf9029332.

Rendeiro, C., D. Vauzour, M. Rattray, P. Waffo-Téguo, J. M. Mérillon, L. T. Butler, C. M. Williams, and J. P. Spencer. "Dietary Levels of Pure Flavonoids Improve Spatial Memory Performance and Increase Hippocampal Brain-Derived Neurotrophic Factor." *PLoS ONE* 8, no. 5 (2013): e63535. doi:10.1371/journal.pone.0063535.

Joseph, J. A., B. Shukitt-Hale, and L. M. Willis. "Grape Juice, Berries, and Walnuts Affect Brain Aging and Behavior." *Journal of Nutrition* 139, no. 9 (2009): 1813S–1817S. doi:10.3945 /jn.109.108266.

Galli, R. L., B. Shukitt-Hale, K. A. Youdim, and J. A. Joseph. "Fruit Polyphenolics and Brain Aging: Nutritional Interventions Targeting Age-Related Neuronal and Behavioral Deficits." *Annals of the New York Academy of Sciences* 959 (2002): 128–32.

Tan, L., H. P. Yang, W. Pang, H. Lu, Y. D. Hu, J. Li, S. J. Lu, W. Q. Zhang, and Y. G. Jiang. "Cyanidin-3-O-Galactoside and Blueberry Extracts Supplementation Improves Spatial Memory and Regulates Hippocampal ERK Expression in Senescence-Accelerated Mice." *Biomedical and Environmental Sciences* 27, no. 3 (2014): 186–96. doi:10.3967/bes2014.007.

Krikorian, R., E. L. Boespflug, D. E. Fleck, A. L. Stein, J. D. Wightman, M. D. Shidler, and S. Sadat-Hossieny. "Concord Grape Juice Supplementation and Neurocognitive Function in Human Aging." *Journal of Agricultural and Food Chemistry* 60, no. 23 (2012): 5736–42. doi:10.1021/jf300277g.

Krikorian, R., T. A. Nash, M. D. Shidler, B. Shukitt-Hale, and J. A. Joseph. "Concord Grape Juice Supplementation Improves Memory Function in Older Adults with Mild Cognitive Impairment." *British Journal of Nutrition* 103, no. 5 (2010): 730–34. doi:10.1017 /S0007114509992364.

CHAPTER 9: THE SPIRIT

Van Wijk, R., and E. P. van Wijk. "An Introduction to Human Biophoton Emission." *Forschende Komplementärmedizin und Klassische Naturheilkunde* 12, no. 2 (2005): 77–83.

Van Wijk, E. P., J. Ackerman, and R. van Wijk. "Effect of Meditation on Ultraweak Photon Emission from Hands and Forehead." *Forschende Komplementärmedizin und Klassische Naturheilkunde* 12, no. 2 (2005): 107–12.

Van Wijk, E. P., R. Lüdtke, and R. van Wijk. "Differential Effects of Relaxation Techniques on Ultraweak Photon Emission." *Journal of Alternative and Complementary Medicine* 14, no. 3 (2008): 241–50. doi:10.1089/acm.2007.7185.

Kamal, A. H., and S. Komatsu. "Involvement of Reactive Oxygen Species and Mitochondrial Proteins in Biophoton Emission in Roots of Soybean Plants Under Flooding Stress." *Journal of Proteome Research* 14, no. 5 (2015): 2219–36. doi:10.1021/acs.jproteome.5b00007.

Winkler, R., H. Guttenberger, and H. Klima. "Ultraweak and Induced Photon Emission After Wounding of Plants." *Photochemistry and Photobiology* 85, no. 4 (2009): 962–65. doi:10.1111/j.1751-1097.2009.00537.x.

Kim, M. "Blue Light from Electronics Disturbs Sleep, Especially for Teenagers." *Washington Post*. September 1, 2014. Accessed September 28, 2015. http://www.washingtonpost.com/national/health-science/blue-light-from-electronics-disturbs-sleep-especially-for-teenagers/2014/08/29/3edd2726-27a7-11e4-958c-268a320a60ce_story.html.

Claustrat, B., and J. Leston. "Melatonin: Physiological Effects in Humans." *Neurochirurgie* 61, nos. 2–3 (2015): 77–84. doi:10.1016/j.neuchi.2015.03.002.

Carpenter, D. O. "Human Disease Resulting from Exposure to Electromagnetic Fields." *Reviews on Environmental Health* 28, no. 4 (2013): 159–72. doi:10.1515/reveh-2013-0016.

EMFs.info: Electric and Magnetic Fields and Health. "Sources." Accessed September 28, 2015. http://www.emfs.info/sources/.

Feychting, M., A. Ahlbom, and L. Kheifets. "EMF and Health." *Annual Review of Public Health* 26 (2005): 165–89.

Miller, A. B., and L. M. Green. "Electric and Magnetic Fields at Power Frequencies." *Chronic Diseases in Canada* 29, suppl. 1 (2010): 69–83.

Kheifets, L., J. Monroe, X. Vergara, G. Mezei, and A. A. Afifi. "Occupational Electromagnetic Fields and Leukemia and Brain Cancer: An Update to Two Meta-Analyses." *Journal of Occupational and Environmental Medicine* 50, no. 6 (2008): 677–88. doi:10.1097/JOM.0b013e3181757a27.

Ferreri, F., G. Curcio, P. Pasqualetti, L. De Gennaro, R. Fini, and P. M. Rossini. "Mobile Phone Emissions and Human Brain Excitability." *Annals of Neurology* 60, no. 2 (2006): 188–96.

Berk, M., S. Dodd, and M. Henry. "Do Ambient Electromagnetic Fields Affect Behaviour? A Demonstration of the Relationship Between Geomagnetic Storm Activity and Suicide." *Bioelectromagnetics* 27, no. 2 (2006): 151–55.

Rohan, M. L., R. T. Yamamoto, C. T. Ravichandran, K. R. Cayetano, O. G. Morales, D. P. Olson, G. Vitaliano, S. M. Paul, and B. M. Cohen. "Rapid Mood-Elevating Effects of Low Field Magnetic Stimulation in Depression." *Biological Psychiatry* 76, no. 3 (2014): 186–93. doi:10.1016/j.biopsych.2013.10.024.

Galace de Freitas, D., F. B. Marcondes, R. L. Monteiro, S. G. Rosa, P. Maria de Moraes Barros Fucs, and T. Y. Fukuda. "Pulsed Electromagnetic Field and Exercises in Patients with Shoulder Impingement Syndrome: A Randomized, Double-Blind, Placebo-Controlled Clinical Trial." *Archives of Physical Medicine and Rehabilitation* 95, no. 2 (2014): 345–52. doi:10.1016/j.apmr.2013.09.022.

Valentini, E., M. Ferrara, F. Presaghi, L. De Gennaro, and G. Curcio. "Systematic Review and Meta-Analysis of Psychomotor Effects of Mobile Phone Electromagnetic Fields." *Occupational and Environmental Medicine* 67, no. 10 (2010): 708–16. doi:10.1136/oem.2009.047027.

Rikk, J., K. J. Finn, I. Liziczai, Z. Radák, Z. Bori, and F. Ihász. "Influence of Pulsing Electromagnetic Field Therapy on Resting Blood Pressure in Aging Adults." *Electromagnetic Biology and Medicine* 32, no. 2 (2013): 165–72. doi:10.3109/15368378.2013.776420.

Sutbeyaz, S. T., N. Sezer, F. Koseoglu, and S. Kibar. "Low-Frequency Pulsed Electromagnetic Field Therapy in Fibromyalgia: A Randomized, Double-Blind, Sham-Controlled

Clinical Study." *Clinical Journal of Pain* 25, no. 8 (2009): 722–28. doi:10.1097/AJP.0b013e3181a68a6c.

Piatkowski, J., S. Kern, and T. Ziemssen. "Effect of BEMER Magnetic Field Therapy on the Level of Fatigue in Patients with Multiple Sclerosis: A Randomized, Double-Blind Controlled Trial." *Journal of Alternative and Complementary Medicine* 15, no. 5 (2009): 507–11. doi:10.1089/acm.2008.0501.

Ganesan, K., A. C. Gengadharan, C. Balachandran, B. M. Manohar, and R. Puvanakrishnan. "Low Frequency Pulsed Electromagnetic Field—A Viable Alternative Therapy for Arthritis." *Indian Journal of Experimental Biology* 47, no. 12 (2009): 939–48.

Meesters, Y., V. Dekker, L. J. Schlangen, E. H. Bos, and M. J. Ruiter. "Low-Intensity Blue-Enriched White Light (750 Lux) and Standard Bright Light (10,000 Lux) Are Equally Effective in Treating SAD. A Randomized Controlled Study." *BMC Psychiatry* 11 (2011): 17. doi:10.1186/1471-244X-11-17.

Pail, G., W. Huf, E. Pjrek, D. Winkler, M. Willeit, N. Praschak-Rieder, and S. Kasper. "Bright-Light Therapy in the Treatment of Mood Disorders." *Neuropsychobiology* 64, no. 3 (2011): 152–62. doi:10.1159/000328950.

Magnusson, A., and D. Boivin. "Seasonal Affective Disorder: An Overview." *Chronobiology International* 20, no. 2 (2003): 189–207.

Blask, D. E., G. C. Brainard, R. T. Dauchy, J. P. Hanifin, L. K. Davidson, J. A. Krause, L. A. Sauer, et al. "Melatonin-Depleted Blood from Premenopausal Women Exposed to Light at Night Stimulates Growth of Human Breast Cancer Xenografts in Nude Rats." *Cancer Research* 65, no. 23 (2005): 11174–84.

Jim, H. S., J. E. Pustejovsky, C. L. Park, S. C. Danhauer, A. C. Sherman, G. Fitchett, T. V. Merluzzi, et al. "Religion, Spirituality, and Physical Health in Cancer Patients: A Meta-Analysis." *Cancer* 121, no. 21 (2015): 3760–68. doi:10.1002/cncr.29353.

Williams, A. L. "Perspectives on Spirituality at the End of Life: A Meta-Summary." *Palliative and Supportive Care* 4, no. 4 (2006): 407–17.

Grant, E., S. A. Murray, M. Kendall, K. Boyd, S. Tilley, and D. Ryan. "Spiritual Issues and Needs: Perspectives from Patients with Advanced Cancer and Nonmalignant Disease. A Qualitative Study." *Palliative and Supportive Care* 2, no. 4 (2004): 371–78.

Martínez, B. B., and R. P. Custódio. "Relationship Between Mental Health and Spiritual Well-Being Among Hemodialysis Patients: A Correlation Study." *São Paulo Medical Journal* 132, no. 1 (2014): 23–27. doi:10.1590/1516-3180.2014.1321606.

Wirz-Justice, A., A. Bader, U. Frisch, R. D. Stieglitz, J. Alder, J. Bitzer, I. Hösli, et al. "A Randomized, Double-Blind, Placebo-Controlled Study of Light Therapy for Antepartum Depression." *Journal of Clinical Psychiatry* 72, no. 7 (2011): 986–93. doi:10.4088/JCP.10m06188blu.

Klerman, E. B., J. F. Duffy, D. J. Dijk, and C. A. Czeisler. "Circadian Phase Resetting in Older People by Ocular Bright Light Exposure." *Journal of Investigative Medicine* 49, no. 1 (2001): 30–40.

Martiny, K. "Adjunctive Bright Light in Non-Seasonal Major Depression." *Acta Psychiatrica Scandinavica: Supplementum* 425 (2004): 7–28.

Loving, R. T., D. F. Kripke, and S. R. Shuchter. "Bright Light Augments Antidepressant Effects of Medication and Wake Therapy." *Depression and Anxiety* 16, no. 1 (2002): 1–3.

Lam, R. W., E. M. Goldner, L. Solyom, and R. A. Remick. "A Controlled Study of Light Therapy for Bulimia Nervosa." *American Journal of Psychiatry* 151, no. 5 (1994): 744–50.

Christakis, N., and J. Fowler. "Connected." ConnectedtheBook.com. Accessed September 28, 2015. http://connectedthebook.com/.

Cheng, C. W., G. B. Adams, L. Perin, M. Wei, X. Zhou, B. S. Lam, S. Da Sacco, et al. "Prolonged Fasting Reduces IGF-1/PKA to Promote Hematopoietic-Stem-Cell-Based Regeneration and Reverse Immunosuppression." *Cell Stem Cell* 14, no. 6 (2014): 810–23. doi:10.1016/j.stem.2014.04.014.

Mendelsohn, A. R., and J. W. Larrick. "Prolonged Fasting/Refeeding Promotes Hematopoietic Stem Cell Regeneration and Rejuvenation." *Rejuvenation Research* 17, no. 4 (2014): 385–89. doi:10.1089/rej.2014.1595.

Hussin, N. M., S. Shahar, N. I. Teng, W. Z. Ngah, and S. K. Das. "Efficacy of Fasting and Calorie Restriction (FCR) on Mood and Depression Among Ageing Men." *Journal of Nutrition, Health and Aging* 17, no. 8 (2013): 674–80. doi:10.1007/s12603-013-0344-9.

Teng, N. I., S. Shahar, Z. A. Manaf, S. K. Das, C. S. Taha, and W. Z. Ngah. "Efficacy of Fasting Calorie Restriction on Quality of Life Among Aging Men." *Physiology and Behavior* 104, no. 5 (2011): 1059–64. doi:10.1016/j.physbeh.2011.07.007.

Liu, J. D., D. Goodspeed, Z. Sheng, B. Li, Y. Yang, D. J. Kliebenstein, and J. Braam. "Keeping the Rhythm: Light/Dark Cycles During Postharvest Storage Preserve the Tissue Integrity and Nutritional Content of Leafy Plants." *BMC Plant Biology* 15 (2015): 92. doi:10.1186/s12870-015-0474-9.

Sutherland, E. G., C. Ritenbaugh, S. J. Kiley, N. Vuckovic, and C. Elder. "An HMO-Based Prospective Pilot Study of Energy Medicine for Chronic Headaches: Whole-Person Outcomes Point to the Need for New Instrumentation." *Journal of Alternative and Complementary Medicine* 15, no. 8 (2009): 819–26.

Lu, D. F., L. K. Hart, S. K. Lutgendorf, and Y. Perkhounkova. "The Effect of Healing Touch on the Pain and Mobility of Persons with Osteoarthritis: A Feasibility Study." *Geriatric Nursing* 34, no. 4 (2013): 314–22. doi:10.1016/j.gerinurse.2013.05.003.

Hart, L. K., M. I. Freel, P. J. Haylock, and S. K. Lutgendorf. "The Use of Healing Touch in Integrative Oncology." *Clinical Journal of Oncology Nursing* 15, no. 5 (2011): 519–25. doi:10.1188/11.CJON.519-525.

Richeson, N. E., J. A. Spross, K. Lutz, and C. Peng. "Effects of Reiki on Anxiety, Depression, Pain, and Physiological Factors in Community-Dwelling Older Adults." *Research in Gerontological Nursing* 3, no. 3 (2010): 187–99. doi:10.3928/19404921-20100601-01.

Bourque, A. L., M. E. Sullivan, and M. R. Winter. "Reiki as a Pain Management Adjunct in Screening Colonoscopy." *Gastroenterology Nursing* 35, no. 5 (2012): 308–12.

Bowden, D., L. Goddard, and J. Gruzelier. "A Randomised Controlled Single-Blind Trial of the Effects of Reiki and Positive Imagery on Well-Being and Salivary Cortisol." *Brain Research Bulletin* 81, no. 1 (2010): 66–72. doi:10.1016/j.brainresbull.2009.10.002.

Díaz-Rodríguez, L., M. Arroyo-Morales, C. Fernández-de-las-Peñas, F. García-Lafuente, C. García-Royo, and I. Tomás-Rojas. "Immediate Effects of Reiki on Heart Rate Variability, Cortisol Levels, and Body Temperature in Health Care Professionals with Burnout." *Biological Research for Nursing* 13, no. 4 (2011): 376–82. doi:10.1177/1099800410389166.

Vickers, A. J., A. M. Cronin, A. C. Maschino, G. Lewith, H. MacPherson, N. E. Foster, K. J. Sherman, et al. "Acupuncture for Chronic Pain: Individual Patient Data Meta-Analysis." *JAMA Internal Medicine* 172, no. 19 (2012): 1444–53. doi:10.1001/archinternmed.2012.3654.

Mackay, N., S. Hansen, and O. McFarlane. "Autonomic Nervous System Changes During Reiki Treatment: A Preliminary Study." *Journal of Alternative and Complementary Medicine* 10, no. 6 (2004): 1077–81.

Buettner, D. *The Blue Zones: 9 Lessons for Living Longer from the People Who've Lived the Longest.* Reprint Edition. Washington, DC: National Geographic, 2010.

CHAPTER 10: HOW TO GET THE MOST FROM YOUR WHOLE DETOX

Kinnier, R. T., C. Hofsess, R. Pongratz, and C. Lambert. "Attributions and Affirmations for Overcoming Anxiety and Depression." *Psychology and Psychotherapy* 82, pt. 2 (2009): 153–69. doi:10.1348/147608308X389418.

Epton, T., P. R. Harris, R. Kane, G. M. van Koningsbruggen, and P. Sheeran. "The Impact of Self-Affirmation on Health-Behavior Change: A Meta-Analysis." *Health Psychology* 34, no. 3 (2015): 187–96. doi:10.1037/hea0000116.

Gelernter, R., G. Lavi, L. Yanai, R. Brooks, Y. Bar, Z. Bistrizer, and M. Rachmiel. "Effect of Auditory Guided Imagery on Glucose Levels and on Glycemic Control in Children with Type 1 Diabetes Mellitus." *Journal of Pediatric Endocrinology and Metabolism* (August 14, 2015). doi: 10.1515/jpem-2015-0150.

Giacobbi Jr., P. R., M. E. Stabler, J. Stewart, A. M. Jaeschke, J. L. Siebert, and G. A. Kelley. "Guided Imagery for Arthritis and Other Rheumatic Diseases: A Systematic Review of Random ized Controlled Trials." *Pain Management Nursing* 16, no. 5 (2015): 792–803. doi:10.1016/j.pmn.2015.01.003.

Kwekkeboom, K. L., and L. C. Bratzke. "A Systematic Review of Relaxation, Meditation, and Guided Imagery Strategies for Symptom Management in Heart Failure." *Journal of Cardiovascular Nursing* (June 10, 2015).

Marchand, W. R. "Mindfulness-Based Stress Reduction, Mindfulness-Based Cognitive Therapy, and Zen Meditation for Depression, Anxiety, Pain, and Psychological Distress." *Journal of Psychiatric Practice* 18, no. 4 (2012): 233–52. doi:10.1097/01.pra.0000416014.53215.86.

Tang, Y.-Y., B. K. Hölzel, and M. I. Posner. "The Neuroscience of Mindfulness Meditation." *Nature Reviews Neuroscience* 16, no. 4 (2015): 213–25. doi:10.1038/nrn3916.

Bhasin, M. K., J. A. Dusek, B. H. Chang, M. G. Joseph, J. W. Denninger, G. L. Fricchione, H. Benson, and T. A. Libermann. "Relaxation Response Induces Temporal Transcriptome Changes in Energy Metabolism, Insulin Secretion and Inflammatory Pathways." *PLoS ONE* 8, no. 5 (2013): e62817. doi:10.1371/journal.pone.0062817.

Dusek, J. A., H. H. Otu, A. L. Wohlhueter, M. Bhasin, L. F. Zerbini, M. G. Joseph, H. Benson, and T. A. Libermann. "Genomic Counter-Stress Changes Induced by the Relaxation Response." *PLoS ONE* 3, no. 7 (2008): e2576. doi:10.1371/journal.pone.0002576.

INDEX